✥

That Jealous Demon,
My Wretched Health

✢

That Jealous Demon, My Wretched Health

DISEASE, DEATH AND COMPOSERS

Jonathan Noble

Foreword by
Petroc Trelawny

THE BOYDELL PRESS

First published 2018

The Boydell Press, Woodbridge

ISBN 978 1 78327 258 7

The Boydell Press is an imprint of Boydell & Brewer Ltd
PO Box 9, Woodbridge, Suffolk IP12 3DF, UK
and of Boydell & Brewer Inc.
668 Mt Hope Avenue, Rochester, NY 14620–2731, USA
website: www.boydellandbrewer.com

A CIP catalogue record for this book is available
from the British Library

The publisher has no responsibility for the continued existence or accuracy
of URLs for external or third-party internet websites referred to in this book,
and does not guarantee that any content on such websites is, or will remain,
accurate or appropriate

This publication is printed on acid-free paper

Printed and bound in Great Britain by
TJ International Ltd, Padstow, Cornwall

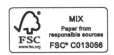

MIX
Paper from
responsible sources
FSC® C013056
FSC
www.fsc.org

To my family, especially my beloved and indulgent wife, Joan. Also to two dear friends, Joyce and the late Michael Kennedy, without whose inspiration and guidance this would have been impossible.

Contents

Illustrations

Figures

Table

Foreword

In my early days at Radio 3 I well remember a veteran producer throwing back a script I'd written for a concert broadcast. 'There's no colour', he proclaimed. 'Bring the composer to life'. It's advice I have never forgotten. Talking about sonata form or key structure is no use to anyone who hasn't studied music theory. But talk about lovers, travels, debts, and above all, health, and a long dead composer can come to life again.

Beethoven's deafness, Schubert's syphilis, and Elgar's acute hypochondria have become part of the shorthand of their lives – even if, as Jonathan Noble reveals, the relevance of each condition to the composer's existence has been rather exaggerated. Until the last century few composers enjoyed serious academic study during their lifetimes; biographies tended to be either self-serving hagiography, the brutally destructive work of an enemy, or a heavily embellished account based on scant information. Few writers would have consulted medical records; loose, generalised descriptions of health conditions quickly became accepted facts. Peter Shaffer's play 'Amadeus' is a masterpiece, but did Mozart really suffer so acutely from Tourette's syndrome? If Sibelius actually was a chronic alcoholic would he have lived to celebrate his 90th birthday?

The number of surgeons and doctors found in amateur orchestras, string quartets and choral societies is raw proof of a close connection between medicine and music. The author, a renowned orthopaedic surgeon, has treated his subject matter as he would a patient coming for a consultation, considering all the information available to him. His treatment of seventy composers provides a series of fascinating and revealing stories. This opportunity to consider their health as a matter of fact, rather than 'colour' burnished by time will surely help us appreciate their lives more, and understand their music better.

Petroc Trelawny

Acknowledgements

To attempt a wholesale review, such as this book, one is very dependent upon and grateful to many wise heads. My family are all gifted and helpful with languages, so that articles in German or French were not a problem. Patience with an ursine chap posting a DO NOT DISTURB sign on his study door has been so generous. My thanks go especially to Martin Holmes at the Bodleian Library in Oxford, and particularly the University of Manchester Medical School Library at Salford Royal Hospital and the Borzoi Bookshop in Stow-on-the-Wold, who all unearthed abstruse articles and books.

Many experts have helpfully pointed me in appropriate directions. They can be divided into the medical and musical. My wife, Joan, has advised regarding disturbances of vision and diseases of the eye and its socket. My son, David, has kept me right regarding renal (kidney) medicine and oncology. My daughter-in-law, Anna, who is tri-lingual, gave advice regarding ear, nose and throat (ENT) conditions, as well as translating articles from the original German. Dr Benjamin Goorney discussed issues in venereology, as Mr John Abercrombie and Dr Wynne Rees did with bowel diseases. Dr Simon Taggart assisted me with respiratory and cardiac medicine, as did Professor Anthony Strong with brain surgery, and Dr Michael Petch with Britten's cardiac issues. I am grateful to John Griffiths, Bruce Phillips, Professor Peter Dickinson and Hamish Halls for helpfully reading my scripts. Their tactful suggestions were all incorporated. Dr Stephen Lock, formerly Editor of the *British Medical Journal*, twice generously reviewed the entire manuscript.

The Salzburg Mozarteum, Troldhaugen in Bergen, the Elgar Birthplace at Broadheath, the Brahms Museum in Hamburg and especially Dr Nick Clark at The Red House in Aldeburgh have been responsive and often generous with their time and archives. Roger Nichols, the late Brian Rees and particularly Roy Howat have helped me with French composers. Michael and Joyce Kennedy advised regarding Elgar, Vaughan Williams, Mahler, Britten and Richard Strauss. Early in my efforts Lord Robert Winston, Professor Eric Clarke, Heather Professor of Music at Oxford, and Michael Steen were most encouraging. Kiffer and Hilary Finzi gave lovely insights into English music, especially Gerald Finzi, as Raymond Head did with

Holst. Colin Matthews and Paul Kildea were helpful over Britten's life and death. The distinguished lawyer Rodger Pannone clarified legal matters. Dr John Harcup very generously shared his own researches into Elgar's medical history with me, as did Professor Barry Cooper with Beethoven and Professor Brian Newbould with Schubert.

Scripts were typed and organised by Virginia Harnden and by Jan Bissell. My greatest thanks go to Joyce and the late Michael Kennedy, who were inspiringly encouraging. They invested their own time and a humbling expertise with extraordinary generosity. I am also extremely grateful to Michael Middeke, Editorial Director at Boydell & Brewer, for his firm and very supportive guidance, and to his colleagues Megan Milan and Rohais Haughton. Lastly I must thank you, the readers, without whom this would have been a pointless exercise.

Jonathan Noble
Naunton, Gloucestershire
2018

Medical Glossary

Acoustic (or auditory) nerve	Nerve that electrically transmits sound from inner ear to brain
Amusia	Musical aphasia
Anaemia	A low haemoglobin level (aka bloodlessness)
Aneurysm	Swelling of, or upon, an artery causing its wall to weaken and even ultimately to burst
Aphasia	An inability to say what you want to say, despite hearing it in your head
Arteriosclerosis	Hardening of the arteries
Ascites (ascitic)	Pathological collection of fluid in the abdominal cavity
Auto-immune	Infers a disease in which certain body tissues become allergic to and are attacked by circulating body cells (e.g. rheumatoid arthritis)
Bacteria	Germs causing infection
Bright's disease	See Nephritis
Bronchi	Airway tubes from the trachea into the lungs
Cardiac	Of the heart
Cataract	A common cause of blindness, due to lens in eye becoming opaque
CVA	Cerebro-vascular accident (See Stroke)
COAD	Chronic obstructive airways disease, due to partial blockage or spasm of tubes into lungs
Conductive deafness	Loss of hearing due to obstruction in the outer ear (e.g. wax) or scarring together of the malleus, incus and stapes

Colon	Large bowel
Cyclothymia	A tendency to marked mood swings
DVT	Deep vein thrombosis (usually in the leg)
Dysgraphia	A partial inability to write down a conceived thought
Dysmusia	Musical dysphasia
Dysphasia	A partial aphasia
Emboli	Pieces of material thrown off into the circulation which can cause serious or fatal blockage of the arteries. Most commonly thrombus (see Pulmonary embolus)
ENT	Ear, nose and throat, in itself a medical speciality (e.g. ENT clinic or surgeon)
Exophthalmos	Protuberance of the eyes associated with thyroid disease
Glaucoma	Condition in which raised pressure in the eye, if untreated, can cause blindness
GPI	General paralysis of the insane
Haematemesis	Vomiting blood
Haematoma	A major bruise or collection of clotted blood
Haemoptysis	Coughing up blood
Haemorrhoidectomy	Removal of piles
Hemiparesis	Weakness down one side of the body
Hemiplegia	Paralysis down one side of the body
Hypertension	Raised blood pressure
Iritis (or opthalmia)	Inflammation of the front segment of the eye
Larynx	Voice-box
Lupus (systemic lupus erythematosus, or SLE)	A complex auto-immune disease affecting many different body parts
Malleus, incus, stapes	Three little bones conducting sound across the middle ear
Myocardial infarct (MI)	A heart attack due to blockage of a main (coronary) artery to the heart (aka 'a coronary')

Nephritis (Bright's disease)	Inflammatory disease of the kidney
Oedema	Abnormal retention of fluid in tissues, especially in the legs (i.e. waterlogging)
Optic nerve	Nerve that electrically conducts light, shape and colour to the brain
Pulmonary embolus (PE)	Sudden blockage of circulation to the lungs, due to a piece of thrombus floating off into circulation
Renal	Of the kidney
Scoliosis	Spinal curvature
Sensorineural deafness	Diminished hearing due to disease of the inner ear and/or acoustic nerve
Septicaemia	Germs and breakdown products in circulation, causing serious illness
Stroke	Sudden affliction of the brain due to thrombosis or bleeding into it, often causing weakness or paralysis and alteration of consciousness (aka cerebro-vascular accident, CVA)
TB	Tuberculosis
Thrombosis	Blockage of a blood vessel due to a solid plug (thrombus) of congealed (thrombosed) blood
TIA	Transient ischaemic attack (aka mini-stroke). A brief episode in which consciousness may be lost, possibly with slurring of speech or transient weakness
Trachea	Windpipe
Uraemia	Abnormal excess of urea in the blood, normally due to renal failure
VD	Venereal disease
WR test	Wassermann's classic test for syphilis

✛

Introduction

Music is the companion of joy, the medicine of sorrow
                            Inscription on *The Music Lesson* (1662–63)
                            by Johannes Vermeer, H.M. The Queen's Collection

IN LATE 1907 THE AUSTRIAN painter Gustav Klimt stood at Vienna's railway station, woefully declaring, 'It's over' as the train taking Gustav Mahler on his journey ultimately to the USA pulled away. Mahler had just suffered the triple hammer blow of his anti-Semitic ousting from the Vienna Opera, the death of his beloved little daughter, 'Putzi', and the news of his potentially fatal heart condition. But it was not over. For his remaining nearly three and a half years, before the train brought him back to die in Vienna, further great music was to come, and in some ways it would be different music. From this vignette, the strong influence of both mental and physical health upon the process of composition is seen. It may be asked how Mahler died and of what disease. We can wonder how he managed at all, as other personal and professional problems overshadowed his remaining life. More questions arise from Mahler's story, as they do from medical accounts of many other great composers. These will be posed, and hopefully answered, within this book. There is, after all, a keen general interest in the influence of ill health upon famous men. The outcome from the meeting of the Big Three at Yalta, so crucial for the world today, might have been very different if Roosevelt had not been close to death. By the same token, this book will consider how prevailing sickness affected both the quality and quantity of composition; was it because of, or in spite of, that illness? The nature of the music and how different Western music would be now if a particular composer had lived longer will be considered. For the person interested in classical composers and their sometimes dreadful deaths, and in the relationship between declining health and creative output, here is an overview.

At the outset it was vital to learn what had already been written on this topic. Not all musical authors have sought medical advice, just as doctors have sometimes neglected musical expertise. Curiously, there are only two books to exclusively address disease, death and great composers, although there are myriad articles in medical and musical journals. John O'Shea is an Australian doctor and medical historian.[1] He treats seventeen 'Great Composers' in a succinct book, focusing on medical interest. Professor Anton Neumayr was distinguished both medically and musically in Austria.[2] His historical and medical accounts of fourteen composers were published in the USA in three volumes. As with O'Shea, one is left wondering about medically interesting composers who were omitted, such as J. S. Bach, Handel, Wagner, Ravel, Debussy, Elgar and Shostakovich. Although O'Shea and Neumayr were probably alone in producing books bridging medicine and musical biography, many primarily musical biographies contain a serious medical input. H. C. Robbins Landon's account of Mozart's last year depended upon the medical opinion of Dr P. J. Davies, an Australian gastroenterologist.[3] Although his work is often sound and well researched, Davies has nevertheless expressed views regarded by colleagues as eccentric and has generated antagonism. One of this book's purposes is to dissect such controversy, thereby leaving the interested reader with a balanced overview of probabilities. Analysing the illnesses and deaths of forty-four composers in depth, with another twenty-six described more briefly, is more illuminating than considering fewer than twenty. With larger cohorts themes emerge and trends can be established more readily. *New Grove* has been a constant reference source, in both the 1980 edition (reprinted 1998 with amendments) and that of 2001.[4] Sometimes the earlier volumes were more informative regarding biographical detail, as is also the case with books cited in the Bibliography. The weight given to biographies in the Bibliography generally reflects how rich a source of medical detail or reflection upon a composer's general habitude a book has been.

Early in my researches a frequent propensity amongst biographies and articles to implicate venereal disease, alcoholism or sexual impropriety quickly became apparent. The media interest since 2013 regarding Benjamin Britten's last illness allegedly having been due to syphilis reveals a public interest in the relationship between sickness and music. It may also demonstrate that such interest can intensify if the subject matter becomes potentially salacious, perhaps beyond an author's original intention. A century after Beethoven's death, Ernest Newman declared him to have been syphilitic, a drunkard and a ruthless cheat,[5] allegations which were to linger whilst continuing to be quoted over subsequent years. Deserving of criticism are those ill-founded, ex-cathedra opinions which, wilfully or carelessly, besmirch reputations. From them the reader may learn more about a writer's tastes than about his subject's life. Accordingly, in an era obsessed with celebrity, both the meretricious and salacious are avoided in the ensuing chapters. The problem is that once a careless or inappropriate statement attaches to a personality, it sticks like proverbial mud, at least some of which hopefully this book will wash away. Stone, commenting on the medical literature regarding Mozart, deplored a tendency to 'pathologise the lives of great men'.[6] That too will be a recurrent theme. Popular opinion can be brutal, and even smutty, whilst simultaneously being hypocritical and censorious. Thereby many composers' reputations have been sullied. An objective attempt is made herein to do justice to reputations.

Just as it seems important to challenge suspect assertions, so it is to question whether Mozart or Tchaikovsky were poisoned. Forensic, and possibly insufficiently forensic, accounts of the alleged suicides of composers as diverse as Tchaikovsky, Schumann or Peter Warlock reinvigorate controversy, and it is important to set the record straight where we can, but by what criteria?

In dealing with case histories from a hundred, let alone two hundred, years ago, research is at the mercy of terms used in the composer's own lifetime. Even today words like 'rheumatism' or 'palpitation' can have several different meanings. In considering treatment long ago it is easy to condemn, as future medical commentators may ridicule much of what we proudly do today. Accordingly, in judging the quality and probity of how composers were treated, a time-honoured legal paradigm, the Bolam Test is invoked throughout this book. It instructs experts, when judging the care of a patient, to consider what a reasonable body of medical opinion would have done at the time of treatment rather than now. Thus, in 2018 we should analyse treatment from 1856 by the standards of 1856, and not 2018. Two other legal paradigms will also be regularly employed. The cornerstone in judging a potentially criminal act is that the evidence is 'beyond all reasonable doubt', which is also applicable to judging the deaths of Mozart or Tchaikovsky. Of greatest help has been the crucial test in civil proceedings, which is to judge whether an event occurred on a balance of probabilities. English law dictates that if the balance of something having occurred is, for example, 52% to 48%, then that event did occur, thereby becoming the basis for all subsequent deliberations. Medical records, with the letters and diaries of composers and their friends, are often vivid and helpful in making clinical decisions today, despite the elapse of time.

Michael Steen's *The Lives and Times of the Great Composers* resonates with the history and geopolitics of each composer's era.[7] His theme of relating musical composition to external influences is well developed, whether these were war, revolution, love, sex or money. Clearly illness needs to be treated in a similar manner. It is always important to entwine life events with the progress of an illness, as a good physician always should whilst assessing a patient. This is especially important in dealing with psychological disturbances. Doctors omitting this basic principle do so at their own risk and that of their patients too. *That Jealous Demon, My Wretched Health* starts by looking at composers who died young, allowing conjecture as to what they might have composed by living to be sixty or seventy. A more crucial question is whether thirty-one and thirty-five, the ages at which Schubert and Mozart died, actually represent death as a 'young' man in 1791 or 1828, when the average age at death then for men was barely forty. Hopefully this question is answered fully in Chapter 1 by describing the average age at death of nearly three hundred composers over four centuries. As well as wondering what masterpiece would have been left had he lived to be sixty-five, I speculate how the composer might have fared had he received modern treatment. Attention to youth is then contrasted in the next chapter, which questions whether apparently triumphant old age really was all fanfares and accolades. Old age is today one of the most hotly debated and worrying medical conditions. Do older composers make musical valedictory statements as they apprehend death's approach? Is there music typically from a composer who knows he is not long for this world? Could a composer's total creative output be a finite entity almost irrespective of age?

A troubling group fall into Chapter 3: those whose medical treatment was harmful. Within the twentieth century three men will be described whose deaths were surgically hastened. For the remainder illness and death have been brought together in broad groups, thereby devoting chapters to heart, respiratory, neurological and psychiatric disease. Syphilis, alcoholism, cancer and deafness are presented on a similar basis. A layman's brief medical explanation introduces each chapter. Hopefully this will make the disease processes more relevant and interesting, but not too facile for medical readers. Each chapter seems to have its own characteristic themes. In places thematic evolution has been allowed to take primacy over simple chronology. One theme was those who died violently and/or accidentally. They are not accounted for in detail, there being little musical correlation. However, that nearly one in five suffered serious accidents is interesting, especially as most were fatal. Moreover, some readers may just want to know how Webern was shot or whether Alkan was fatally hit on the head by his Talmud. These were deaths which were more difficult to totally exclude than to briefly include. Thus, there is the brief Appendix summarising these violent deaths. A few stories creep in because, as well as holding a medical interest, they are entertaining, hence Gounod or Gesualdo.

Much which follows comes from a major review of appropriate biographies and a literature search of musical and/or medical publications, as well as from more primary research. Generally there can be two approaches to research and coming thereby to an informed judgement. One is to objectively and impartially gather all the evidence of reputable provenance and then to propose a conclusion. An alternative is to formulate a hypothesis and then to select pieces of confirmatory evidence. The latter risks disregarding other evidence whose inclusion might contradict the conclusion with which the study started rather than ended. The point is exemplified in Chapter 4 relating to Schubert, with whom Maynard Solomon appeared to have been selective,[8] only to have his views deconstructed in an analysis by Rita Steblin.[9] She proclaimed that 'It does not speak well of our critical faculties that we are blind to the deficiencies of the argument.' That became a compass to guide us through many other proclamations, often from writers of great repute but still capable of questionable judgement. An enthusiasm to attribute human frailty to composers was exemplified recently in a paper which declared seventy-seven of them to have been 'substance abusers'.[10]

Despite these reservations about medical aspects of the musical literature, there remains much medical good sense intertwined with musical biography in many publications. This has been abstracted and summarised within the terms of these studies. Some may wonder how these seventy composers were selected. Criticism is foreseen concerning why there is so much about Delius and little about Vaughan Williams. Firstly, most of the principal forty-four, as well as revealing a strong medical interest, would, I believe, be almost universally accepted as great composers, which hopefully defines for these purposes what I subsequently mean by 'great'. When relating music to illness, few composers are more revealing than Delius and less interesting than Vaughan Williams.

Whereas plagiarism has been earnestly avoided, many authorities will be openly and gratefully quoted, especially those who were generous with their help. Occasionally references have been made to concert programmes and to TV or radio broadcasts. By their very nature, these pronouncements are out in the public domain and thus are cited for corroboration or discourse. Above all else, throughout these studies the mantra of, 'If in doubt – ask,' has been invoked, recollecting J. K. Galbraith's caution that 'The conventional view serves to protect us from the painful job of thinking.'

In considerations of many conditions, psychological or organic, issues arise regarding music and the brain. Since the publication of a benchmark book by Critchley and Henson,[11] musical neurology has become topical, and further understanding may come by considering the output of composers with brain disease. A related topic is whether geniuses are mad, and whether madness itself may fuel musical creativity. Similarly alcohol, whatever it does to poets or actors when taken in regular excess, is assessed for its effect upon musical composition. The question as to whether illness itself can stimulate composition is also addressed.

It was difficult to judge how much purely medical analysis to include in this book, which is intended to be one of general and musical interest. This is especially so with Mozart, Beethoven and Tchaikovsky. However, my stated purpose of unravelling controversy and attempting conclusions is impossible without accounting for previous often conflicting claims. Medical description and conclusion are not strangers to musical writings. Sustaining opinion on a balance of probabilities is possible only by presenting the evidence before reaching a new conclusion to survive the test of time. Hopefully this will then enable us to reject much rumour, eristic speculation and occasionally absurd claims. In biography we are inevitably custodians of reputation. To these ends I have used my own varied professional experience over four decades in which exposure to both internal medicine and psychiatry preceded surgical practice. My conducting research for many years and an involvement with civil litigation have been bedrocks underlying these studies. Use of the first person has been eschewed except where its avoidance became contrived.

There is probably no better case with which to start than that of Mozart, with whom myth, legend and the absurd will all be encountered. His case illustrates the kindly awfulness which was eighteenth-century medicine but, above all, it will reveal the man's extraordinary determination to carry on almost until his last breath. Such courage and drive will re-appear with many subsequent composers, becoming perhaps the entire book's unifying theme, as triumphantly exemplified by concluding with Beethoven.

✛ Chapter 1 ✛

The Frailty of Youth

Almost everything that is great has been done by youth
Benjamin Disraeli, *Coningsby*, 1844

I N SOME MINDS COMPOSERS, like poets, die young in cold attics. Thirteen composers who died before they were forty are dealt with herein. They are:

Mozart	Chapter 1
Bellini	Chapter 1
Bizet	Chapter 1
Pergolesi	Chapter 1
Purcell	Chapter 1
Gershwin	Chapter 3
Schubert	Chapter 4
J. Clarke	Chapter 6
Warlock	Chapter 6
Mendelssohn	Chapter 7
Weber	Chapter 9
Chopin	Chapter 9
Butterworth	Appendix

This seemed reasonable evidence for the frailty of youth, which is accordingly examined further. Dorling Kindersley published brief sketches of over 300 composers, 293 of whom are now dead.[1] From this the average ages at death were calculated for each century until the present (Fig. 1). That average age remained fairly constant from the time of Hildegard of Bingen until the Second World War and, as Fig. 1 shows, composers generally have been survivors, despite Chopin or Mozart. The graph also shows the average age at death in the UK taken from the internet for the same periods, accepting that data before 1800 is very sketchy and that it is severely depressed by the inclusion of infant mortality, so rampant until modern times. That only 6.6% of the 303 composers died before reaching forty supports the view that the deaths of Mendelssohn and Schubert were of tragically young men. During their epoch the average age of a compos-er's death was sixty-five.

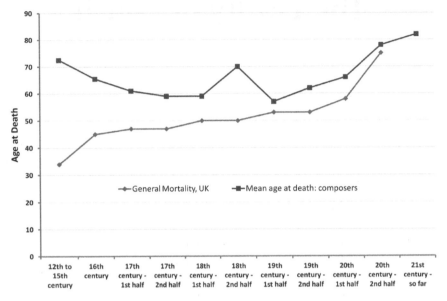

Fig. 1 Composers' average ages of death from the twelfth century until the present day

To Mozart we now turn.

✢ WOLFGANG AMADEUS MOZART ✢
(1756–1791)

Patience and tranquillity of mind contribute more to cure our distempers than the whole art of medicine.

W. A. Mozart, 1787

Just before Christmas 1790 two friends dined together in Vienna. One, a small man in his thirties, was energetic and wore his fair hair in a pigtail. The other was approaching sixty, looked it, and in the manner of the day wore a wig. The older man was about to set forth for London later that month, at the invitation of Salomon, the London impresario. When the younger man, W. A. Mozart, bade 'Papa' Haydn, older by twenty-three years, a tearful farewell, he said, 'I fear Papa, this is the last time we shall ever see each other.'[2] It seems a strange remark as Salomon's plan was for Mozart to join Haydn in London during 1792. Later Haydn's pupil Sigismund von Neukomm related that Mozart had a premonition of death,[3] although he explained that Haydn had assumed the remark to derive from the rigours of the imminent journey and his being the older man. Less than a year later, Mozart was dead and Haydn was to outlive him by a further eighteen years. Robbins Landon discarded the 'premonition of death' implicit in von Neukomm's account because Mozart was energetic, usually optimistic, and had thereunto enjoyed relatively good health, having vigorously survived numerous illnesses, including small-pox.[4] We should approach the 'greatest tragedy in the history of music' as an acute illness, about which the outpouring of variable opinion reaches almost industrial proportions.[5]

Mozart was a frequent letter writer, especially to his wife Constanze and his father. He also kept in regular touch with friends and colleagues. In 1938, Emily Anderson edited the Mozart family's correspondence into an invaluable source of information. With this, and the biographies of Deutsch, Jahn, Holmes and Glover, we have a firm basis for Mozart research. Ruth Halliwell's account of the Mozart family is assiduous in assessing the reliability of source material. Constanze's second husband, George Nikolaus von Nissen, late in life wrote a biography of his wife's first husband, published posthumously in 1828. The earlier biography, upon which Nissen drew, was that by Niemetschek.[6] The Salzburg Mozarteum's *Answers to the 111 Most Common Questions* is a useful source of opposition to fallible hearsay.[7] Furthermore, they have no recent additions to Mozart's correspondence. Mozart was a character about whom many recorded their dealings and meetings. Thus we are reasonably well served with material regarding the comings and goings, dates of composition or performance and illness, although much of it comes with the benefit of hindsight.

Although the basic facts of Mozart's life are familiar to many people, they are obfuscated by more controversy and diametrically opposed views than with almost any other composer, clouding a real appreciation of the man and his achievement. Peter Shaffer, whom some might hold partly at fault, put it well, saying, 'Nobody has suffered more than Mozart from sentimental misjudgement.'[8]

As we will see, many people have latched onto Mozart's amusement in farting and his earthy, but loving letters to Constanze and earlier to his cousin, known as the 'Bäsle', to the exclusion of what should be the main picture.[9] Perhaps it is we, the demotic public, who are responsible for these diversions. The Mozart lifeline is a well-trodden path which most biographers follow until they stop to discuss it, which is when controversy often sets in. Therefore, what are these controversies, and how may we reconcile them?

1 Did Mozart's father Leopold exploit his son's prodigious talent, thereby blunting his development, adversely affecting the boy's general health?
2 Was Mozart essentially robust or was he always a sickly lad?
3 How normal or abnormal was Mozart's appearance? Did he have a congenital abnormality of his left ear and if so did that have an association with kidney disease? Was his head deformed?
4 Is the 'Mozart skull' Mozart's, and was it fractured?
5 Did Mozart exhibit features of Tourette's syndrome?
6 Did Mozart have syphilis?
7 Was Mozart poisoned or self-poisoned?
8 What do the known facts surrounding Mozart's last illness lead us to conclude regarding his most probable cause of death?

Leopold Mozart

In a letter dated 30 July 1768, Leopold wrote of his son declaring, 'God has let a miracle see the light in Salzburg.'[10] Wolfgang was twelve at the time, and his verdict on Leopold was 'Next to God comes Papa.'[11] Loyalty and affection were Mozart's most endearing characteristics. As a child he said that when he grew up he would put his father in a glass case to protect him.[12] Davies suggests this was evidence of infantile omnipotence, which he added to other characteristics including narcissism, immaturity and obsessional behaviour: all very questionable.[13] His father was acutely aware of the genius he had sired and promoted his son so that, from the age of six, Mozart and his father, often with his talented sister, Nannerl, were on the road travelling throughout Europe. The Mozarteum Foundation has calculated that he spent a third of his life travelling;[14] no wonder he and Nannerl had a portable practice keyboard. It is from this daunting programme that the criticism of Leopold has arisen. That his children were ill on several occasions during these travels is well recorded, most notably in The Hague during 1765.

Obviously travel on unmade roads was slow and treacherous, but it is difficult to agree with O'Shea, who claimed that Mozart's chief medical biographers conclude that it was the ramifications of cumulative stresses of his early years, combined with overwork and poor self-care, that led to his early demise.[15] That illness sometimes occurred *during* his travels is undoubted; whether they were caused *by* his travels or demanding schedules of performance is dubious. Moreover, there is no evidence that had he stayed at home he would have been fitter and stronger. O'Shea writes of 'the pathos of a unique and awesomely gifted human being adrift in an often harsh and uncomprehending world'. Surely Mozart, during his travels with Leopold, was not adrift, but quite the opposite: possibly over-organised and over-worked. So let us consider what he might have done had he taken time out with other children. He was a small, highly intelligent, emotionally uninhibited, extrovert genius. One might argue that getting him to play the piano to acclaim and admiration amongst Europe's elite nobility was ideal for this unique child and young man. One suspects that laddish rough and tumble would not have suited the diminutive Wolfgang as well as the courts of Europe seem to have done.

Leopold was not wealthy so, pragmatically, he was probably correct to exploit the rewards for his son's talents, in the boy's interests as well as those of the family. This exposure seemed to be the best investment for Wolfgang's long-term security and professional progress. What would Mozart have done had his parents been 'enlightened' enough to insist on periods of rest and recreation? The answer is probably that this creative genius would have been utterly frustrated and, in O'Shea's words, 'adrift in an often harsh and uncomprehending world'.[16] Mozart himself should have the last word on his being pushed around by his father allegedly stunting his growth, for he wrote to his father, 'People who do not travel

– that is, those who are interested in the arts and learning – are miserable folk indeed.' In another letter from Italy, he declared what 'fun' it was to travel.[17]

The literature expands the charge sheet. Deutsch quotes Jean-Baptiste Suard, who attributed Mozart's 'stunted growth' and 'frail constitution' to the stresses of his childhood.[18] Provided that he was not malourished, and there is no evidence that he was, then medically there is nothing to suggest that travelling around Europe in a coach to play the piano would stunt skeletal development. Dr J. Barrault in 1905 observed that 'Mozart must have had an exceedingly robust constitution.'[19] He based this sensible assertion on the fact that, as others have testified,[20] Mozart was quite robust until the autumn of 1791, when it is clear that his preoccupation was with impecunity.[21]

A Robust or Sickly Constitution?

The notion that Mozart was sickly or puny has grown from his past medical history. This has been summarised by several authors, who have given varying weight and direction to their conclusions,[22] as follows.

1762   Upper respiratory tract infection (URTI), presumably
        streptococcal with possible associated tonsillitis*
            Later in 1762 another streptococcal infection with mild
        rheumatic fever, including appearance of red nodular patches
        (possibly erythema nodosum). May have had rheumatic fever
1764   Whilst in Paris and London experienced both tonsillitis and
        sinusitis
1765   Further tonsillitis and sinusitis. In December, whilst Mozart was
        in The Hague with Leopold and Nannerl, both children became
        gravely ill with recorded clinical features said to be typhoid,
        endemic there at the time. Made a full recovery
1766   In Munich: 'Further attacks of rheumatism'. Presumed to be

---

* Streptococcus is a germ which can lead to a number of infections, some serious, most notably of wounds, the respiratory tract, but also leading to kidney disease and/or rheumatic fever. L. R. Karhausen ('Mozart's Terminal Illness: Unravelling the Clinical Evidence', *Journal of Medical Biography* (2001) 9.34–48) has rightly pointed out that the literature's easy acceptance of streptococcal infections is without the firm foundation of a laboratory diagnosis, which remained unavailable for another century.

rheumatic fever, which can cause damage to the lining and valves of the heart (endocarditis)

1767 Smallpox whilst at Olmütz

1771 To recurrent URTI we can add jaundice, probably viral hepatitis A

1772 Tonsillitis

1774 Severe dental abscess

1778 and 1780 RTIs

1784 Bad attack of violent vomiting and colic as well as 'rheumatic inflammatory fever'

1787 and 1790 'Rheumatic pains'; headaches

So was he little better than a chronic invalid? It appears not, as he made staunch recoveries from many illnesses.[23] That he had thrown off and survived smallpox, possible rheumatic fever, probable recurrent streptococcal throat infections, and a severe infection in 1765 said to be typhoid reveals a young person who, had he been of a weaker constitution, might not have survived. The supposed typhoid in 1765 is often quoted, although Halliwell's researches reveal a condition whose description is more suggestive of pneumonia than of typhoid.[24] Overall, today he would have had antibiotics and his tonsils removed, potentially to great advantage. It was only when probable chronic kidney disease overtook him in his last weeks that we encounter a man whose moods veered towards depression without his customary frenetic energy.[25] Before then, his attitude to illness was epitomised whilst convalescing from smallpox, when he took up fencing. On 3 July 1791 he wrote that he was well in a letter to Constanze, and three months later he talked of hard work and a huge appetite. His letters of October 1791 are not those of a sick man.[26] The inference here is that, until 'the final illness', Mozart was generally vigorous.

Glover has chronicled Mozart's last few months, concluding that he was by then grossly overworking. Being a workaholic and having the output to prove it essentially precludes a feeble constitution or severe depression. His diminutive physique has led some to regard him as sickly. Keynes suggested he may have been as small as 4ft 11in or as high as 5ft 5in,[27] a stature consistent with the recent presidency of France. Dwarfism apart, there is little correlation between height and health, an exception being rickets and a variety of congenital syndromes such as Down's, none of which Mozart exhibited. Karhausen, normally a champion of assiduous Mozart research, has suggested that Mozart may have had rickets, which he states was endemic amongst children in late eighteenh-century cities such as London or Vienna, with a prevalence of 50–80%.[28] I am uneasy as to how such statistics emerge. Rickets could be consistent with Mozart's diminutive stature and his allegedly large head, although it was described by others as a short head.[29] Karhausen believes that Mozart's fingers may have been crooked because of rickets. The Nepomuk portrait shows Mozart and his sister with their right fingers straight and the left ones bent, as is normal at the mid-finger joints. Rickets affects bones, not joints. The typical deformity with rickets is bow-leg, not crooked fingers. Mozart had neither and we should dispense with this theory. Dr Barrault's view in 1905 that 'Mozart must have had an exceedingly robust constitution'[30] is surely correct.

Appearance

Much written has been too fanciful and fashioned into polarised views. In 1970 Carp, a surgeon, wrote 'Mozart: His Tragic Life and Controversial Death', opening his account with the view that 'his physical stature was against him'.[31] Dr Peter Davies, an Australian physician, tells us, 'Mozart suffered a great deal from his unattractive appearance.'[32] Keynes, an English surgeon, wrote similarly.[33] Carp opined that Mozart was, 'unimpressive, short and thin, with a disproportionately large head', and that 'his ears were deformed'.[34] It sounds like Tolkien's Gollum, but this was Dr Carp's view regarding Mozart, who, he wrote, evidently 'squandered a good deal of his income on clothes', and 'Jewellery was another fetish of his.' So strident are these opinions that the manner of their expression might undermine their veracity. The biographical literature hardly supports these judgements, although Nannerl did write, 'His physiognomy did not show his genius or the spirit which our great God has given him.'[35] From contemporary accounts, despite his being small, his charm, energy, quick wit, intelligence and affectionate nature secured his position in society, being threatened only by his tactlessness and the jealousy of others.

The fifteen authenticated portraits of Mozart do not reveal a handsome man, nor is his countenance displeasing.[36] Neither does his head seem to be unduly large or misshapen, although his nose may be a little prominent at the expense of his chin, and his brow steep. Nevertheless, we are looking at one of the greatest musical geniuses of all time, not casting for the next 'Superman' film. We do know that his face was pockmarked by smallpox.[37] A key to some of these claims may lie in the 'Mozart skull' in the Salzburg Mozart Museum.

The Mozart Skull and Mozart Ears

Mozart was buried in a standard communal, not a pauper's, grave.[38] A skull was supposedly retrieved by Joseph Rothmayer, a grave-digger, whilst reorganising the graveyard ten years after he had buried Mozart.[39] Rothmayer claimed to remember where he had buried Mozart and recognised the remains.[40] One wonders how. Gravediggers were badly paid and perhaps sought gratuities. A more generous view is that he kept the skull as a holy relic. In 1842 the brother of Joseph Hyrtl, a Viennese anatomist, obtained the skull from Rothmayr's successor.[41] It remained in the Hyrtl family until 1901 becoming, after two years of legal proceedings, the property of the city of Salzburg and thereafter reposing in the museum. There is further confusion because there are two Mozart skulls, one with seven teeth, the other with eleven.[42]

In 1989 a Franco-Austrian group with an interest in skull morphology reported on the Mozart skull from the Salzburg Mozarteum.[43] Their studies included taking X-rays and CT scans, as well as twenty-three morphometric measurements from the skull. They also made tracings and related them to pictures of Mozart. A problem there is that there is no good portrait of Mozart.[44] They also studied ten south German skulls which had a congenital abnormality known as premature synostosis of the metopic suture (PSMS), as well as male inhabitants of an Austrian village where that condition may be in-bred. In simple English, PSMS means that the parts of the skull, normally separate in children, become prematurely joined in adolescence. This may lead to a recognisable syndrome with a steep forehead, a prominent upper face and nose when related to the jaw (missing from the Mozart skull) and oval, shallow eye sockets. They concluded that Mozart had PSMS,[45] and claimed that the various correlations they had made further verified the Mozart skull as having once been Mozart's.[46]

They made another much more important observation, for the skull exhibited a 10cm fracture which crossed the line of the middle meningeal artery, a feature notorious for causing potentially fatal intracranial bleeding (extra-dural haemorrhage) after skull fractures.[47] Moreover, there was on the inside of the skull an actual footprint-like impression of where such a haemorrhage had been. This was no serendipitous finding. For a fracture to have occurred, serious violence would have been necessary and, as there had been no trephining of the skull to relieve the haemorrhage, one would, on a balance of probabilities, have expected a coma to precede inevitable death. This group does recount that for several months in 1790

Mozart was prone to bandage his aching head.[48] A haemorrhage sufficient to leave a bony imprint would obviously have been a serious entity. Since there is absolutely no record or suggestion of a fall or blow to the head, we can be all but certain that the fracture, and therefore the skull, was not Mozart's. DNA analysis of material from this skull, carried out in 2006 for Austrian TV, was 'inconclusive'.[49] The Mozarteum do not know whether the skull is Mozart's,[50] and accordingly lines of research based on this relic, favoured by tourists, would be upon a very uncertain basis.

What remains interesting is the perplexing case of 'Mozart's ear', in itself today an eponymous clinical entity. This is an inherited abnormality of the external ear, whose outline is rather square with an underdeveloped lobe just behind the jaw and a narrow helix (outer rim). Researchers concluded that Mozart ear is a very unusual abnormality.[51] They studied various pictures of Mozart and/or his children. In the well-known Knight of the Golden Spur portrait, we can see only the lowest third of his right ear, the rest being covered by hair, very much as in the Barbara Krafft painting of, admittedly, 1819. However, the famous Nepomuk family portrait of 1780 shows the lower half and may reveal a square configuration. Davies claims that congenital ear malformations occur in 1:3,800 live births, and 90% of them are one-sided.[52] He shows a lithograph from Nissen's biography illustrating a drawing of Mozart's ear. The famous silverpoint drawing by Dorothea Stock of 1789, like other pictures, reveals more hair than ear, but Davies suggests that the auricular lobe is absent. Moreover, Gerber said there was no drawing of Mozart's left ear in Nissen's first edition of his Mozart biography of 1828.[53]

The reader's pulse is unlikely to have quickened with these deliberations. Do they matter? Davies believed that Mozart was very self-conscious about it and covered it with a carefully tailored wig. There is little good evidence that Mozart was sensitive about his ear, and if the ear was covered, how did they know it was deformed? He was proud of his own usually well-coiffured fair hair.[54] So the problem would be solved or discarded as an utter triviality, were it not for the question as to whether there is an association between congenital abnormalities of the external ear and of the kidneys,[55] something rejected by Davies,[56] relating the alleged Mozart ear deformity to polycystic kidneys.* Mozart probably died of chronic renal disease, to which a number of congenital abnormalities can lead. Thus Mozart's ear invites the question of whether his kidney failure

---

* One of the commonest renal congenital abnormalities.

was secondary to a congenital abnormality of his renal tract,[57] to which his ear may be a clue.

Karhausen, something of a Davies opponent,[58] showed that the chance of someone with an external ear abnormality having a congenital abnormality of the urinary tract was a hundred times higher than in the general population.[59] One would be more impressed with Mozart's ear were those little bits of ear poking through his hair examples of it. As with the skull, we fall at the first fence. The postulates are all interesting, only providing that the ear was abnormal and the skull was Mozart's.

Tourette's Syndrome

In 1983 it was first suggested, at the World Congress of Psychiatry in Vienna, that Mozart had Tourette's syndrome,[60] which is said to prevail in 2% of the general population,[61] perhaps because today many milder cases are diagnosed, possibly over-diagnosed, than were in the past. The diagnostic characteristic of Tourette's is multiple involuntary tics which wax and wane, one of which must be vocal and all lasting beyond one year to sustain a diagnosis. Copromania or coprolalia (an abnormal tendency to talk or exclaim about excrement) is reported in 10% of cases,[62] but neither this nor uttering profanity is essential to a diagnosis.[63] The commonest tics are eye blinking, coughing and throat clearing, often like a bark. The cause is unknown, beyond a tendency for inheritance,[64] although no gene has been identified. A recent suggestion is that the cause may be a previous streptococcal infection,[65] a point of interest as Mozart is presumed to have suffered from many assumed 'strep throats' since childhood.[66]

Dr Benjamin Simkin's book '*Medical and Musical Byways of Mozartiana* is well researched, medically and musically.[67] One quickly grasps that Dr Simkin has a simple thesis: Mozart exhibited Tourette's syndrome. His paradigms are the unshakable fact that Mozart was scatological in his conversation, his writings and, in the case of the B flat major Canon (K231), in his composition, this piece being subtitled 'Leck mich im Arsch' ('Lick me in the arse').[68] Of Mozart's letters at least 10% are said to be scatological.[69] Bottoms and their product were clearly a Mozartian preoccupation.

But he was not alone. 'Leck mich im Arsch' derives from Goethe's *Götz von Berlichingen* and, as yet, Tourette's syndrome remains unascribed to the courtly German poet. Another curiosity is the famous *Bäsle-Briefe*,[70] the 'Bäsle' being Mozart's younger cousin and an early lady love. His letter to her of 5 November 1777 is quoted by Simkin.[71] He gives us the English translation in full, to illustrate repetition of word sounds and rhyming as well as mirror imaging, word scrambling and, of course, scatology. Associations such as 'my uncle carbuncle', like the hope that there will be no serious 'consequences, excrescences', illustrate his point perfectly, with one problem: they work in English but, translated back into German, in which the Bäsle letter was written,[72] the mechanism does not work as well. There are various translations, as a comparison between Simkin's and Emily Anderson's translation of the 5 November 1777 letter to his father reveals.[73] Clearly, 'I shit on your nose', as Simkin reports Mozart wrote to 'Coz Fuzz',[74] comes unexpectedly, although it is absent from the translation given by Anderson.[75]

The Canon in A major (K561) is a sweet thing, with lullabies in five different languages. At the end in Viennese, Mozart pops in the line 'Shit in bed until it creaks', an unseemly exhortation, but one even made by his mother.[76] Such vulgarity was commonplace in both Bavaria and Salzburg in the late eighteenth century. Although this is not diagnostic of Tourette's, it is the uttering of obscenities which most people still associate with its diagnosis. This, however, was the time of *Bölzschiessen* – target practice sometimes at pictures of people's bottoms, evidently a game for all the family.[77]

Dr Simkin accommodates Mozart's repetitive retreat into the lavatorial by describing two types of Tourette's syndrome. The *stereotypic* form is that already described. The second form he terms *phantasmagoric*, a concept coming from Oliver Sacks, the famous neurologist.[78] In this condition mimicry, playfulness, having an exceptional memory, being inventive and with a tendency to dramatisation and emotional incontinence are the classic features and coincide well with many people's picture of Mozart's personality. No wonder one in fifty of us are said to suffer from Tourette's, without necessarily knowing about it! Swerdlow likened a neurologist and a psychiatrist discussing this neuropsychiatric disorder to two blind men discussing the appearance of an elephant.[79] There is no good clinical reason to base a diagnosis of Tourette's on the complex wordplay beloved of Mozart and described by Winternitz.[80] Karhausen reminds us of Mozart's love of challenging taboos.[81]

The tic aspect of the diagnosis seems very unclear from what we know of Mozart's eccentric behaviour. Being garrulous, profane or jumping off the stage may be irritating for others, even bizarre, but medically these are not tics. Karoline Pichler, one of Mozart's circle, described a rehearsal by Mozart with the Mannheim orchestra when he 'meowed like a cat, leapt over tables and turned somersaults'.[82] This could be regarded as Tourette-like behaviour, but on questionable grounds.

Mozart's hyperkinesis and strange lapses into scatology do not support a firm diagnosis. Uttering profanities is so much at odds with the sublime music of *Figaro*, or the Requiem and much else, that people need to attribute these aberrations to a disease process, for how else could such a beautiful composer say such vulgar things? But do we really need the supporting appellation of a syndrome? As for uttering profanities, if that makes a diagnosis of Tourette's then I had never realised how many of my pleasant, sometimes ribald, acquaintances may be suffering from this disorder. As Sacks said, it seems to be all about 'Exploiting the Ticcy Witticisms and Witty Ticcicisms'.[83]

An even more complex subject evolved by Dr Simkin was the issue of Mozart's 'musical Touretteisms'. He says that the very early D major Symphony (K19) contains chromaticisms, major-minor shifts and, to quote, 'herky-jerky base rhythms', as well as 'an offbeat held A-sharp unison at the onset of the development'. These he believes are all examples.[84] Whether they would be recognised by the Tourette Syndrome Association must be uncertain. Meanwhile, Karhausen advises us, 'Beware of psychiatrists who analyse jokes, instead of laughing at them.'[85] Before we leave this subject it is salient to reflect that, had Mozart lived in the twentieth century, he would probably have been saved from death due to kidney and/or heart failure. But he might also have been treated with haloperidol for his alleged Tourette's syndrome, which could have suppressed his creativity.

Kammer, a German psychiatrist, observes that Tourette's syndrome is an 'inventive but implausible diagnosis' with Mozart which fails to meet diagnostic criteria.[86] Neither was Sacks entirely convinced either.[87] We should judge Mozart's odd behaviour in two principal lights. Social custom determined then, as it does now, what is and is not acceptable. Secondly, Mozart was always a bit of a jester. My two final authorities on Mozart's Tourette's are Humpty Dumpty, who said that when he used a word, it meant what he wanted it to mean, and Leopold Mozart, who frequently observed that his son was a bit of a scamp.

Syphilis

We are seldom far from syphilis in historical musical considerations. An article suggesting Mozart may have had syphilis appeared in Germany as recently as 2005.[88] Stafford reported Katner and Kerner's claim that Mozart may have misjudged the dose of mercury which he was taking, presumably, for syphilis and accordingly and accidentally poisoned himself.[89] The signs of mercurial overdose were well known in 1791. Suffice it to say that no sound clinical evidence of those signs is recorded, despite Kerner's views, with which Stafford then disagrees. Writing of 'Syphilis in Composers', Franzen exonerates Mozart,[90] as Fluker, a venerologist, did over thirty years ago.[91] There is no retrospective, let alone contemporaneous, account leading to a suspicion that Mozart suffered from the first or second stages of syphilis. Analysing his final illness, we can be entirely confident that he did not die of, or with, tertiary syphilis. Doctors depend upon signs and symptoms and, of those for syphilis, contemporary and early accounts in the case of Mozart are notably absent.

Murder and Poison

Conspiracy theories abound about the death of Mozart, and we should first consider whether he was *murdered* by being struck on the head. The improbability of this beyond all reasonable doubt has been dealt with in relation to the Mozart skull. Dr Closset was a respected physician in late eighteenth-century Vienna who regularly attended Mozart until the end. He also called in Dr Matthias von Sallaba from the Vienna General Hospital, and they conferred with other eminent colleagues.[92] Significantly, neither at the time when Mozart was dying nor subsequently did either of them suspect foul play, but Dr Closset is reported as having said that Mozart had a 'deposit to the head' ('un deposito alla testa').[93] The language is curious in the use of the word 'deposit'. Hirschmann infers that implicit in the German literature is that 'deposits' and 'determinations' to the head are vernacular from eighteenth-century medicine.[94] However, nothing in the later accounts of Constanze, her sister Sophie or his son Karl suggests that Dr Closset or Dr Sallaba was concerned that there was any evidence of Mozart having sustained a blow to the head or worse. The nature of his passing was totally inconsistent with a head injury.

A more promising line of investigation is into *poisoning*, whether medically prescribed or administered with nefarious intent. Just before he died Mozart told Sophie, 'I already have perceived the earthy taste of Death on my tongue',[95] which is sometimes thought to mean the taste of poison. It was more probably a metaphor of foreboding, as many disease processes, including uraemia, lead to unpleasantness in the mouth. Rebuttal of this theory rests upon two facts. Firstly, his immediate family, close friends and doctors were in constant attendance during the final illness. Ease of access for those of murderous disposition would have been very difficult. Yet Carp reported that, during a performance on 23 May 1824 of Beethoven's 'Choral Symphony', circulars were passed around the auditorium saying that Salieri had placed poison by Mozart's bedside.[96] By early December 1791 Dr Closset was in daily attendance, which, as he put it himself, was 'as much the solicitude of a friend, as the attention of a medical man',[97] and there is no evidence that either he or Dr Sallaba ever suspected poisoning. This was recorded later by Dr Eduard Vincent Guldener von Lobes in his correspondence with Giuseppe Carpani, Haydn's biographer, with whom Dr Closset had communicated during the final illness.[98]

Kerner has been a leading proponent for death by poisoning.[99] He suggested that Mozart received two doses of mercury, one in the summer of 1791 when he was still well, and a second larger one on 20 November 1791, two days after his return from the Masonic dinner. Administration of mercury was commonplace in those days for many conditions. Kerner even suggested that Mozart may have unwittingly poisoned himself with one of the potions prescribed and/or self-administered in the late eighteenth century, a view demolished by Stafford.[100] Nevertheless, just once before he died he confided to a friend that he had been given aqua tofana six months earlier.[101] Aqua tofana was a commonly prescribed 'medicine', to be found on many bedside tables, based upon a seventeenth-century formula. It contained lead, antimony and bismuth. The clinical features over his last six months or during the last few weeks do not suggest poisoning from these substances.

According to Constanze, Wolfgang unburdened himself to her in the Prater on 20 or 21 October 1791, 'I am only too conscious that my end will not be long in coming for sure, someone has poisoned me.'[102] Death by poisoning over two months or more would be unusual. Although basically cheerful, Mozart always had been subject to mood swings and, according to some, was manic-depressive.[103] When low, Mozart tended to muse about death and mortality, but then many of us do, and he always quickly bounced back.

Professor Jenkins summarises Mozart's medical history and death,[104] quoting from Anderson that in July 1791 Mozart had written, 'As for my health I feel pretty well.'[105] Six weeks before he died he confided, 'I have a voracious appetite today.' Mozart by then was working prodigiously hard, once saying that he had worked until he was ill as he composed *La clemenza di Tito* in eighteen days.[106] Completion of the Clarinet Concerto followed, along with a cantata, before the fateful embarkation upon the Requiem. People either die immediately from poisoning or succumb incrementally to more surreptitious dosage over a longer period of time. Being 'pretty well', hungry and dashing off great operas makes poisoning highly improbable.

Popular impetus to the poisoning theory came from Peter Shaffer's play *Amadeus* with its strong imputation that Salieri, eaten by jealousy, poisoned Mozart. There is an accord that at least superficially the two men were on cordial terms, but possibly there were undertones, perhaps because the idea for *Così fan tutte* had originally been Salieri's. A letter from Leopold to Nannerl in 1786 is worth quoting: 'It will be surprising if it [*The Marriage of Figaro*] is a success, for I know that very powerful cabals have ranged against your brother. Salieri and all his supporters will again try to move heaven and earth to bring down his opera.'[107] The word 'again' is especially interesting. Paradoxically, Mozart had written to Constanze that Salieri had congenially accompanied him to a performance of *The Magic Flute* in October 1791.[108]

By 1791 Salieri's professional star was in the ascendant and Mozart's in decline, bringing motive into question. The contrasting diplomatic skills of the two composers may have been critical to their career development. Shaffer's play implies that Salieri recognised Mozart's genius better than most. However, he also had a good opinion of his own abilities, and he was the Court Composer. Although Mozart was appointed Music Director of St Stephen's Cathedral just before he died, Salieri's position was pre-eminent, so motive is questionable. During 1829 Franz said that his father had not been poisoned by Salieri, but imputed that his *life* had been.[109] In so saying, perhaps Franz finally laid the Salieri poisoning theory to rest.

Probably the greatest substance for the legend emanates from Salieri himself. In the early 1820s the by now old and frail Salieri was in an institution, starting to develop dementia. One of his claims is said to have been that he had poisoned Mozart. One person to take great interest in this was Beethoven, whose secretary, Schindler, noted that 'Salieri is again in a very bad way. He is quite ruined. He has fantasies that he was responsible for Mozart's death and gave him poison.'[110] As ever, the pendulum swings with claim and counter-claim, for in October 1823 Beethoven's pupil Moscheles visited the sick and senile Salieri in hospital. This meeting concluded with Salieri saying, 'Although this is my last illness, I can assure you on my word of honour that there is no truth in that absurd rumour; you know, that I am supposed to have poisoned Mozart. But no, it's malice, pure malice, tell the world dear Moscheles, old Salieri who will soon die has told you.'[111] Soon after this, Salieri unsuccessfully attempted suicide. He eventually died on 7 May 1825. Those attending Salieri affirmed that they had never heard his famous confession. Perhaps, in the way of the senile,

Salieri may have rambled on that he did it, or he may have rambled on about people who *said* he had done it. Mary Novello believed that Salieri's self-accusations were born out of a sense of guilt for his earlier duplicity towards Mozart.[112]

In conclusion, although the conspiracy theories of poisoning are not totally without foundation, as Davies has outlined, most are flawed, and there are others that are essentially without foundation. Other alleged culprits have included Constanze, Süssmayr and the Freemasons.[113] We will see from the next section that there are several good explanations for Mozart's death, based upon known facts and opinions from people who were there at the time, or who had known him. It is probably no coincidence that the poisoning/Salieri school had its acme not in Austria, but in Hollywood, where we should leave it.

The Cause of Death in the Final Illness

A definitive history of Mozart's last year is that of H. C. Robbins Landon, despite reservations regarding the purely medical aspects, where we need to be circumspect in assessing the evidence. For example Robbins Landon, relying heavily upon Dr Peter Davies, affirms that in 1762 Mozart had a 'streptococcal throat' infection.[114] Our problem in seeing 'streptococcal throat' in black and white is that it appears so authoritative. But there is no way of positively affirming that it was a streptococcal infection, tests for which did not exist at the time, although different infections can present with a typical clinical picture.

Circumspection is also due with medical terms from the late eighteenth century. For example, 'rheumatic' or 'rheumatism' does not necessarily refer to either rheumatic fever or rheumatoid arthritis. Then it was generally a synonym for aching pain, and it still is. So an assertion of rheumatic fever due to streptococcus without corroborative evidence may mean little more than general aching in someone with a sore throat, possibly with a fever. From this we will now work assuming, as many authors appear to have done,[115] that Mozart was generally well until his last few months, whereafter authors diverge. So we go to the beginning of the end.

On 6 September 1791 Mozart attended *La clemenza di Tito* in Prague as part of the celebration for the coronation of Leopold II. Then he conducted the first few nights of *The Magic Flute*, as well as being busy composing. Davies quotes from Mozart's friend Niemetschek the story that it was then when 'Mozart fell ill and dosed himself ceaselessly, his colour was pale and countenance sad, although his merry sense of humour often bubbled into jesting.'[116] Whether this is a picture of an overworked man or one drifting into mortal decline we cannot know. Authorities may fit their judgements around their own presumed diagnoses.

At this time Mozart also escorted Constanze to Baden, where she went for cures and he went over to their son Karl's school. By these and other accounts, until October 1791 Mozart was usually well and worried far more about his wife's health than about his own.[117] There is some evidence that 'Mozart was depressed' – a clinical term. Davies quotes a letter from Wolfgang to Constanze dated 7 July 1791 when she was away as evidence of depression.[118] Mozart spoke of 'aching for you', 'emptiness' and 'longing' and said even playing the piano stirred his emotions too much. Such florid language is not typical of serious depression; it seems to be a letter from a lovesick artist who was missing his adored wife.

We cannot detail the final illness without considering the Requiem. In July 1791 Anton Leitgeb, a gaunt stranger, came to Mozart's apartment to solicit the anonymous composition of a requiem mass and for a substantial fee. Leitgeb was sent by his master, Count Franz Walsegg-Stuppach, who had been widowed earlier that year. Mozart, driven at this time by money worries, accepted the commission. When Leitgeb returned to Mozart in October 1791 he saw that Mozart seemed unwell. His friend the Abbé Stadler wrote in 1826 to Mozart's publisher André that in October 1791, Mozart was working with love, diligence – and difficulty.[119] Davies and others have suggested that by now Mozart was tormented by the thought that sinister forces were conspiring to cause his death.[120] He believed that he might have been commissioned to compose his own requiem,[121] a popular theory subsequently. This stems from the story given first by Niemetschek and then Nissen of his unburdening to Constanze when they drove to the Prater on 20 or 21 October.[122] It may be argued that even as he dined with Haydn in December 1790 Mozart may have had a premonition of his own death.[123] For all his customary vigour, Mozart had by then been complaining of recurrent headaches and loin pain, 'swooning' and being enervated. Rochlitz reported in 1798 that, during composition of the Requiem, Mozart often sank into complete exhaustion and 'fainted'.[124] Too much might be read from translation after two centuries into words like 'faint' or 'swoon'. Today people say that they are 'shattered'. One hopes that in two hundred years' time experts will not suspect that all such persons had been found in many bloody pieces.

On Mozart's return to Vienna at the end of September 1791 *The Magic Flute* was produced, quickly followed by the Clarinet Concerto (K622) with its plangent middle movement and lastly the Masonic Cantata (K623), to which Constanze had tried to divert him in order to deflect thoughts of composing his own requiem. If we are to accept the sadness implicit in K622 as foreboding of future tragedy, then we should make similar application to many earlier compositions with sad themes, such as the Piano Concerto No. 21 (K467). Surely in much of art beauty is betrothed to sadness.

Then there comes Mozart's last visit to the Masonic lodge on 18 November. The suggestion first appearing in Jahn's biography of 1891, that he may have been poisoned there, was regarded by Guillery as 'Nazi propaganda'.[125] To this outing, from which Mozart had returned cheerfully, Davies and thus Robbins Landon have attributed the acquisition of an assumed streptococcal infection from which all else stemmed.[126] By 20 November Mozart was so ill that he retired to his bed, from which he never significantly arose again.[127] Therefore we contemplate a fifteen-day illness, Mozart remaining conscious until two hours before his death.

Available clinical information comes from those in attendance, namely Constanze, her sister Sophie, his older son Karl Thomas, Dr Closset and Dr Sallaba. To the accounts of these final days we may add the memoranda of Vincent and Mary Novello of the Novello publishing family. Sophie had earlier corresponded with Mozart's biographer Georg von Nissen, by then her second brother-in-law. Distinct patterns emerge. On retiring to bed Mozart developed painful swelling of the hands and feet, which might suggest some form of inflammatory arthritis. The headaches, nausea, vomiting and fainting worsened. He was said to have had a rash,[128] although accounts of direct observation, as opposed to supposition of such a rash, are hard to come by. Karhausen suggested it could have been due to 'prickly heat', which was discounted by Keynes.[129] Everyone noticed that Mozart had become increasingly swollen, which we can safely assume was due to generalised oedema. So swollen did he become that Sophie and her mother made him nightshirts that would open at the front; as she wrote to Nissen, 'He was very swollen and therefore movement was difficult.'[130] She also noticed his making such heavy weather of completing the Requiem that he deputed his pupil Süssmayr to complete the work 'after I have gone'. There was also a stench, which was due to 'putrefaction';[131] this was possibly why an autopsy was not performed. Therefore the ghoulish notion of Mozart literally rotting in bed grew up. The most probable explanation for the rotting smell is that the immobile Mozart had developed infected bedsores.

Death and Funeral

In early December 1791 the pale, grossly swollen patient lay painfully in bed, miserable and hardly able to move. There had been some projectile vomiting and there was a foul odour in the room, but Mozart's son, his wife and her sister were kindly, attentive and distressed by his obvious suffering. The young musician Süssmayr had taken down the master's final musical offerings to the incomplete Requiem and Dr Closset visited daily, although when called on the evening of 4 December he was delayed at the theatre, despite Constanze correctly believing that the end was nigh. Early on the morning of 5 December 1791 Mozart died, perhaps the greatest tragedy in the history of music.[132] Despite rumours and conspiracy theories, the funeral and subsequent burial were routine and in keeping with the recently introduced statutes of the time.[133] Within them is the obvious assumption of infection.

The Cause of Death: Fact or Fiction?

Medically the key points are the following:

1 Mozart was probably of previously robust constitution despite a number of past illnesses.
2 He had suffered from many URTIs and throat infections for which the likely germ was streptococcus. It is well recognised today that other diseases which streptococcus may cause include rheumatic fever, bacterial endocarditis, Bright's disease (glomerulo-nephritis of the kidney) and Henoch-Schönlein purpura, of which more soon.
3 At the end Mozart was grossly swollen with oedema.
4 There may have been earlier swelling of joints (inflammatory arthritis or polyarthritis).
5 There is said to have been a rash, the evidence for which is scant.
6 There are vague intimations suggesting an epidemic at the time.
7 There was weakness, immobility, headache, lassitude and paleness (assumed to be anaemia) worsened by draconian blood-letting.
8 There are descriptions of pain, of variable distribution.
9 Mozart remained conscious until almost the very end.
10 The cheek-puffing at the end is probably mythical, although picturesque.
11 There were probably foul-smelling bedsores.

12 Mozart complained of a nasty taste in his mouth.

Diagnosis: Possibilities and Fallacies

1 **140 different diagnoses** have been advanced so far.[134] As Mark Twain once quipped, 'Researches of many scholars have already thrown much darkness on the subject.'

2 **Syphilis and head injury** have been discounted beyond all reasonable doubt.

3 **Alcoholism**, as attributed by Breitenfeld,[135] has little foundation, like his improbable suggestion of brucellosis, a largely agricultural disease. He then went on to suggest that paintings of Mozart showed exophthalmos (protruding eyes), which may be associated with an overactive thyroid gland. This is a fair suggestion in a thin hyperkinetic patient, with possible exophthalmos. We are at the mercy of portraits, and I am far from persuaded that his eyes were abnormal, having discussed all the pictures with a surgeon experienced with thyroid eye disease.*

4 **Bronchopneumonia** is believed by Dr Peter Davies to have been the final cause of death; it is the Great Reaper's calling card with many seriously ill people. On a death certificate today the secondary cause of death would probably be kidney failure.

5 **Dr Peter Davies and Professor L. R. Karhausen**, two prominent doctors in Mozart research, have often been adversaries. It all gets quite personal, as Karhausen says of Davies, 'There is a striking contrast between the discerning line of reasoning he makes against alternate hypotheses and the extreme laxity with which he justifies his own proposals.'[136] Davies and Karhausen even write papers 'contra' the other.[137] Davies's excellent contributions have been overshadowed by the antagonism he has sometimes stirred, although the Mozart Museum was unaware of Dr Davies's work.[138] However, his deconstruction of the various poisoning theories is probably pre-eminent. To take a purview of medical Mozartology, the writings of Karhausen are sensible, thorough and usually hard to contest.

6 **Dr Carl Bär**, a Swiss dentist, was regarded as the leading authority on Mozart's death,[139] until Davies first published in 1983.[140] In his definitive book about Mozart's last year, Robbins Landon said, 'All

---

* The author is grateful to Mrs J. L. Noble FRCSE, DO for her expert opinion.

an amateur can do in the circumstances is to summarise Dr Davies's findings and express admiration for their lucid presentation', whence he introduces Henoch-Schönlein purpura, hypertensive encephalopathy and even a stroke, as Bär recedes from attention.

7   **Heart failure:** Bär's diagnosis of rheumatic fever was based upon the known past medical history, the likelihood of streptococcal infection and hearsay about an epidemic. This and the death in gross oedema led him to the reasonable conclusion that it had been heart failure secondary to acute rheumatic fever. He went on to suggest that Dr Sallaba's bleeding of Mozart hastened the end by adding the strain of haemorrhage to an ailing heart. That and the variation upon the rheumatic fever diagnosis, namely bacterial endocarditis (which is an infection of the lining of the heart), are all plausible arguments.[141] However, they were rejected by Davies on several grounds.[142] Firstly, neither typically cause the gross oedema, which is one of the few absolutely firm facts in our possession. That, however, may be a twentieth-century view, because the resolution of untreated rheumatic fever or endocarditis was very different when there were no antibiotics, diuretics or drugs to stimulate the heart. Rheumatic fever still fits the available facts better than many alternative theories. Keynes 'ruled out' rheumatic fever, without fully elucidating his reasons.[143] Karhausen infers that Mozart did not have arthritic joints.[144] He may be right, but consider this. He himself writes of Mozart's swollen hands and feet and even went on to say that his hands were 'probably crippled'. Oedema can stiffen, but does not cripple the hands; arthritis does. Davies's other reasons for rejecting rheumatic fever or endocarditis were that they did not come within an epidemic, or account for the 'neurological crisis' described by Davies alone.[145] So both are now considered.

8   **An epidemic:** Open to debate is whether there was in Vienna, at the time of Mozart's death, an epidemic. Von Lobes had written many years after the event that many of the inhabitants of Vienna had been labouring under the same complaint.[146] From such recollections perhaps epidemics may spread. Mozart died in gross oedema, which is principally seen with kidney or heart failure. Zegers et al. looked at deaths in men under forty from 'oedema' registered in Vienna from November to January in 1790, 1791 and 1792.[147] There was a small, significant increase in 1791, the year of Mozart's death: a cluster, but not of epidemic proportions. Karhausen reported on the registration of 656 deaths in Vienna at that time and could find only

one individual with whom 'severe miliary fever' (*hitziges Frienfieber*) was given as the cause of death.[148] That one individual was Mozart: hardly an epidemic. It must be conceded that *hitziges Frienfieber* is a very non-specific diagnosis.[149] In the epidemiological records available for that period, there is only a 17% increase in the anticipated death rate during November and December 1791.[150] It all calls into serious question whether Mozart was victim of an epidemic said to have been rife in Vienna.

9　**Neurological crisis**: Davies advanced the diagnosis of chronic kidney failure as the most likely cause of death.[151] So far so good, but Davies then said this led to a stroke which caused paralysis. But let Davies, again extensively quoted by Robbins Landon, explain: 'It may be concluded that Mozart at this time suffered a hemiparesis and was paralysed down one side of his body', (i.e. a stroke), then warming to the subject: 'His partial paralysis was a hemiplegia'. He continues: 'About two hours before he died, he convulsed and became comatose.'[152] Coma accords with most accounts, but Davies continues: 'Then an hour later he attempted to sit up, opened his eyes wide and fell back with his head turned to the wall, his cheeks puffed out.' Davies then concluded, 'These symptoms suggest paralysis of conjugate gaze, and facial nerve palsy, consistent with massive cerebral haemorrhage',[153] to which I will return. The cheeks puffing out seem to be the part of this myth to attract most interest. Sophie Haibel's explanation was that he was trying to suggest drums for the incomplete composition of the 'Lacrymosa' for his Requiem. It evokes a cinematographic picture, but generally has little clinical resonance with the final passing of those who are desperately ill. As Karhausen implied, that he wept is a more plausible scenario.[154]

I take issue with hemiparesis or hemiplegia. This explanation for Mozart's immobility does not fit the facts. His weakened, debilitated state, worsened by being waterlogged as well as having painful, swollen joints, all features for which there is consistent evidence, are more than ample reasons for him being immobile. Nothing in the various accounts suggests that he had suffered the stroke which Davies imputes. Karhausen refers us to Jahn's biography,[155] saying that 'almost complete immobility' (in Geman) was mistranslated then as 'partial paralysis' (in English). In 1845 Edward Holmes translated Nissen upon this point as 'an almost total incapacity of motion'.[156] This is the key: inability or incapacity is undoubted; paralysis certainly is not. Yet to support his theory of paralysis due to a stroke,

Davies cites Schack, quoted by Holmes, who, many years after Mozart's death, said that he had helped Mozart to move in bed.[157] Eybler wrote likewise.[158] Davies argues that Mozart's inability to sit up without assistance was due to 'muscular paralysis'. He attributed Mozart's 'violent shuddering' to a sequence of events more in keeping with a convulsion due to a stroke as a result of a massive brain haemorrhage, followed by coma. More simply, Dr Wheater believes the shudder to have been 'slight', occurring when a cold compress was applied to his brow.[159] During a forty-year career in hospital medicine, I encountered thousands of patients unable, if only for a time, to sit up without assistance, and only a tiny proportion had suffered strokes. There is a temptation to ask Davies if Mozart suddenly sitting up with both cheeks puffed out is consistent with the profound paralysis and facial weakness which he describes as Mozart's lingering fate.

These neurological features were introduced by Davies, not least to accommodate his own suspicions regarding raised blood pressure (hypertension) leading to hypertensive encephalopathy, a condition where hypertension goes out of control causing a disorder of the brain: indeed, a likely stroke. Davies's introduction of hypertensive encephalopathy is suspect, because it should not be called to account for undoubted headaches or dubious fainting fits, from which Mozart is said to have suffered intermittently for his last weeks. Hypertensive encephalopathy, once started, is relentless, rapidly becoming fatal unless quickly and effectively treated, which obviously it was not.

When we consider the last few hours, even less plausible is the 'paralysis of conjugate gaze, and facial nerve palsy', which should be assessed, like facial weakness, at the time in an awake, cooperative patient. Clearly that did not happen and it is not capable of retrospective diagnosis and accordingly should be dismissed. It is tantalising to reflect that one of the reasons for Davies rejecting Bär's view that Mozart died of rheumatic fever was that it does not explain the neurological symptoms which Davies himself promotes.[160] That too may be questioned because endocarditis (inflammation of the lining of the heart) secondary to rheumatic fever may cause emboli to be thrown into the circulation, from which they may cause a further blood clot in the brain and thus a stroke.

To finally reconsider Mozart's alleged stroke, he was lucid and capable of conversation until two hours before his death and was assisting with composition the day before, making the chance of a stroke causing immobility remote. On those grounds alone strokes can be struck off the record, along with hypertensive encephalopathy. But let Dr Davies have the last word, for he believes that the final cause of death was bronchopneumonia, which is very probable.[161] Indeed the fever, with bronchopneumonia and then possible brief delirium turning to coma and death, possibly was 'una deposito alla testa'.

10 **Depression:** Mozart was sometimes moody, although usually cheerfully energetic. Nonetheless it has been suggested that he was also depressive on occasions.[162] Anderson's collection of letters reveals little evidence for a diagnosis of bipolar depressive disorder, rather the opposite. Davies also avers that uraemia (see the next section) caused him to be clinically depressed. Mozart was generally cheerful until mid-1791, when his disposition intermittently became more morbid.[163] That said, his last letter of 14 October 1791 was a cheery one.[164] Steptoe's psychiatric review of Mozart's correspondence did not support a clinical diagnosis of depression.[165] Davies, as well as describing Mozart as an obsessional immature personality, also regarded him as depressive,[166] a view shared by Reichsmann, who also argued that his 'immature personality was particularly vulnerable to object loss'.[167] One hopes that we may be spared the future case of Mozart and his missing rattle!

To adopt, as doctors should, an objective approach to diagnosis, especially of psychological illness, and then to accept an organically based depression is more difficult. Analysing the signs of depression, we need to balance the expressions of gloom and foreboding against the reports of more positive sentiments which persisted until the last fortnight. Indeed, after Mozart's gloom in the Prater he cheered up again. In that respect we have already seen Mozart's busy musical and domestic schedule until the start of the final illness. That is not the diary of a significantly depressed person, not least with composition maintained until the very end.

11 **Chronic renal failure (CRF) and uraemia:** Davies's assertion that Mozart died in uraemic chronic kidney failure is sound,[168] likewise his suggestion that it may also have subdued his normally cheerful mood in the last months. Uraemia is an excessive accumulation of urea, a waste product, in the blood. It can cause depression. Urea is normally cleared into the urine by the kidneys, so kidney failure, whatever its cause, has a common end point with uraemia. But what caused renal failure? Davies has an original explanation. His links were the assumed streptococcus and its

dissemination by an epidemic, the evidence for which is meagre.

The two conditions which link streptococci and the kidney most obviously are glomerulonephritis (Bright's disease) and Henoch-Schönlein purpura (HSP).* Davies intriguingly believes that Mozart had HSP caused by an earlier illness which was exacerbated by a streptococcus, allegedly picked up on 18 November at the Masonic lodge. We can accommodate fever, swollen joints, malaise, oedema and vomiting in this speculative diagnosis. As his kidneys failed, allegedly because of HSP, he became more oedematous. There are weaknesses in this train of thought too. From those present the evidence for a rash is scant, although Sophie may have implied one, and we may speculate as to what 'inflammation' (well recorded) meant in 1791.[169] Treves says there was one without presenting his evidence.[170] A diagnosis of HSP without a rash is possible, but is rather like a pub with no beer. Davies attaches much importance to the causal relationship between streptococcal infection and HSP. Karhausen quotes two studies showing that the association was weak,[171] but a more recent study does suggest a link between streptococcal infection and subsequent HSP,[172] so that and the 'cluster' of cases which was not quite an epidemic do give Davies so far a case to hang on to.

Nevertheless, an alleged epidemic was crucial to some of Davies's reasoning. His enthusiasm is for HSP rather than more plausible conditions such as Bright's disease caused by the presumed streptococcus and leading to chronic nephritis and the final pathway of uraemia and renal failure. Lastly, HSP is a rare disease with an incidence of one in 100,000 in the general male population and with a low mortality, although that is to judge 1791 in 2018. Meanwhile, HSP is relatively rare in people of Mozart's age, being a disease of children and adolescents, only 1% of whom progress to kidney failure. The balance of probabilities is against Mozart dying of a rare childhood condition that today is rarely a killer during a suspect epidemic, with a recondite rash.

CRF, which could be due to chronic urinary tract infection, also common with or without a congenital abnormality or Bright's disease, even HSP, is the probable cause of death. All or any ultimately

---

* Features of Henoch-Schönlein purpura (HSP) include the following: children and adults under twenty-five are typically affected; haemorrhage in the wall of the gut causing it to obstruct; painful swelling of the joints; fever; and/or purpura (a mottled or speckled blood-stained rash) of the skin. When purpura is secondary to streptococcus, then acute nephritis (inflammation of the kidneys) is the most dangerous complication.

caused renal failure as bronchopneumonia finally took over. Beyond this discourse we cannot unravel the mystery any further, and are unlikely to in the future.

So perhaps prosaically we can conclude:[*]

1 He was neither murdered nor poisoned, although Dr Sallaba's lancet may have hastened the inevitable end by exsanguination.

2 'Deposits' and 'determinations' to the head are a vernacular mystery. We can, however, be very confident that he suffered neither a head injury nor a brain tumour, nor meningitis. The Court Counsellor Dr Eduard Vincent Guldener von Lobes had corresponded with Dr Sallaba.[173] He had feared a fatal result from 'a determination to the head', going on to say it was impossible to prevent it. Deposits or determinations, in translation over 200 years, were probable figures of speech for illnesses ending in coma.[174]

3 He did not have syphilis.

4 He was not clinically a depressive, until cast down by terminal uraemia.

5 TB, brucellosis, epilepsy, Tourette's syndrome and probably hyperthyroidism can be safely disregarded.

6 That he had a rare craniofacial abnormality remains unsustainable unless the Mozart skull is proved scientifically to be that of Mozart.

7 Evidence that swelling was of a joint (e.g. the knee), as opposed to being general swelling such as oedema of the legs, is questionable.

8 The histories of entirely presumed streptococcal infections and the weak epidemiological data could accord with HSP, glomerulonephritis or endocarditis. All of these afflictions conveniently converge upon ultimate kidney or heart failure, or even both.

9 On a strong balance of probabilities a stroke should be disregarded as a cause of death. There is no good evidence for hypertension, which could only be assumed anyway.

10 We are left with a desperately ill young man who succumbed finally to bronchopneumonia and who, above all else, was grossly waterlogged. The cause for that was probably kidney failure or, less probably, heart failure.

11 In a young man, kidney failure having been due to urinary tract infection, in the absence of a congenital abnormality, is improbable.

[*] I am grateful to Dr David Noble MA, MB, MSc, MRCP, FRCR, a physician in Cambridge, for helping with the clinical analyses in this section.

    Presuming that he did have one, then if it affected both kidneys he would have been unlikely to live to be thirty-five, whereas if only one kidney was affected, then he might well have lived longer.

12   The route by which infection may have killed him is much more likely with a streptococcal infection, for which there is only circumstantial evidence. It can trigger auto-immune conditions, including kidney disease and even HSP.

13   Heart failure (instead, or even as well) following endocarditis remains as an unlikely cause of the final illness.

14   Today probably all of these diagnoses would be treatable. To take an improbable, if not extreme, position, kidney transplantation could have averted for many years the greatest tragedy in musical history.

15   When asked for their view regarding cause of death, the staff of the Mozart Museum's answer was simple: 'We don't know.'[175]

An Afterthought

Other theories abound, but there is one which recently seemed plausible. Mozart's favourite meat was said to have been pork,[176] which he may even have enjoyed at the Masonic dinner on 18 November. There is a particularly horrid worm infection called trichinosis which can be caught by eating undercooked pork, first fully described in 1860 but probably implicitly understood since ancient times. The salient clinical features are an incubation period of eight to fifteen days, fever, lassitude, anorexia, vomiting, muscle and joint pain as well as generalised swelling. Throughout the illness, intellectual capacity is preserved, although coma may supervene shortly before the patient dies. A stroke or convulsions can occur latterly. This fits the known facts much better than most of the other theories already outlined. Just as Schubert may have died as a result of a suspect fish supper, so Mozart may have died after enjoying a simple pork chop. It is not my purpose to re-inflame a popular and not always very objective debate but, apart from fitting the facts, trichinosis reminds us of the utter frailty of unfettered genius. Once more the Mozart Museum had no view regarding trichinosis or 'deposits to the head'.[177]

    The banality of this death is hard to reconcile with the beauty of the Requiem, especially when we realise that today he would probably have been saved. This leads to the only useful conclusion. Extravagant, unfounded, unattributable opinion should be disregarded in future. The exchange of academic invective clouds Mozart's memory and little else.

We should accept working hypotheses for which evidence can be produced. One hopes that further medical writing regarding this genius will be soundly based.

We will now pass from a detailed account of Mozart to briefer accounts of some other composers who died young.

✣ VINCENZO BELLINI ✣
(1801–1835)

I never believed you would fade so soon, oh flower.

Vincenzo Bellini, *La sonnambula*, 1831

The German poet Heine declared Bellini to be 'noble and good'.[178] He also described him as 'a sigh in dancing pumps'.[179] Bellini's ascent to fame and fortune, although rapid, had been uneven. After the very successful premiere of *La straniera* in 1829, he developed alleged gastroenteritis and recuperated by Lake Como.[180] After his recovery, the period 1830–31 saw success with *I Capuleti e i Montecchi*, *La sonnambula*, his masterpiece, *Norma,* and finally *I puritani*. Rossini later wrote, 'I am delighted to be able to tell you that Bellini's opera *I puritani*, composed expressly for Paris, has just had a brilliant success.'[181] At this time Bellini found it congenial to leave the city of Paris to visit the villa in Puteaux, now a Parisian suburb, of his 'close English friend, Mr Levys'.[182] Orrey, Galatopoulos and Rosselli, in their biographies of Bellini, refer to a young, rich, English, Jewish gentleman and his lady, Mme Levys, to others Mlle Oliver. She was possibly what the Scots call a 'bidey-in'. Orrey tells us that Levys (or Lewis or Levy) was a financier,[183] while Galatopoulos describes him as a banker. Today the difference seems academic, and perhaps it was then. Rosselli has researched Levys thoroughly, describing him as a sweatshop-owning mass-producer of garments.[184]

After the Paris premiere in January 1835 of *I puritani*, completed two months earlier, he composed nothing new apart from two canons whilst directing and supervising operatic production.[185] This could reflect a worsening of his bowel condition, preceding the terminal decline. In mid-May, Bellini moved to Levys's villa at Puteaux, suffering a 'gastric fever' shortly thereafter.[186] On 1 September, Bellini wrote that he was unwell with his 'usual diarrhoea',[187] as well as fever, which he had experienced before.[188] After three days he wrote to his friend and first biographer, Florimo,[189] that he was much better, and went up to Paris on business. When he returned, he relapsed. The Princess Belgioso was sufficiently worried to detail Dr Montallegri to attend upon the sick composer, which he did on 9 September, opining that his condition was 'not serious'.[190] Bellini's nineteen-year-old friend, Augusto Aymé,* was more resourceful, writing

---

* Aymé did not become the Baron d'Aquino and a minor diplomat until a decade or more later.

on 11 September that 'a few days ago' he had seen Bellini at Puteaux, where he had been rebuked by Mme Levys for disturbing the patient who, she declared, needed rest.[191] On 12 and 13 September Aymé was barred entry by a difficult gardener, but on the 14th Aymé's uncle Carafa gained entry by posing as a doctor.[192] It was then that Dr Montallegri returned, issuing daily bulletins from 15 September. Galatopoulos chronicled these from papers now in the museum at Catania.[193] The patient was deteriorating, passing both blood and mucus from his bowels. Montallegri was encouraged on the 22nd by the passage of much less blood and mucus, saying that Bellini had become calmer. This was the quiet before the storm, for on the 23rd he became very ill and delirious, passing away that same evening. Now the gardener told Aymé that the Levyses were in Paris.

Within twenty-four hours, news of Bellini's death was circulating in Paris with speculation as to what could have been the cause. Conspiracy theories included poisoning, perhaps by Levys because Bellini and Mme Levys might have become intimate.[194] This is as unsubstantiated as are claims for Sicilian vendettas. Fortunately, Professor Dalmas undertook an autopsy within thirty-six hours of the death. The original report was initially made available to Rossini and described all body parts to have been in good condition, apart from a large abscess in the liver and ulceration throughout the entire large intestine.[195] From this we can confidently conclude that the cause of death was not poison, nor was it likely to have been epidemic, particularly as this illness was an exacerbation of a long-standing disease process. Of various diseases proposed only two merit serious consideration:

1 Amoebic dysentery was said by Sir Ronald Bodley-Scott, a distinguished physician, after examining Dalmas's report, to be 'beyond any doubt' Bellini's cause of death.[196] One can no more disregard so eminent a diagnostician than Sir Ronald should view an autopsy report from 180 years ago and conclude 'beyond any doubt'. Sometimes eminent opinion plus 'beyond any doubt' become grounds for further research. Sir Ronald's views were similar to those of another eminent doctor, Victor de Sabata from Milan, who said, 'Bellini quite obviously died from chronic amoebiasis.'[197] Well, did he?

2 The second possibility is ulcerative colitis, an auto-immune disease, first described in 1859.[198]

The long-remitting course that is well documented in Bellini's case would be more probable with ulcerative colitis than with amoebiasis. Ulcerative colitis is a more probable diagnosis, not least because Professor Dalmas's report reads like a textbook description of that disease. Moreover it is the commoner condition in northern Europe, although we cannot gauge whether that was the case in 1835. Today either disease is treatable. In 1835 ulcerative colitis was unknown; amoebic dysentery was only vaguely rec-ognised.* Sometimes ulcerative colitis can come to a dramatic crisis which, if not quickly aborted, usually by surgery, is quickly fatal. This condition, toxic megacolon, fits well with the accounts of Bellini's last days and his autopsy. Apparently this has not deterred the conspiracy theorists in their criticism of the Levyses or of Dr Montallegri, mainly on the basis that Bellini did not receive best attention or benefit from a second opinion. We may ask what that hypothetical second physician would have offered the patient: perhaps some energetic blood-letting, killing him a few hours sooner. The Levyses may have misapprehended the malaise as typhoid or cholera and cared for him until it was clear that Bellini was not long for this world, whereupon they established a cordon sanitaire maintained by the surly gardener. They probably harmed their own reputations by writ-ing a delayed and then very brief answer to Bellini's distressed father, who had wanted details about his son's final days.

The conclusion must be that once the final illness commenced, Bellini's case was hopeless, and would have remained so until the introduction in the twentieth century of intravenous fluid and electrolyte replacement therapy, antibiotics, steroids and modern surgery. In 1876 Bellini's remains were re-interred at the cathedral in Catania, Sicily. Happily, bel canto glo-riously lives on.

---

* Gratitude is due to Mr John Abercrombie MD, FRCS, a consultant colorectal surgeon at the University of Nottingham, for advising upon the surgical pathology in Bellini's case.

✢ GEORGES BIZET ✢
(1838–1875)

I foresee a definitive and hopeless flop
> Bizet on the opening night of ***Carmen***, 1875

Sadly, the premiere of *Carmen* on 3 March 1875 at the Opéra-Comique in Paris was a failure. Critics lambasted it as a work being 'devoid of colour', 'undramatic' and 'undistinguished in melody'. One wonders if they had actually attended the performance. The theatre was half-full for the second night. The production's gestation had been lengthy and troubled. Later that March, Bizet developed a quinsy, described as 'angina of the throat'.[199] He had a history going back to 1858 of throat complaints, with many treatments ranging from gargles to leeches. On this occasion he retreated to bed, observing that it was taking longer to recover from than previous similar attacks.[200] He also became depressed, worried that the critics might have been correct about *Carmen*. The librettist Gallet, in his memoirs of 1891 observed that, even when well, Bizet harboured fears of catastrophe and early death.[201] Curtiss attributed these to the indifferent state of his marriage to Geneviève Halévey.

In a bizarre episode shortly after *Carmen*'s premiere, Bizet had some friends round, including a promising young soprano.[202] Whilst she was singing songs from *Carmen*, he suddenly interrupted and played the funeral marches of Chopin and Schumann.[203] There lingers a suspicion that Bizet may have had the taste of impending death. On 28 May, contrary to Geneviève's advice, he decided to go to their house at Bougival outside Paris, by the Seine, even though he was still suffering from a recurrence of the quinsy and an attack of 'rheumatism'.[204] The description is also (or instead) very suggestive of a middle ear infection. On arrival, husband and wife enjoyed a walk together. Then Bizet, who was feeling better and was a keen swimmer, rashly decided to bathe in the river.[205] On 30 May he had a 'violent and incapacitating attack of rheumatism', with pain, immobility, gloom and a 'fever'. On 1 June (the date remains a little uncertain) he suffered a 'severe heart attack'.[206] A doctor attended and quite reasonably advised calm and rest. The following day Bizet was restless with an alleged fever, although when his two sons visited him later he seemed somewhat better. He became concerned as to the affect his death might have on his family. Then he suffered a second heart attack and lost consciousness.[207] By the time the doctor returned, Georges Bizet, aged only thirty-seven, had died, on his sixth wedding anniversary. Four thousand people attended his funeral a few days later.[208] Had he been spared, he would have added a second to his only symphony and realised plans for a piano concerto, over which he had cogitated for several years.

His cause of death remains mysterious. Just before his wife died in 1926 she told her biographer that Bizet had died of an inoperable tumour of the ear. Blood and pus had been noted on his pillow just after he died.[209] A tumour of the ear is very unlikely. Quite probably his throat infection had spread to the middle ear: the common condition of otitis media, of which there was an earlier history. If such cases remain untreated then the eardrum (tympanic membrane; see Fig. 7, Chapter 11) ruptures and the ear discharges blood-stained pus. He had become deaf in the left ear in late May according to his friend the composer Ernest Guiraud.[210]

Both Dean and Curtiss quote from two accounts by Eugène Gelma, once Professor of Psychiatry at Strasbourg, one published in 1938 and the other a decade later.[211] Gelma believed the quinsy was an unlikely cause of death, unless there was evidence of Bizet choking to death, which there was not. He suggested that Bizet died of 'a cardiac complication of articular rheumatism'. That is both speculative and improbable. In March 1875 he had complained of 'angina of the throat' at the same time as 'muscular rheumatism'. It is probably there that this inappropriate conflation arose. Today 'angina' instantly relates to the heart, and it is common for cardiac angina to radiate into the neck, hence mention of the throat. Then 'angina' was a word used more generally. Theories were also mentioned which relate his death to a state of depression and stress over *Carmen*. These should be disregarded as we stick to the facts, such as there having been a focus of infection with the quinsy and that he had a fever. To then jump into cold water and exercise violently would adversely affect someone who by then might have had germs in the bloodstream (septicaemia). The latter condition is often attended by alarming falls in blood pressure, sometimes fatal in themselves, in compromising an ailing heart. He had complained earlier of breathlessness on climbing stairs and also an irregularity of his pulse (heartbeat),[212] both sound evidence of heart disease. That history plus the swim would alone have been enough to kill him, even at the age of thirty-seven. A potentially compromised heart is always vulnerable to activities such as suddenly swimming in cold water. Today the possible septicaemia would be treated with antibiotics and Bizet's heart rhythm would have been stabilised, with any coronary artery blockage stented. Professor Gelma was side-tracked in his analysis by 'rheumatic attack'.

Giovanni Battista Pergolesi (1710–1736)

Pergolesi was only twenty-six when he died in a monastery at Pozzuoli. His health had deteriorated in 1735, and in early 1736 he donated his few possessions to an aunt.[213] There is the image of an impecunious young genius coughing his way to an early grave, the ultimate frailty of youth. A cruel lithograph of him when he was twenty-four reveals his left leg as clearly shorter and thinner than the right, causing him to walk on tiptoe.[214] There were two siblings who had died in infancy, and Pergolesi himself was sickly. Perhaps, like Schubert, he was a man for whom divine creation did few favours beyond a sublime musical ability, for, in a short life, his output was prodigious. TB, the likeliest cause of death, is also an explanation for the limping short leg, which may have affected his hip since childhood. In the summer of 1735 Pergolesi's health deteriorated further, and his last success was with the comic opera *Il Flaminio*, with whose completion the assistance of Nicola Sabatino was required.[215] The final composition, for which today he remains justly famous, was the lovely *Stabat mater*, written for a church in Naples as a replacement for Alessandro Scarlatti's *Stabat mater*. Pergolesi may have sensed a closeness to death and infused his greatest work with grief for a life soon to be cut tragically short.

Henry Purcell (1659–1695)

Purcell died aged thirty-six and, like Mozart and Schubert, he still produced a prodigious output. King lists five operas and semi-operas, including *Dido and Aeneas* and *The Faerie Queen*, as well as the incidental music for forty-five plays.[216] Eight of these were composed in part or totally during the year of his death. There were hundreds of anthems and songs, many of which, like 'Sound the Trumpet', remain popular today. He was a composer resonant with his epoch. The list of instrumental music is similarly prodigious.[217]

Purcell had become very feeble before death took him.[218] Like Mozart, he had been grossly overworking just before he died. This included composing music for the allegorical poem 'Lovely Albina's Come Ashore', said to symbolise a reconciliation between William III and the future Queen Anne. Zimmerman discounts Hawkins's view that Purcell caught a chill, having been locked out by his wife, Frances, after a night of revelling, despite which he told of a lingering death.[219] Records reveal that November 1695 was unseasonably mild anyway, and the marriage between Henry and

Frances was warm and loving.[220] Although his final demise was rapid,[221] Westrup believed that Purcell had been in declining health for several months.[222] This supports the general supposition that TB caused his demise. It may have been of the miliary type, which spreads and disseminates rapidly and fatally. Purcell apprehended his swift terminal decline, hardly able to hold the pen, as he made his will only hours before death.[223] Today Purcell, like Pergolesi, would have had a good chance of cure with antibiotic therapy. He had been a good-humoured, witty man, very much in harmony with the enlightenment of his time. It is fitting that this early death was followed by a funeral in Westminster Abbey, where he is buried and where his music lives on today.

In other chapters we will encounter leading composers who also died young. Weber (Chapter 9) succumbed to TB, as Chopin probably did (Chapter 9). Gershwin (Chapter 3) never recovered from surgery for a brain tumour, whereas today Mendelssohn (Chapter 7) might well have successfully undergone brain surgery for an aneurysm (weakness in a blood vessel wall) beneath his brain. Although Schubert (Chapter 4) probably had the first two stages of syphilis, antibiotics for that and for the gastroenteritis which killed him might have significantly extended his life.

We cannot know what might have been composed had these lives been significantly longer. We have seen composers who lived much longer, but retired from composing. Mendelssohn's composition may have started to decline, like his health, a couple of years before his death, as suggested by Hans von Bülow, who said he started as a genius and ended as a talent.[224] It could just be that within each composer there is a finite amount of music whose expression, if not conception, is finite.

✢ Chapter 2 ✢

A Triumphant Old Age

Old age is the most unexpected of all things that happen to a man
Leon Trotsky, *Diary in Exile*,1935

WE HAVE SEEN both the pathos and the tragedy of young deaths, and yet there was an extraordinary body of work from that group and the eternal question as to what might have been had they lived longer. So what happened with those who survived beyond their seventh decade? Was it all autumnal contentment? But perhaps the key question is whether some may have just laid down their pens because they ran out of ideas and, if they did, were there underlying medical reasons for that or did they just reasonably retire? In relating health to composition, old age, not least today with its anxieties about senile degeneration, is an important condition to consider. It has become a clinical entity and takes people in diverse ways.

✢ JOSEPH HAYDN ✢
(1732–1809)

Life levels all men; death reveals the eminent
> George Bernard Shaw, *Man and Superman*, 1903

On Haydn's seventy-sixth birthday in 1808, Antonio Salieri conducted *The Creation*. In the audience was a former pupil, who tearfully came forward to embrace the equally lachrymose Haydn.[1] That pupil was Beethoven. By 1808 Haydn was the doyen of composers, to whom Mozart, Beethoven and Schubert had variously paid their obsequies. His long career as Kapellmeister to the Princes Esterházy at Eszterháza, rather than his probably loveless marriage, was the bedrock of his security. His wife, Anna Maria, was barren, to his eternal sadness, as well as being unsympathetic to music, especially Haydn's, whose manuscripts she used to roll pastry upon.[2] He may have fathered a child with his mistress, an Italian singer, Luigia Polzelli.[3] The Swedish composer Johan Fredrik Berwald suggested that his unhappy marriage was why he composed so much.[4] Haydn was not only a stable personality, but he was agreeable, pragmatic and with his wits about him.

Like other allegedly triumphant old ages, Haydn's was less easy than popular supposition might have us believe. From 1803 until his death in 1809, Haydn composed almost nothing, and Neumayr believes he was ill for his last ten years.[5] Even before that he had struggled to compose *The Seasons*, possibly because of his problems with Baron van Swieten's translation of James Thomson's original English verse. But by this time he was in both mental and physical decline.[6] Haydn had said that '*The Seasons* broke my back' as he complained of declining powers from as early as 1793.[7]

Part of this infirmity may have been due to a nasal polyp, which probably predisposed him to the sinus infections from which he suffered. Neumayr gives a colourful account of this ailment which he derived from Haydn's original biographer, Dies.[8] He had undergone surgery, unsuccessfully, in Vienna, by Dr Bramhilla, who, in his surgical enthusiasm, inadvertently and very painfully removed part of the nasal bone. When Haydn was in England in 1792, the great surgeon John Hunter had been keen to re-operate, affirming to his patient that 'The polyp would be repugnant to ladies.' He clearly understood Haydn's little weakness, not least because Haydn was perhaps a little smitten with Mrs Hunter. The account of Haydn then sturdily repelling Hunter's assistants, who came to hold him down so the master could operate, is amusing and derives from Dies.[9] Sadly, increasing infirmity cannot be solely attributed to the polyp, although Neumayr quotes Griesinger's observation that it impaired his breathing.

In December 1803 his last public performance was with *The Seven Last Words from the Cross*, and that year he had wearily abandoned completion of his D minor Quartet Opus 103.[10] During Haydn's last four or five years he upheld a punctilious routine and maintained a courtly appearance, but found it difficult to draw on his boots and breeches over his swollen legs.[11] He had increasing difficulties in trying to compose or even write and, despite provision of a small piano, he now made simple mistakes whilst playing, which distressed him, and he tended to weep,[12] although his moods had always been labile. By the early 1800s he was probably in chronic heart failure, which was associated with disease of his peripheral circulation, including early senile dementia, due to hardening of the arteries (arteriosclerosis) to the brain. By 1806 he was noticeably forgetful.[13]

So at the end we can empathise with Haydn spending his days still elegantly attired, reading the newspaper, checking household accounts, chatting and playing cards with neighbours or riding out in a coach. He remained mentally alert, although forgetful, until his death at home on 31 May 1809.[14] Outside his house in Vienna, that city's invader, Napoleon Bonaparte, had only two weeks previously placed a guard of honour.[15] His life and even death were marked by charm, good sense, humour and freedom from either acrimony or melodrama.[16] His declining years were a little sad, perhaps graceful, but not triumphant.

Perhaps inevitably, in common with Mozart, Handel, Bach and others, there is the usual ferment of speculation regarding human remains and the possibility of their having been Haydn's.[17] A familiar cast of suspect gravediggers, wily anatomists and imaginative scholars ultimately produced charming pictures of skull parts, revealing prodigious mental and musical talents which had lain therein. They need have looked no further than the late string quartets for abundant evidence of that.

✠ CAMILLE SAINT-SAËNS ✠
(1835–1921)

He knows everything, but lacks in experience

Hector Berlioz of Saint-Saëns, 1863

As a child prodigy Saint-Saëns was composing at three and making his professional debut when he was ten;[18] he died seventy-six years later. By seventy his old age had become far from triumphant, although to the end he preserved his keen intellect and sharp wit, remaining busy as a pianist, conductor, producer, composer, poet, amateur scientist and compulsive traveller. His life became punctuated by personal tragedy. After his somewhat capricious marriage in 1875 came the deaths within six weeks of each other of his two little sons, ending his illusions of childhood and his fragile marriage.[19] Shortly after this he precipitously left his much younger wife, Marie, and from thenceforth his life became nomadic.[20] In Russia, shortly after disappearing from Marie, Saint-Saëns famously danced with Tchaikovsky, inevitably evoking suggestions of homosexuality, as had his friendship with Reynaldo Hahn, an opinion voiced by Harding in his biography of 1965.[21] This has been dispassionately analysed by Rees, who concluded that we should not draw too much from a sometimes lonely man enjoying the company of Proustian young men,[22] any more than we should from his obvious delight with the slender curves of well-corseted young ladies, as noted by John Philip Sousa in San Francisco during 1915.[23]

There are various indistinct accounts of his health during his last four decades.[24] Studies of Saint-Saëns are as elusive as he often was. Few wrote in English during the nearly eighty-year gap between Hervey or Lyle in the 1920s and then Rees in 1999, Harding during 1965 being the exception.[25] Shortly after his mother's death he simply disappeared, as he had done after leaving Marie. He was said to be plagued by insomnia, fears of madness and 'a night feeling in my mind'.[26] Rees has, however, failed to trace sad events in his music. He attributed Saint-Saëns's liking for southern France and North Africa to afflictions of his health, which may have been chronic bronchitis or asthma. Concerns over his health had emerged in 1873 and 1883–84, when he was 'too unwell for public appearance'.[27] In 1888 he had been grief-stricken by his mother's death, and there followed a period of 'collapse and recovery'.[28] He was often a disturbed and unhappy man, sometimes 'disgusted with life'. In 1890 he had a liver complaint. As the word 'jaundice' is absent from the reports, the 'complaint' was unlikely to have been serious. But so frail was he at the outset of his first American tour that there were doubts as to whether he would survive the schedule.[29] He did.

Late in life Saint-Saëns complained of pain in his legs and their 'near paralysis'. There is no good evidence of him ever being partially, let alone fully, paralysed. Medically one is tempted to question arteriosclerosis in the legs or even osteoarthritis of the hips or knees. But aged eighty-four he at last went to Greece, writing, 'I have mounted the Acropolis myself', despite lung congestion on the journey there.[30] However, a year later, because of 'congestion of the lungs', musicians from the Opéra came to his apartment to prepare for *Hélène*.[31] His last concerts at the piano and with the baton were only four weeks before his death. As to composition, the last opera, *Déjanire*, was premiered a decade before his death. In the year of that death he composed sonatas for oboe in D, for clarinet in E flat and for bassoon in G, along with some piano works. Even so, his best work was very largely nineteenth-century. The ever popular *Carnival of the Animals* and the Third Symphony ('Organ') both came in 1886.

Saint-Saëns's constant wanderings, emotional dependence on his two valets and diminution in the quality of his work point to an old age in stark contrast to the autumnal sunshine of Verdi or Richard Strauss. He may have been a lonely old man, but he had been callous in his dealings with colleagues such as Debussy and especially with his poor wife, Marie, for all his generosity to servants and urbanity with young women who had brains and good figures. In 1951 Martin Cooper wrote tellingly that 'Saint-Saëns died full of years and malice.'[32]

Just before Christmas 1921 Saint-Saëns was again in Algiers for health reasons, staying as usual at the Hôtel de l'Oasis. Just before bed on 16 December he leant over a balcony as a dance band played below. He muttered, 'A foxtrot – what a pity', and collapsed. Rapidly, his second valet and friend, Laurendeau, attended the groaning old man. Saint-Saëns opened his eyes and murmured, 'I believe this is the end', and so it was.[33] He died an atheist, leaving instructions that there be a minimum of obsequies at his funeral, which in fact became a state funeral.

Today in such circumstances the victim is sometimes fortunate that some public-spirited individual, accomplished in simple cardiopulmonary resuscitation, recognises the probability of a heart attack, even cardiac arrest, as he or she keeps the patient ticking over (literally) until the paramedics arrive. But in an ailing 86-year-old this surely was the best conclusion for him. In many ways Saint-Saëns is an exception to themes in this book. So prodigiously talented was he that his life was one of under-achievement and intrepid restlessness. Verdi, who had lost not only two young children but also a beloved first wife, is a stark contrast. With resolution Verdi soldiered on as one masterpiece after another flowed from his vivid imagination. Some might say that Verdi had the great good fortune to be supported into a triumphant old age by a loyal second wife and Saint-Saëns did not, but that surely was his decision. Despite professions of agnosticism from both men, their final commemorations differed; Saint-Saëns went sceptically into the unknown, whereas Verdi seems to have accepted a religious experience. That Saint-Saëns usually took the often tortuous, lonely road was largely his own choice.

✦ EDWARD ELGAR ✦
(1857–1934)

His music has a heroic melancholy

W. B. Yeats, 1911

Like that of his approximate contemporary Rachmaninov, Elgar's music often has a melancholy about it, but then they both were masters of music's yearning nostalgia. We should consider disorders of his mind as well as body. Elgar lived until 1934 and, after the death of his wife Alice in 1920, he composed much less and seems to have been a rather tortured soul, saying of his late wife, 'All I have done was owing to her.'[34] Michael Kennedy recalled that during this period he wrote to a friend, 'I am so desperately lonely.' The harrowing Cello Concerto was first performed shortly before Alice died. It was perhaps a requiem for his great music too. Kennedy described it as music of autumn with the sadness of disillusion, beneath which he became submerged during the 1914–18 war.[35] This can be starkly contrasted with earlier and cheerful successes, notably *In the South* (*Alassio*), *Cockaigne* or the mischief enshrined in the *Enigma Variations*, although with 'Nimrod' Yeats's point is apposite, for in 1911 Elgar said that *Enigma* was started in a spirit of humour and continued in seriousness.

His friend Richard Strauss dubbed him 'the first English progressive'.[36] Perhaps such a description, and the ambition beneath it, demanded excessively of his inner creativity and hung heavily upon him. The sometimes common image of a patriotic, slightly blimpish hack is nonsense, even though Siegfried Sassoon once described him as a 'club bore'.[37] In 1922 the neurologist Sir Henry Head described Elgar to Sassoon 'That little provincial music master'.[38] despite the problem having probably been Ménière's disease. Today such ill-mannered pomposity would be regarded as defamatory and unprofessional, and correctly so. Mercifully, strutting pin-stripes are no longer the medical fashion. Sassoon's description is gratuitous, but that is partly Elgar's fault as, like many successful but basically insecure people, he surrounded himself with a carapace against public scrutiny, which Alice could always penetrate. Elgar needed her to lead him out of his shell, and so after her death he became spritually incarcerated. During the 1920s there was a decreasing interest in, or taste for, his music. Anyway, Kennedy reminds us that, as Alice's demise drew down the curtain on Elgar the composer, he himself went on to say, 'I have gone out and I like it.'[39] He reflected that he had 'settled into servile slipperdom very easily', which is acquiescence, not clinical depression.

Behind the tweeds or frock coats, amongst the great and the good, there still remained a creative genius stopped in his tracks, and overshadowed by resentment and insecurity because of his humble origins. This persisted even when he became famous. Rosa Burley, a friend from his days as a young music teacher, said, 'He was a shy, frustrated, moody man' and that he was subject to sudden mood changes, not least whilst composing.[40] Here we must consider whether Elgar's health had extinguished his creative flame. For much of his adult life he experienced various medical complaints, possibly engendered by stress. A crucial account is that of Harcup, a general practitioner in Malvern and an Elgar scholar, after careful examination of all surviving correspondence and diaries.[41] He asks whether Elgar was a 'victim of medical mistakes' and 'the paucity of medical knowledge at the time'. As we will see, he was.[42] His troubles included swallowing difficulties, indigestion, bowel irregularity and 'eye weakness'. He has been regarded as a hypochondriac.[43] For his digestive complaints a barium meal X-ray was undertaken in January 1918. Thereupon his medical advisors declared that he had gastroptosis (i.e. dropped stomach).[44] Various treatments were prescribed including electrotherapy and corsets. Gastroptosis, like G. B. Shaw's 'nuciform sac', does not exist. It was a misconception due to the different positions of the stomach in a live and erect person in comparison with the recumbent formalin-stiffened corpses from which anatomical learning derives. Harcup believes that Elgar's painful eye complaints, following a scratching injury, were probably due to a corneal abrasion, which can be notoriously painful. Furthermore, his throat complaints had persisted for thirty-eight years.[45] He was seen by a variety of distinguished ear, nose and throat (ENT) specialists. That he had severe chronic tonsillitis, unresponsive to the paints and tonics of Sir Maurice Abbot Anderson, culminated in his submitting to having his tonsils taken out (tonsillectomy) in March 1918, aged sixty, by Mr Herbert Tilley, who had recently devised a safer technique for the procedure.[46] Sixty is an advanced and unusual age for tonsillectomy. Within ten days of this operation Elgar was back at work again on his String Quartet;[47] this was not a neurotic's convalescence. Also at this time he conceived the beginnings of the Cello Concerto.[48] Nevertheless, Alice pampered and cosseted him physically as well as spiritually now, as before. He once caught a chill, which was quickly staved off by this formidable woman armed with knitted bed socks and five hot water bottles.[49]

There are photographs and film of Elgar into his old age, usually without glasses and with a back like a ramrod. They suggest no obvious physical problem, being comfortable, reassuring pictures. Until close to his end, he had been a cyclist, walker and golfer. Like William Wordsworth, he often composed in his head whilst walking in the countryside, committing the results to paper upon returning home.[50]

Shortly after Elgar's resurgence following tonsillectomy, the indomitable Alice fell sick and, on 7 April 1920, she died in Elgar's arms of previously undetected lung cancer. He was utterly devasted, pathetically saying that now his poor wife had gone he could no longer be original. In 1925 he consulted a physician, Arthur Thomson, who proclaimed that Elgar was a 'neurotic, who most of all wanted reassurance'.[51] Most of us do. Regrettably some doctors fail to differentiate keen observation from gratuitous, ill-mannered judgement of their patients. The patient pays any doctor a compliment by confiding in him or her at all. Although not without its own pitfalls, it is both a pleasure and privilege to be able to reassure patients that little or nothing is seriously wrong. Thomson clearly recognised this in Elgar, saying that 'Again and again he would come in depressed, as if all useful life was over, and after reassurances he would brighten up perfectly.'[52] This is one of those short anecdotes acquainting us with a great deal. Kindly reassurance is all in a doctor's day's work, and the extent of Elgar's needing reassurance is revealed by his 'coming again and again'. Patients who enter the consulting room from their world's end and who then 'brighten up perfectly' are not seriously depressed. Despite the professed loneliness, Elgar enjoyed the theatre, the races, parties and the company of young people, especially ladies. He wrote to the young Yehudi Menuhin, 'You have given me a new zest for life', and it was Menuhin who, many years later, said how free of self-importance the old man had been.[53] Latterly, Elgar was interested in recording his own music.

It remains difficult to judge Elgar's state of health in his last two years. His stick by then may betray the worsening low back pain, of which he had complained since 1903,[54] and left-sided sciatica, which first developed in 1929. That ultimately proved to be due to inoperable malignancy of the lower large bowel (carcinoma of the rectum) invading the roots of his sciatic nerve, concluding his long, silent coda. But photographs reveal that his stick had been long-standing, probably just a fashion accessory and no more indicative of ill health than his military moustache.

Harcup's first thesis is one we may apply to other composers, namely that the clinical diagnosis of depression is sometimes made too freely.[55] That Elgar had periods of misery with a cyclothymic personality is undoubted. He mentioned suicide to the discomfiture of his daughter,

Carice, on several occasions.[56] Sadly, some people who commit suicide never talk about doing so before their tragic deaths. After the disastrous premiere of *The Dream of Gerontius*, he wrote to his friend Jaeger, saying, 'I really wish I were dead over and over again – but I dare not, for the sake of my relatives, do the job myself.'[57] Later in the same letter he went on to say, 'We are all very well and jolly', declaring himself to be 'riotously well'. Burley was right about those sudden mood swings! At Christmas time in 1925, he had emergency surgery for haemorrhoids (piles),[58] presumably because there had been serious bleeding. Few people opt to have a haemorrhoidectomy on Christmas Eve without good reason.

Then at the age of sixty-nine he told his friend and supporter Frank Schuster, 'I don't seem to get tired these days.'[59] In 1933 he started sketching plans for his first opera, *The Spanish Lady*, based on Ben Jonson's *The Devil is an Ass*, and his partial and now controversial Third Symphony. Whilst close to death saying, 'Billy, this is the end',[60] he asked his friend Billy Reed to ensure that no-one would tamper with or perform this incomplete symphony after his death, saying that they would not understand it. He even suggested that Reed should burn it,[61] although Reed does not relate this to us in his book. A few days earlier he had told his surgeon that if he didn't complete it someone else would. It is beguiling to speculate as to how much this late return to composition was evoked by his very close relationship with Lady Stuart of Wortley – 'Windflower'. Elgar was probably one of those men for whom intimate female companionship was essential. By the time of his final illness, he had became besotted again, with a young violinist, Vera Hockman.[62]

In October 1933 he was admitted to the South Bank Nursing Home in Worcester under the care of Mr Norman Duggan because of the recent increase in the severity of his painful left sciatica, weight loss and abdominal symptoms. He had written to Sir John Reith at the BBC to say that he had a 'sudden problem' and was to undergo surgery the next day, although two months earlier, whilst he was conducting his Second Symphony, the *Evening Standard* had noted how ill he looked.[63] At surgery, inoperable cancer of the rectum was revealed. Elgar's doctor, Moore-Ede, sought out Billy Reed to give a prognosis of survival for less than six months. His belly was simply opened and closed, and large doses of morphine were subsequently administered.[64] Carice Elgar told Kennedy that the surgical wound suppurated until his death.[65] It is hard to understand why a colostomy (stoma) was not performed, whereby the bowel is brought out to a surgical hole in the abdominal wall, where it empties into a colostomy bag. It is a routine procedure which can endow much greater comfort upon the unfortunate patient dying in this manner. Debussy had undergone that procedure nearly twenty years before, and techniques improved during and after the First World War. Both the surgical and pathology records probably no longer exist, although the death certificate does. It unequivocally gave Sir Edward Elgar's cause of death as carcinoma of the rectum.[66]

In correspondence with his friend Dr Buck, a general practitioner in Settle, Elgar had complained of his bowels for several years,[67] something he also tended to talk about loudly at his club! It is doubtful that, during the surgery for piles in 1925, an internal examination (sigmoidoscopy) of the large bowel (rectum and lower colon) was undertaken, because a tumour at an early stage might have been revealed then. Today, and even looking back fifty years, a patient complaining of weight loss and altered bowel habit, and who has experienced previous rectal bleeding and left-sided sciatica for several years, should first be investigated with a high degree of suspicion that the symptoms, apparently unrelated, might unhappily be all too closely associated. That was an opportunity which earlier could have made a difference to the end of Elgar's life with completion of the Third Symphony. Then his old age assuredly would have finally become triumphant, if only musically so.

It was probably the huge quantities of morphine which brought him close to death before Christmas 1933. That he had intolerable pain is revealed by the surgical consideration given to surgically dividing pain tracts in his spinal cord (tractotomy),[68] which unpredictable operation was contemplated to allow completion of the Third Symphony, using Billy Reed as an amanuensis. It is probably as well that it was not done. At Christmas 1933 he wrote to Delius saying he had incessant pain,[69] although music was the letter's apparent prime theme. He had refused the last rites, only to receive them a little later, whilst semi-comatose.[70] Elgar had told Arthur Thomson that he had no faith in the afterlife, nor in the church's 'mumbo jumbo'.[71] For someone brought up as a Roman Catholic, such apostasy must have been a desolate realisation close to death. He could be a tortured soul, and some of the beauty of the Cello Concerto is a strange emptiness.

There was a final rally, revealing an indomitable spirit. We meet the real man when Dr Thomson came to visit him, saying that he admired Elgar because 'After all his years of worrying about imagined troubles, he displayed magnificent courage in the face of great adversity.'[72] As most of these 'imagined troubles' were very real medical conditions, it was an inappropriate misjudgement. Elgar had endured not only invasive cancer of the bowel, causing intractable pain, but thirty-eight years of chronic tonsillitis, haemorrhoids, Ménière's disease and a painful corneal abrasion, certainly not 'imagined troubles'. In 1912 an eminent neurosurgeon had diagnosed gout of the eyes and head![73] There is a final enigma about Elgar, which appeared in the *Sunday Times* in 1955.[74] Ernest Newman, the music critic, revealed that in February 1934, he had visited Elgar when he was very close to death. Newman claims that Elgar made a remark about himself of allegedly five words, which Newman had never disclosed to anyone, and said he had no intention of ever doing so.[75] He explained that Elgar's distressing remark 'would lend itself too easily to the crudest of misinterpretations', because these few words were 'too tragic for the ear of the mob'. De-la-Noy's judgement of studied arrogance here appears just.[76] Carice Elgar told Kennedy that she believed her father had been too 'drugged up' for this conversation to have been likely anyway.[77]

It is sad to see how far Elgar had departed from his original roots and the solace of his religion. His finale is far removed from the imperial grandeur of the late Verdi or the reflective sunset of Richard Strauss. Perhaps W. B. Yeats best described the dying Elgar, entirely unwittingly, in a poem published five years after Elgar's death:

> All that I have said and done
> Now that I am old and ill
> Turns into a question 'til
> I lie awake night after night
> And never get the answers right

The composer of the *Enigma Variations* was himself an enigma, a concoction of contrasts, not least in matters medical and psychological. He was solitary but gregarious, both petulant and generous, miserable and self-pitying, as well as cheery, witty and, at the end, brave. Elgar's response to ill health is contrasted with that of Delius in Chapter 4.

✝ JEAN SIBELIUS ✝
(1865–1957)

Silence ruled this land. Out of silence mystery comes, and magic, and the delicate awareness of unreasoning things

Eleanor Dark, *The Timeless Land*, 1941

At ninety-one Sibelius must have been the ultimate grand old man, but here perhaps was another tortured soul. His final major composition, *Tapiola* (1926), written thirty-one years before he died, is a desolate piece. This accords well with the middle-aged and elderly photographs of an always unsmiling Sibelius, which seem to convey austerity. He looked like that terrifying elderly uncle to be avoided if possible at Christmas. Evidently he was camera-shy and experienced stage fright.[78] Yet this was the man who, when he visited London with Busoni, had led the cheery Sir Henry Wood to remark that they were like two irresponsible schoolboys on an outing.[79] In contrast, Christopher Nupen's biographical film is suffused by Nordic gloom.[80] Privately Sibelius was a witty man who enjoyed jest and joking. Nevertheless, there had been periods of depression, as when he was in Berlin around 1889–90 with Joachim and von Bülow.[81] They may well relate to his relinquishing ambitions to be a solo violinist and thereafter becoming a composer. But there could be another reason. Of controversial interest is his hospitalisation in Berlin during 1889, when Goss infers that Sibelius had syphilis.[82] Although Goss's account is a good review of prostitution in Finland in the late nineteenth and early twentieth centuries, little corroborative evidence is presented to support such a diagnosis in Sibelius's case. There is no description of possible features of syphilis, nor of any treatment or its side effects. Goss suggests he may have received the Jauregg therapy, to be described in Chapter 4. No evidence for this occurring is adduced. A year later Sibelius became engaged to Aino Järnefelt, a lively girl who became his wife for the next sixty-seven years and the mother of his six children.

Medical reasons put forward for his 31–year musical silence include clinical depression and alcohol.[83] Undoubtedly he drank far too heavily on occasions. In 1920 he declared alcohol to be his truest friend,[84] but he had managed to give it up for seven years in 1908 on medical advice when a benign throat tumour was diagnosed,[85] an eventual cure for which was achieved only after multiple surgery. It may have been related to his intermittent partial deafness from 1901–05, with which his mood continued to fluctuate concurrently with patterns of composition.[86] The question is how much the chronic throat problem was due to a tumour and how much had been the heritage of chronic infection. Karl Ekman explained why there were thirteen operations.[87] Sibelius had consulted an ENT professor in Berlin after surgical failure in Helsinki. This elderly surgeon had tried twelve times to remove the 'malicious tumour', which he nevertheless said was not cancer.[88] Each attempt failed and so, for the fateful thirteenth, the great man invited his assistant to operate, which clearly was successful.[89] It may be that the bleakness of the Fourth Symphony composed in 1910–11, which came after throat surgery in Berlin, reflected his concern that he might have cancer of the larynx. In 1912 Sibelius declined the chair in composition at the Vienna Conservatoire, for he wanted to remain in Finland. The years after surgery were musically active as his reputation spread internationally. There were then more fallow years from 1914 to 1918, when he worried about money and the approach of old age. But the war years were when he composed and revised the Fifth Symphony, finally realised in 1919. Once more he sought refuge in whisky but also in composition.[90] In 1918 he and Aino were, for a time, forced out of their home by the Red Army.[91] Amidst the privations and food shortages, he had lost forty-five pounds by the time they were relieved by the Germans. Following the People's War, his heavy drinking resumed and musical activity declined.[92]

In March 1923 he went to Gothenburg to conduct his Fifth Symphony, arriving five days before the performance. Come the moment, he disappeared, eventually being found in a bar consuming oysters and champagne and rather the worse for wear.[93] Ekman, writing when Sibelius was still alive, observed that, as performances approached, his self-confidence ebbed and flowed, as did the alcohol, but there is no compelling evidence that chronic alcoholism was the cause of his nearly final retirement at sixty-one. Chronic alcoholics seldom live to celebrate ninetieth birthdays. Neither, typically, do they pursue a quiet and seemingly ordered life with their wife of many years. Perhaps prosaically, by 1927, when the 'silence' began, Sibelius had finally paid off all his debts, which had preyed on his mind for so many years. Perhaps that is no coincidence in judging his retirement. But he became depressed again in 1927, despite resolving once more to reduce his alcohol intake, which he logged daily.[94] After completing *Tapiola* he said, 'Now that my youth is past, my work and whole development are on a different plane. Formerly I longed to go out into the world and I have indeed lived a good deal in the great world abroad. Now it is the quietude up here that is dearest to me';[95] this probably explains the retreat to 'Ainola', his country house outside Helsinki, which he had built in 1904 and subsequently loved.

Upon reading accounts of Sibelius's last three decades, one is struck by some apparent harmony as he engaged in correspondence, received guests, played recordings on the gramophone and listened to the wireless.[96] He had long since become an internationally respected celebrity, although after his ninetieth birthday he became apparently depressed and socially withdrawn.[97] In earlier years visitors to 'Ainola' had been surprised by his wit, charm and interest in current events. His fall from musical grace after the First World War was at least in part because he had not followed the musical trails set by Stravinsky, or those of the Second Viennese School. He went out of fashion, despite the devotion of conductors such as Beecham and Koussevitzky, his music re-emerging from the shadows in the decade after his death. He had become a legend in his own lifetime, but what Goss described as his 'inward turn' had musically become established in the early twentieth century.[98] Death came quite suddenly, after lunch on 20 September 1957, when he arose feeling dizzy and quickly collapsed, dying of a massive stroke, said to be a cerebral haemorrhage,[99] later that same day.[100] His heritage is above all seven great symphonies. Harold Schonberg's judgement that 'He deserves to occupy an honourable place amongst the minor composers' as 'a prolific composer, mostly of ephemera'[101] is silly.

Looking at Sibelius's health and retirement, we should not expect to see all composers writing or dictating final bars from their deathbed. There is absolutely no reason for them not to feel that their contribution has been made, and that the time has come for what Elgar had called 'servile slipperdom'.

The story of the Eighth Symphony is complex and elusive, possibly reflecting Sibelius's state of mind, and thus relevant here. Its conception coincided with an increase in his already rigorous predisposition to self-criticism. After *Tapiola*, his diary records that he had 'suffered' because of it and that he was 'physically not strong enough for all of this'. He was sometimes lonely and again drank too much whisky, saying in 1928 that he was 'abused, lonely, all my real friends dead. Just now my prestige here is non-existent. Impossible to work.'[102] But he had promised Koussevitzky and Beecham the Eighth.[103] Accordingly, he went to Berlin in order to compose, writing to Aino in April 1931 that he was making good progress – 'I must get it finished whilst I still have my mental strength.'[104] He made further promises in 1932 and 1933 to Koussevitzky and Basil Cameron.[105] There is evidence that at least the first movement was delivered by Aino to Sibelius's usual copyist.[106] In 1927 he had told Olin Downes that he had completed the first two movements and that the rest was in his head.[107] Then there is silence, although the popular view that after 1927 he was musically inactive is not quite accurate. Layton enumerates eleven compositions after 1926, including *The Tempest*.[108] There can be no doubt that the stumbling composition of the Eighth Symphony was a reflection of his state of mind and, above all else, his self-confidence.

In the early 1930s, he engaged a secretary, Santeri Levas, who remained with him until his death. Towards the end of the Second World War Sibelius put many old scores in a laundry basket and then burned them.[109] Aino believed the Eighth Symphony was amongst the ashes, and she observed that after this pyre he seemed happier.[110] So why did he destroy it, as seems likely? Perhaps it fell short of his standards or he realised that after the Seventh Symphony he had said nothing new? Goss speaks of Sibelius conceiving 'real, private composition, not meant for the people'.[111] Anyway we cannot convincingly attribute the demise of the Eighth to health issues. Maybe he feared a resumption of the adverse criticism he had endured before. In old age there is much to be said for a quiet life.

We leave Sibelius with Levas in the autumn of 1957. His diary records that 'During his last months the master's home seemed strangely altered. The life force of its owner no longer irradiated the place. He was in retreat from life and he knew well that his last hour would soon strike.'[112] This advanced old age was a paradox: in many ways triumphant to outward appearances, but musically it became a personal resignation.

Claudio Monteverdi (1567–1643)

Monteverdi may be safely said to have enjoyed a triumphant old age. This followed chronic difficulties with his health and with parsimonious and excessively demanding masters for much of his life. Headaches, exhaustion, eye problems and a chronic irritating rash,[113] probably eczema or neurodermatitis, hung over many of his middle years. In 1608 he wrote to Chieppo, treasurer to the Duke of Mantua, saying that his treatment at court had made him ill-disposed and not friendly. He predicted his own early death, should his grievances not be addressed.[114] Despite the death of his much-loved wife, Claudia, in September 1607,[115] he was rapidly coerced into a mammoth programme of composition for the nuptials of the Hereditary Prince Francesco Gonzaga, and in 1608 he suffered 'great nervous depression' and a 'nervous breakdown'.[116] This was at least a state of mental and physical exhaustion, probably adumbrated by grief. He left Mantua for Cremona in June 1608. Later that year his father wrote to the duchess, pleading for his son's release on health grounds.[117] We should not be surprised that cautery, purgatives or blood-letting contributed only to the patient's misery.

Although after his return to Mantua in September 1609 composition became more prolific, including the premiere of *Orfeo* in 1609 followed by *Arianna* and the *Vespers of 1610*, he was happy to accept an appointment as *Maestro di Cappella* in Venice, moving there in 1612.[118] Despite much better and less demanding conditions in Venice, his headaches, breathing difficulties and eye problems continued.[119] But he then had to strive intensely, and ultimately successfully, for the release by the Inquisition of his doctor son – the authorities had disapproved of one of the books he read.[120] Monteverdi survived plague in Venice, smallpox in Mantua and both the Thirty Years War and the War of the Mantuan Succession. Sadly, many of his manuscripts perished in the Siege of Mantua.

His health seems to have improved as he grew older.[121] Redlich describes him 'plunging into a vortex of intensive activity as a composer' when he turned seventy.[122] This glory was crowned by *The Coronation of Poppea*, composed and produced when Monteverdi was seventy-five. Herein affection and ecstasy first enter music drama.[123] After completing *Poppea*, perhaps presciently he sought leave, travelling for six months to scenes of his earlier life. Then came the final return to Venice, where after nine days he died of a 'malignant fever', about whose precise nature little is known or inferred.[124] The fact remains that he overcame mixed health, personal sadness and worry, and in the Gonzaga days exploitation and meanness.

He was a truly original composer and deep thinker about musical directions. His old age was truly triumphant with composition sustained until the end. By what it was sustained remains a mystery.

Giuseppe Verdi (1813–1901)

Verdi's influence in old age extended all over Italy and far beyond music. One mystery has been the lengthy musical silence between *Aida* in 1871 and *Otello* in 1887, apart from the Requiem in 1874, for which there are no ready medical or psychological reasons. Conati had reported that Verdi, conducting *Falstaff* at the age of eighty-one, was a 'dynamo' and 'a force of nature'.[125] Phillips-Matz referred to reports of his extraordinary physical strength, energy and soundness of mind at that time.[126] Nevertheless, he may have suffered a minor stroke or transient ischaemic attack (TIA) in 1883.[127] After the triumph of *Otello* and then *Falstaff* his friend and librettist Arrigo Boito suggested that they next tackle *King Lear*. Ever perceptive, Verdi's second wife, Giuseppina Strepponi, took him aside saying, 'For Heaven's sake Boito, Verdi is too old and too tired.'[128]

Shortly before Giuseppina died in November 1897, she had found him 'paralysed' in bed and unable to speak.[129] Despite these afflictions, and never one to waste words, he demanded pen and paper; thereupon he wrote 'coffee' and promptly got it, whereafter he was quickly himself again. This was surely a transient expressive dysphasia (wanting and knowing what to say, and then being unable to do so) due to another TIA. The following year Boito visited 'the old man, who plays the piano, eats as he pleases, walks, argues with a youthful vivacity. He is as merry as a lark.'[130]

Verdi spent Christmas at the Grand Hotel in Milan in 1900, ordering that two crates of early compositions be destroyed.[131] Just after reaching Milan, he received some music to look over. He replied, 'I have not read for some time, I no longer write and even less can I look at musical compositions, no matter what they are. It is not my fault.'[132] Were it not for that final disclaimer, this would appear a reasonable rejection from a tired old man, but there lingers a suspicion that by now he realised a physical deconstruction amongst his most critical faculties. In May 1899 he arranged to meet Boito, on condition that they did not discuss music.[133] He had not composed for his last two years and wrote that he badly needed quiet.[134] After Christmas he remained in Milan and on 20 January 1901 Toscanini visited, finding him a little confused.[135] The following day Verdi arose as usual, and whilst buttoning up his shirt he collapsed. Six days later, aged eighty-eight, he died of a stroke.[136] It is probable that circulation to his brain had been in decline for the previous two years.

A month later his and Giuseppina's remains were removed to be finally laid to rest at the Casa di Riposo. This was a home for aged musicians, founded and funded by the Verdis, who regarded it as the vital project of their mature years. His generosity was free of ostentation and, as Budden put it, often discreetly so, by stealth. Three hundred thousand people followed the cortege.[137] His will decreed that he and Giuseppina should be attended by one cross, two candles and two priests. Was this because of a late spiritual contract with Roman Catholicism, or was it out of love and respect for his Catholic wife, to whom he had not always been the easiest of husbands? But he had been a triumphant old man.

Johann Strauss II (1825–1899)

Johann Strauss II had a life of hard work and, at first sight, effortless success as he wrote music of mass appeal. It was said in Vienna that the Emperor Franz Josef reigned until the death of Johann Strauss.[138] It was he above all others who took operetta from its French origins to being intrinsically Viennese.[139] But it came as it always does at a price. The stress of merging concert, composition and impresario demands for a time proved too much for him, and he was said to have had a 'nervous breakdown' in 1853.[140] In 1871, because of a 'chronic ailment' whose nature remains obscure, he begged to be released from his post as *k.k. Hofballmusikdirektor.*

Strauss told his third wife, Adele, that she was queen of his happiness, and it was to his happy home that Strauss returned from conducting on Whit Monday, 22 May 1899. Feeling a little sweaty and giddy, he settled to play cards with a couple of friends.[141] Two days later he felt well enough to attend the fashion parade in the Prater.[142] Once more he became sweaty and unwell and retiring home, where it was noted that he had a fever. By the beginning of June what had at first been regarded as a chill was clearly more: it was double pneumonia.[143] On 3 June his wife mopped his brow and beseeched him, 'Go to sleep dear.' He quietly replied, 'I will, whatever happens.' So with no pain, distress or death throes he gently slid away with a smile, to lie permanently opposite Schubert and next to Brahms,[144] who had so admired him. Today, with antibiotics and oxygen, he would probably have survived.

Strauss's old age was triumphantly glorious. He was also admired by Wagner, Verdi, Mahler and Richard Strauss. He loved to walk in Vienna, where he was a national treasure. He admired the pretty ladies admiring him. He worked, often overworked, with a conductor's baton or composer's pen, until the end of his life. Although he died in triumph, it was gently, as a happy man.

Leoš Janáček (1854–1928)

Janáček enjoyed one of the most triumphant of all musical old ages. At twenty-five, when he walked out of the Vienna Conservatoire, his studies were ended,[145] but he had produced almost nothing. Nevertheless, he became a good administrator and teacher, and later a beloved one. Lock has reviewed Janáček's illnesses in Tyrrell's mighty biography.[146] Generally, they were slight. He complained of 'gout', but the symptoms do not resonate with that diagnosis. His 'depression' was likely to have been exhaustion. Interestingly, he underwent sinus surgery in 1903 and again in 1908. The greatest influence upon his musical composition came late in his career and was probably due to his long-term passion for, if not obsession with, Kamila Stösslová. She was already married and thirty-seven years his junior. He wrote constantly to her, most days, for eleven years.[147]

Tyrrell implies that the new independence of Janáček's country may also have been a stimulus to his extraordinary creative surge of composition after the age of sixty.[148] He was an impressive figure. A bold head with flashing eyes was crowned by a mane of white hair. At last musically a major figure, he was energetic, loved and feared. This autumn of his life contained most of his masterpieces: *Mr Brouček's Excursion to the Moon* (1921), *The Cunning Little Vixen* (1924), *The Makropulos Case* (1926), the *Glagolitic Mass* and the Sinfonietta (1927). *From the House of the Dead* was not premiered until eighteen months after his death. Nature's renewal is perhaps the final note of *Little Vixen*. Janáček's brooding upon the nearness of his own death may be a reason for finally killing off Elina Makropulos, aged 337. Then, as Hollander points out, his last opera was infused with Christian metaphysics.[149]

In the summer of 1928 Janáček and Kamila went with her son to the countryside, which he loved. They were to be joined later by Kamila's husband, with whom friendly relations continued. Then the boy got lost in the woods and Janáček caught a chill looking for him.[150] Back at the house he rapidly became unwell and was admitted to the local hospital, where pneumonia was diagnosed. He relapsed with a gentleness that had not been his own life's attendant. On 12 August 1928 he quietly slipped away before his wife, Zdeňka, could arrive.[151] Such had been much of their marriage. Today antibiotics, oxygen and supportive care would probably have pulled him through. But he had the satisfaction, in old age, of an attractive young woman on his arm, and of that extraordinary burst of creative energy in his seventh and eighth decades being recognised and applauded in his own lifetime. It would not have been predicted less than twenty years earlier during the various rejections of *Jenůfa*.

Richard Strauss (1864–1949)

Perhaps Richard Strauss, more than any other composer, epitomises the glow of a triumphant old age. In his eighties, whilst with his friend Thomas Beecham Strauss is supposed to have said that if he wasn't a first-rate composer, he was a first-rate, second-rate composer.[152] Perhaps such sayings, tinged with self-parody, are the acme of triumphant old age, with its comfort zones and in satisfaction of things well done. Strauss was, after all, a universally respected and self-confident man. When asked, during that last visit to London in 1947, about his future plans, he laconically replied, 'Well, to die.'[153]

In many ways, life was good to Strauss, although Ronald Harwood's play *Collaboration* dramatically reveals that he had to compromise his principles with and subvert his own ego to those of his rather strident wife Pauline, then of his librettist Hofmannsthal and lastly of the Nazis. His son-in-law was Jewish, and it was suggested that Strauss may have had some protection from Baldur von Schirach.[154] If ever there was a perfect musical ending, tinged with autumnal sadness, it is his *Four Last Songs*. Perhaps no man has so exquisitely realised in music the joys and the pain of advancing years. Possibly his prosperous bourgeois life, with a long and devoted marriage, enabled him in old age to encompass passion, reflection, joy and sadness all in one character, such as the Marschallin in *Der Rosenkavalier*, or in a song like 'Im Abendrot'. The *Symphonia Domestica* and *Ein Heldenleben* are clearly autobiographical, but perhaps subtly his wonderful last works were even more so.

After his successful de-Nazification, he entered a Lausanne hospital in December 1948 to have a large bladder stone removed.[155] Shortly after this he wrote: 'I ask myself why they have brought me back to an existence in which I have actually outlived myself.'[156] This was the time of his final composition, the *Four Last Songs*. He was eighty-five and his energies ebbed as his heart failed, there having been a heart attack in the summer of 1949.[157] He last conducted, with an episode from *Capriccio*, during July 1949 in Munich. He was a frail old man until the baton was raised, then composure and authority.[158] His final illness overcame him the day after he finished his last, very appropriate, composition, *Besinnung* (*Reflection*). He approached death with apparent equanimity. He once said that Mahler was always seeking redemption, but he himself did not know what he was supposed to be redeemed from.[159] Close to the end, he told his daughter-in-law, Alice, that dying seemed 'just as I composed it in *Death and Transfiguration*',[160] although he told Hartmann, 'There is still so much I would still have to do.'[161] After Hartmann left, he told Alice that with that final interview he had passed on his artistic legacy, and he became serene. He died peacefully at home on 8 September 1949 after another heart attack,[162] and possibly kidney failure. He remained an agnostic, declaring that he did not fear death.[163]

Ralph Vaughan Williams (1872–1958)

Vaughan Williams defies generalisation. For many years he coped with the ascetic withdrawal of his increasingly disabled first wife, Adeline. After her death aged eighty in 1951 he seemed liberated, initially almost violently so.[164] Few composers have enjoyed a creative Indian summer like that of Vaughan Williams. Many compositions flowed in his ninth decade including the last three symphonies and *Pilgrim's Progress*, and he showed a new energy with song. Good health, an honourable life and a loving, late second marriage to the much younger Ursula Wood all nurtured his glowing maturity and happiness. He did become partially deaf and possessed numerous hearing aids. Although he had developed prostate cancer, he died painlessly and peacefully in August 1958 of a heart attack aged eighty-five, just four months after the premiere of his Ninth Symphony.[165] He had become a national treasure.

With a telling phrase Michael Kennedy, who knew Vaughan Williams well, described him as an 'extraordinary ordinary man'.[166] This is perhaps epitomised by his having sat on the bed, the night before he died, scoffing bananas and biscuits.[167] Sir John Barbirolli observed, 'VW had the youngest mind of anyone I knew.'[168] His was a life of virtue rewarded. Perhaps the greatest testimony to his undoubtedly triumphant old age comes from his biographer James Day: 'The time he required had been exactly allotted him and he had not wasted it.'[169] Perhaps that is the parent of contentment.

*

There are other composers who lived beyond seventy, to be found in other chapters. It is worthwhile looking at them briefly in terms of their old age, glorious or otherwise. Bruckner's passing (Chapter 6) was gradual and rather sad as he succumbed to a failing heart and his overriding obsessive-compulsive disorder. Composition of the unfinished Ninth Symphony lasted for five years. Fauré (Chapter 11) was belatedly lauded in his own lifetime. His last years were overshadowed by deafness and a weakening chest and heart, but he composed almost until he died. Stravinsky (Chapter 9) defies summary, for he lived until he was almost ninety, surviving endless serious and often life-threatening conditions. Although he remained more or less mentally intact, his ability and wish to compose tailed off, but into his last year he travelled extensively and clearly enjoyed society and his prestigious position in it. His old age was triumphant, as were the medicine and surgery which kept saving him.

Gluck's ending (Chapter 7) was also one of steady decline with three successive strokes. He last composed seriously six years before his death, which suggests that inspiration had dried up, or more probably that his brain became diminished by increasing atherosclerosis. But like so many of the other elderly men in these pages, he maintained his courtly station in society until the day of his passing. Gounod (Chapter 7) also succumbed to a stroke and did so as he sat composing a requiem for his grandson. After farcical disorder in England he returned to Paris under the supervision of his wife. Composition resumed, and great folk paid their respects. For Liszt (Chapter 8) late old age was a sad business. He travelled until the very end, dying in great distress from cardio-respiratory failure at Bayreuth. For all his geriatric appearance, musically he remained intact as a performer, but composed little in his declining years and nothing apart from two piano works in the year of his death. He had run out of puff and probably inspiration too. Handel (Chapter 3), whilst maintaining his exalted position in London society, not least as an organist, composed nothing of note in the years after the surgery which finally destroyed his vision. Rossini's 'retirement' (Chapter 10), although the longest (forty-six years), was not absolute. Songs, instrumental pieces, hymns and incidental pieces all slipped out after the premiere in 1829 of *William Tell*, his last opera. Of his two late sacred works, the *Stabat mater* was finished just before he was fifty, and the *Petite messe solennelle* in the year before his death. So to the public the old age of Rossini, like that of Handel, was something of a triumph, beneath which compromises and concessions were inevitable.

The one overriding characteristic to emerge from this collection of elderly gentlemen is that they almost all carefully preserved their position in society. Of greater interest is that few experienced new impulses to continue composing a significant quantity or quality of music once they had stopped. Some were assiduous in destroying earlier work, notably Sibelius and Verdi, revealing a relentless persistence of exacting standards until the very end. Vaughan Williams and Richard Strauss are clearly glorious exceptions here. Another noteworthy feature was that most of these men were very dependent, if only for their contentment, upon the loving care of a good woman, usually a long-suffering wife, in Bruckner's case a housekeeper and homemaker (as we will also see with Brahms), or sometimes a new lady friend. Monteverdi and Saint-Saëns would appear to be the solitary exceptions, with their itinerant ways of life. Once we have deliberately juxtaposed these survivors with the young geniuses snatched from us tragically young, there is some substance in the thesis that a great output of musical composition correlates badly with age at death.

✛ Chapter 3 ✛

Iatrogenic Afflictions

First do not harm the patient

Hippocrates, c.400BC

THE TERM 'IATROGENIC', used of illness and/or death, simply means that they were hastened or caused by medical treatment. Sadly, the biographies of many composers are replete with the iatrogenic.

Potion or Poison?
Good Music and Bad Medicine

The stark fact is that, until the era of aseptic surgery with anaesthesia, doctors did not really have much at their disposal with which to treat patients. These two advances came in the mid-nineteenth century, followed in the twentieth by intravenous fluids and antibiotics, as well as insulin, steroids and drugs to treat failure or irregularity of the heart rate and raised blood pressure. Then came chemotherapy and radiotherapy to treat cancer. Before the 1840s there were generally half a dozen or so treatments which became somewhat rigid blandishments for most and diverse conditions. Because those therapies applied initially usually failed, others would relentlessly follow. The sick composer was in many cases saved from worse medical remedies only by the felicitous intervention of nature, or by his professing scepticism regarding further medical torture with alternative practitioners. Of these 'treatments', the application of leeches and especially bleeding are probably the most notorious although, in fairness, there are today very occasional uses for both leeches and blood-letting. They are specific and beyond the scope of this book. Blood-letting achieved little apart from making patients anaemic, placing a great strain on the heart, which was sometimes the root of the problem originally. This was despite Harvey having explained the circulation in the seventeenth century.

Poultices, often dirty, were applied to open wounds and sores, introducing further infection. Bed rest and mountain air were benign and, for the tuberculous patient (TB sufferer), removal from smog-bound, overcrowded and insanitary conurbations could be genuinely beneficial. One encounters with many case histories practitioners wedded to one particular treatment. Little wonder that Beethoven famously referred to 'bumbling doctors and medical asses',[1] for many of them did literally continue regardless. In so doing, perversely, they generally encountered less opposition than did Semmelweis or Lister introducing asepsis, and Simpson pioneering anaesthesia.

Leaving surgery, we should consider those medicines which were available in the eighteenth and nineteenth centuries, if not before. Our gallery of composers often received cocaine or opiates (laudanum, morphia, heroin), which are still in use today for pain relief, as are cocaine derivatives for surgery under local anaesthesia. Coughing from TB could be suppressed only by opiates. Arsenic, like mercury, became the treatment for syphilis. Mercury was given until signs of toxicity became overwhelming.[2] To spot this, however, required some clinical intuition. Many medical advances have been based upon just that. Intuition led William Withering to discover and then use digitalis, which was extracted from foxgloves in the eighteenth century, but it was not until the last century that digoxin 'caught on'.

Meanwhile it is fundamental, in assessing whether sub-standard medical care has occurred, to judge the plaintiff's treatment by judging what a reasonable body of medical practitioners would have done then, not now. Being wise after the event is no valid case in law. So it does seem that by one legal paradigm most of the quacks were not guilty. It sometimes seems that, if nearly all the doctors practised bad medicine, then legally there was safety in numbers! One can understand Voltaire quipping 250 years ago that the art of good medicine consists of keeping the patient amused whilst nature cures him.

✠ JOHANN SEBASTIAN BACH ✠
(1685–1750)

> I smoke my pipe and worship God
>
> J. S. Bach, 1725

John Eliot Gardiner has recently tried to enliven the dour, sometimes humourless, image, enshrined as it is in wig and statue.[3] But how does this Protestant demi-god find himself in a chapter of afflictions visited upon the musically great by medical practitioners who were not great, except perhaps in their own estimation? The answer in three words is John 'Chevalier' Taylor,[4] of whom his biographer, Henry Jones, said, 'Never was the art of puffing displayed to such perfection.'[5]

Taylor was no 'Chevalier'; he was a quack,[6] and he practised all over Europe as an itinerant ophthalmic surgeon.[7] To quote Taylor himself: 'But to proceed, I have seen a vast variety of singular animals, such as dromedaries, camels etc., and particularly at Leipsick, where a celebrated master of music, who already arrived to his 88th year, received his sight by my hand.'[8] Well, wrong, and wrong again. Bach was a reasonably robust 64-year-old and never recovered his sight after Taylor operated twice.

Baer rightly rehearses for what indications this pedlar operated, although we do not know Taylor's exact diagnosis. There was said to be a family history of blindness.[9] We know from Forkel's early biography that Bach's blindness become painful for the three months before surgery.[10] Uncomplicated cataract is usually painless, whereas glaucoma is painful. Boyd quotes Emanuel Bach as saying his father had been vigorous in both mind and body until his involvement with Taylor.[11] Wolff, in a detailed account and depending upon Forkel, Bach's first biographer, describes a weakness of the eyes, worsening in his later years, although he surmised that his general health was robust until April 1749.[12] Williams reports a deterioration in his handwriting starting at the end of 1748,[13] inferring a parallel decline in his vision. Bach's second visit to Potsdam in 1747 had been his last public performance.[14] A hint of declining powers may be evident in the late compositions, but also when the authorities in Leipzig discussed in 1749 with whom they should replace Mr Bach, should he die.[15] During that year, over five months Bach created his *Musical Offering*, which was to be on sale in Leipzig by Michaelmas; money and security were of constant concern. Boyd indicates that Bach's last years were occupied with completing the organ preludes BWV 651–7 and the B minor Mass, and starting on *The Art of Fugue*.[16]

In 1750 Bach said that he wanted to continue to work for 'God and my neighbour'.[17] This wish is the embodiment of a Protestant work ethic, of which J. S. Bach is a paragon. Williams and Wolff believe it was that work ethic and a wish to resume work as before, plus the recent onset of pain, which persuaded Bach in 1750 to undergo surgery with Taylor.[18]

It is likely that Taylor's operation was for a cataract, which is not necessarily to say that Bach had one (or two). The usual surgical treatment for cataract in 1750 was 'couching'.[19] This involved sticking a sometimes blunt knife, or needles, into the eye and laying down (hence 'couch') the opaque lens below the visual axis of the eye, all with neither anaesthesia nor cleanliness. Ideally, this procedure prevented the opaque lens obscuring the visual pathway. Baer actually believes that, clinically, Taylor differentiated between cataract, which he described quite well, and glaucoma, which he did not fully understand.[20] In an article in the *Vossische Zeitung* of 1 April 1750, it was reported that Bach briefly recovered his eyesight after surgery, but that a few days later a second operation was undertaken.[21] Baer's account, deriving from Taylor's 1750 paper on glaucoma, implied that Taylor's recommendation for two-stage surgery was for glaucoma and not cataract. Or was it both and was he sure? Both Ober and Baer offer explanations for there having been two operations. One is that Taylor did one eye and then the other a few days later. The other is that, as sometimes occurred, the couched lens popped back into the front chamber of the eye, which would then have caused painful glaucoma. In Taylor's practice a double procedure could have been for glaucoma anyway.[22] Taylor may also have attempted a repeat couching resulting in the eye becoming painfully infected.

The unhappy fact is that, after the second operation, Bach remained totally blind, except for one possible brief interlude, and suffered from an obstinate, painful inflammation of the eyes for the rest of his life.[23] Wolff describes Bach's health falling into disarray after the second operation.[24] Baer quotes Elias Friedrich Heister, another contemporary, who claimed that Taylor's methods 'endangered the very lives of his patients'.[25] So it was that Bach retreated to a dark room, from which the dictation of the chorale BWV 668 may be anecdotal. Anyway, it was a resetting of an earlier composition.[26] He quickly went downhill, and Taylor's post-operative remedies, which included bathing the eyes with Peruvian balsam,[27] would have worsened his post-operative infection and the poor man's misery. At the end, Bach became frail and bedridden. One inexplicable curiosity is the account that, after the second operation and ten days before he died, Bach's eyes briefly improved, so that he was able to endure the light for a short time.[28] Following this, he was said to have suffered a stroke, that is about ten days or so before the second stroke which killed him.[29] His obituary said: 'Despite all possible care by two of Leipzig's most skilled doctors, on 28th July 1750 after quarter past eight in the evening, in the 66th year of his life, he passed away gently and peacefully, through the merit of his Redeemer.'[30] A stroke was the stated cause of death, a view upheld by Baer.[31] The original source of most of this information regarding Bach's last few weeks comes from his student Mizler.[32]

It is unlikely that his eye condition itself brought about his death, although his eyes and general health deteriorated in tandem. So what clinical conclusions may we sensibly draw? This was a burly man, whose prodigious energies ebbed towards his life's end. His final illness was heralded by blindness and worsened by post-operative infection. There is one common disease which in 1750 was neither understood nor treated, as it is now, possibly linking all these diverse facets, including infection. Wolff has studied this issue thoroughly and has concluded that diabetes seems to explain Bach's medical decline,[33] a view with which Williams concurs.[34] The seminal article today is that by Kranemann in German,[35] which is quoted by Wolff. Stroke is more common amongst diabetics than in the general population; so is post-operative infection. Previously, Terry diagnosed Bach as having died of Bright's disease.[36] That is reasonable, but as a diagnosis it does not wrap up the loose ends as diabetes does. Both cataract and glaucoma, common conditions in themselves, are more prevalent in diabetics than in the general population. The importance of whatever ailed him is that for some time it diminished the devout zeal which was the engine of Bach's creativity.

Today cataract and glaucoma are routinely and successfully treated, as is diabetes. Even in the case of the more ubiquitous cardiovascular disease, then today treatments ranging from statins to surgery, which unblock clogged-up arteries, are conferring very senior citizenship upon many of us. With Bach surely here was a man whose entire being was filled by his domestic contentment and expressing his genius to the glory of his Maker, until blindness, declining health and John Taylor took their final toll.

✛ GEORGE FRIDERIC HANDEL ✛
(1685–1759)

And the people will rejoice

Messiah, 1742

Some composers resonate loudly with their times. Beethoven's is the Napoleonic, Elgar's the Edwardian. Handel's is the Georgian, showing many characteristics from that era of order, elegance, confidence and the burgeoning of the bourgeoisie. He first went to England in 1710 and was naturalised in 1726. He was a tall, corpulent man, energetic, sometimes bad-tempered, resilient and persistent, as well as courageous and generous.[37] He had a mighty appetite for food and drink, and his mood vacillated.[38] Handel once went to an inn, ordering dinner for three. The waiter asked if he should wait for the other two diners. Handel gruffly indicated that dinner for three was just for him.[39] An original main source of biography has been the Rev. John Mainwaring,[40] whose own source was John Christopher Smith, an amanuensis after Handel became blind. But how does Handel find himself in the iatrogenic section of this book? The answer is that any lingering hope of restoring even a modicum of visual acuity to Handel was cut away after his third and last operation by John 'Chevalier' Taylor in 1758.[41]

Handel was a fast and prolific composer, often impatiently overtaking his librettists. His English reputation was quickly founded upon *Rinaldo*, *Acis and Galatea* and *Esther*. Then, in November 1736, his health was said to be deteriorating, with 'an indisposition due to rheumatism'.[42] In the spring of 1737 he had a 'paralytic disorder of the right arm', with a 'disorder of the senses'. Keates quoted Lord Shaftesbury, who recorded that

> Great fatigue and disappointment affected him so much that he was this Spring 1737 struck with the palsy, which took entirely away the use of the four fingers of his right hand and totally disabled him from playing. And when the heats of summer came on, the disorder seemed at times to affect his understanding.[43]

Mainwaring wrote of a 'useless' right arm caused by a 'stroke of the palsy'.[44] His Lordship shortly thereafter concluded that 'It is certainly evidence of great strength of constitution to be so soon getting rid of so great a shock. A weaker body would perhaps have hardly born ye violence of medicines, which operate so quickly.' Probably a shrewd case analysis. Never one to tarry for long, Handel was up and off to Aachen (Aix-la-Chapelle) to splash amongst the curative waters. For this confirmed Protestant it was an apparent and rapid success; he was playing the organ within a few hours.[45] Handel returned in full vigour, whilst the nuns debated whether it been a miracle.

Great success with *Samson* and *Messiah* followed. The latter, composed in only three and a half weeks, was premiered in Dublin in 1742. A year later Horace Walpole noted that Handel 'has a palsy and can't compose'.[46] A 'disorder of the head and speech', as well as his 'being delirious with fever', were mentioned by Jennens.[47] The fact is that five weeks later he was busy writing *Semele. Joseph* quickly followed. Following these episodes in 1737 and 1743, there were no similar paralytic problems and he remained generally well until the onset of his blindness, with no lasting impediment of his handwriting. There was, however, said to be a 'disorder of the head' in 1745.[48] There were no lasting sequelae, and Handel could be a volatile man. Both Keates and Frosch recount maladies to which the 1737 and 1743 episodes were attributed.[49] The descriptions are vague, but include recurrent muscular rheumatism, nervous exhaustion, colic, lead poisoning from drinking excess port, psychological distress and gluttony or comfort eating.

The modern diagnosis has been that he suffered two strokes, from which he made excellent recoveries. Slater and Meyer commented that, contrary to their usual course, 'The strokes had been insidious in their onset and rapid in their recovery' and accordingly unusual in sustaining a diagnosis of a typical stroke.[50] However, today we recognise people as suffering transient ischaemic attacks (TIAs), generally known as mini-strokes, whose course may be very brief, with full or nearly full recovery of all faculties. Keynes and Frosch both incline if only in part to a musculo-skeletal or rheumatic disorder,[51] rather than to a neurological one. This would be more plausible were it not for Walpole's reference to disordered speech.

We skip a few years, punctuated by success after success, including Handel's appointment as a governor of the Foundling Hospital, which his prosperity and generosity after *Messiah* established. Then, in early 1751, there was a deterioration in the sight of his left eye.[52] O'Shea's claim, that Handel was almost totally blind by 1743,[53] does not withstand research. Handel had written a note upon his own score of *Jephtha* regarding the start of his eye trouble on 13 February 1751,[54] although there had been a suggestion of visual deterioration in 1749. By the end of 1751 he was almost completely blind, whereupon Samuel Sharp, a respected surgeon, operated unsuccessfully for a cataract.[55]

Sharp suggested that he might find help and solace in the company of the well-known composer John Stanley who had been blind since the age of two. Somewhat sternly, Handel remarked, 'Mr Sharp, have you never read the scriptures? Do you not remember that if the blind lead the blind they fall into the ditch?'[56] Handel was recommended to go for further surgery by couching from William Bromfield, surgeon to the Prince of Wales, and this took place in November 1752, again unsuccessfully. Handel was almost totally blind by January 1753.[57] John 'Chevalier' Taylor finally operated, painfully and unsuccessfully, in 1758. Dr Samuel Johnson said that the career of the 'Chevalier' was 'an instance of how far impudence will carry ignorance'.[58] It seems this reputation was justified, although he introduced a blunt couching knife whose principle was to avoid rupturing the opaque lens. He is also said to have made the first good clinical description of staphylococcal infection of the eye, possibly on the basis of his own considerable post-operative experience.

It is noteworthy that, in 1748, a French surgeon, Jacques Daviel, described an actual removal of the opaque lens as a better alternative to couching. Today, replacing the diseased lens with an artificial one is commonplace. There stands in Cordoba, Spain, a statue to a Moorish physician, Mohamed Al-Gafequi, who undertook successful cataract surgery in the twelfth century.

This all presupposes that the cause of Handel's blindness was cataract. Ober questions whether the original diagnosis was cataract.[59] Sharp gave it as 'amaurosis gutta serena', which infers that no cataract could be seen.[60] The sudden onset reported on 13 February 1751, however, also casts some doubt upon cataract. Cataracts are due to the material within the lens turning from transparent to opaque, and generally develop slowly. A more advanced cataract can be seen as an opacity by an observer simply looking the sufferer in the eye. So commonplace are cataracts that it is seductively easy to assume they are the cause of the patient's loss of sight. However, other conditions leading to blindness may lurk with or behind a cataract, such as glaucoma, as suspected with Bach. Disease of the retina, at the back of the eye, may be caused by a thrombosis. So other underlying causes of blindness can draw attention to cataracts, which were initially assumed to be the cause of the blindness. With Handel we encounter a gluttonous gentleman who may have suffered from cardiovascular disease such as raised blood pressure and/or diabetes, the latter especially predisposing to all the eye conditions already outlined.* It also may be that Taylor did little surgically, but falsely claimed considerably more.

Other conditions have been suggested as causes of Handel's declining health.[61] Young spoke of Handel fighting a nightmare of mental disturbance, although he generally seems to have been a very rational man.[62] Hunter is keen to have Handel exhumed to test Frosch's theory that lead poisoning may have caused the various neurological impedimenta already outlined,[63] as well as headaches, abdominal and rheumatic pain. [64] The suggestion that he improved at Aachen because of a dramatic reduction in lead ingested with cheap wine is implausible.[65] Furthermore, the symptoms preceding his visit to Aachen did not recur when Handel returned to the taverns of London.

Despite permanent blindness, Handel continued to engage in many musical activities, especially playing the organ. Although he directed his works with authority, his powers of innovation waned. He lived another seven years after becoming blind. During this period it is clear from accounts by Shaftesbury and others that his general health varied greatly.[66] His overall history is of a late-increasing frailty in a once robust man. By April 1758 he was clearly deteriorating. During these declining years, collaboration with John Christopher Smith was often one of reworking pieces, songs and arias that he composed before blindness overtook him.[67] It seems that total blindness ended the previously relentless flourish of his creative genius, but this may additionally have been due to other afflictions of his health.

His last public appearance was on 6 April 1759, when he attended a performance of *Messiah* at the Foundling Hospital.[68] He was 'seized with deadly faintness' and returned home to bed, never rising again.[69] He had permanent carers, as he had been ailing for a few months. He dictated a new will only three days before he died on 14 April 1759. His last moments were chronicled for us by his friend James Smyth, a Bond Street perfumier, who tells us that Handel was sensible to the last moment, having taken leave of his friends. Smyth says, 'He died as he lived, a good Christian.'[70] He requested burial in Westminster Abbey, and so it was. He had always

---

* The author is grateful to consultant eye surgeon Mrs Joan Noble FRCSE for guidance in describing the eye afflictions of both J. S. Bach and Handel. She counsels that having one eye normal and the other with cataract may for a time go unnoticed by the patient, who one day casually covers the good eye with his or her hand, suddenly realising that he or she cannot see with the other. So a perception of 'sudden onset' of blindness may be born.

been well aware of his own worth. The cause of his final demise is more elusive, although Lord Shaftesbury commented that shortly before his end he appeared 'much better'. Maybe this elderly, overweight man succumbed to a sudden stroke, as was assumed at the time, although that is suspect in that Smyth would have been likely to have noted the signs of it. Furthermore, his mind seems to have been clear until the end, so heart failure is a more likely cause of death, perhaps owing to a heart attack or raised blood pressure.

In Handel's will, numerous charitable bequests were made. He died a very rich man. What matters is that the English seem to have taken him to their hearts to this day, just as he embraced England. How fitting, therefore, that Charles Dickens now lies at his feet in Westminster Abbey.

✣ GUSTAV HOLST ✣
(1874–1934)

The planets in their station list'ning stood,
While the bright Pomp ascended jubilant

John Milton, Paradise Lost, 1667

Holst, despite his name, originally von Holst, which was a problem during the Great War, was a very English man born in Cheltenham to a middle-class family coming from a genetic pool which mixed Sweden with Spain. As a youngster he was a very good pianist but, by the time he was admitted to the Royal Academy of Music, he had problems with 'neuritis' in his right arm and hand, which persisted intermittently for the remainder of his life.[71] Accordingly, he transferred from piano to trombone to accommodate his neuritic pain and attached a nib to his right index finger in order to write and compose more comfortably.[72] His daughter and biographer, Imogen, attributes his rather 'juvenile' handwriting to his teaching himself to write left-handed,[73] and so he also came to conduct, as his statue in Cheltenham reveals today.

As a young man Holst was shy, frugal, self-consciously intellectual, a vegetarian and a socialist. In the mid-1890s he had the two most important meetings of his life: in 1895 with Vaughan Williams, and two years later with Isobel Harrison, who, according to Imogen, tidied him up and got him eating properly and even eating meat.[74] They married in 1901. Like so many English composers, Holst and Vaughan Williams were powerful walkers, which is a salient point, for we hear of his weak physical health only to find that sometimes he walked over from Cheltenham to Oxford (about forty miles).[75] This alleged quasi-invalid would arrive to conduct soaked with mud after coming on foot.

In 1908 his neuritis become so severe, relieved only by heat, that he was advised to take a long holiday in the sun.[76] So he went cycling in Algeria, which inspired *Beni-Mora*. This was the first of many solitary holidays taken for health reasons. In 1913, after a first success with the *St Paul's Suite*, he became interested in astrology and astronomy, whence came immortality with *The Planets*, his laboured completion of which in 1916–17 was in part by dictation.[77]

In 1914 his application to enlist had been rejected because of his myopia and the ongoing neuritis. He could hardly pick up a musical instrument, much less a rifle. During the war the Holsts purchased a country property in Thaxted, as a retreat from their base in London. Thaxted, once a medieval Essex wool town, became in the early twentieth century a centre for Christian Socialism. It was intermittently to be his home for the remainder of his life. Nonetheless, he found having two homes a strain.[78] Holst seems to have found quite a lot a strain, but not the holidays to relieve that strain, which would have exhausted many a lesser mortal!

Shortly before his first visit to the USA in 1923, which he enjoyed, he banged his head. It is clear that Imogen has attributed much subsequent symptomatology to this injury.[79] The medical advice was for him to give up all work and to live alone at Thaxted for nearly twelve months.[80] I asked the Holst scholar Raymond Head whether there been a breakdown in Holst's marriage.[81] If there had been it might have been difficult for his daughter and prime biographer to dwell too much upon it. Head was much more of the view that they were both rather strange and often solitary people, and that Mrs Holst just accepted that sometimes Gustav went away by himself. In contrast, reading many years of correspondence between Holst ('Gussie'), his wife ('Iso') and Imogen ('Imo') reveals a decent and affectionate family.[82] What the medical basis was for separating a sensitive, possibly self-engrossed man from his family and beloved work is today completely beyond medical comprehension.

Doubtless it was on doctor's orders in 1925 that he retreated to Switzerland, unable once more to work or sleep. There he met Dr William Brown, by whom he was successfully psychoanalysed.[83] By 1926 his fear of crowds, as well as insomnia and headaches, all improved, the latter according to Imogen because he was 'allowed to wear stronger spectacles'.[84] In that one word 'allowed' we perhaps encounter a key to 1920s medicine. Doctor knew best then, and orders or 'allowances' were beyond question or reproach, even the strength of spectacles.

In 1927 Holst was invited to become conductor of the Bach Choir, but he quickly resigned on doctor's orders (again) for fear that his duties might put too great a strain on his heart. It might become 'too much' for him.[85] Just before this he successfully conducted *The Planets* at the Cheltenham Festival, albeit with his friend Adrian Boult waiting in the wings, baton in hand – just in case. There followed another period of weakness only to be resolved physically and then musically with his exploration of *Egdon Heath*, his own favourite composition. When given under Monteux in Paris it was hissed,[86] although Holst always claimed to be indifferent to criticism. How are we to apprehend this in any performing artist; was this not English stiff upper lip? On returning from Paris he sank into a numb, grey isolation of utter despair.[87] Holst clearly was a neurotic man with predispositions to anxiety and depression, with consequent swings of self-confidence and self-esteem. After a successful and prestigious trip to Yale in 1929 he returned in good spirits and full vigour. He revisited the USA in 1932, at the invitation of Harvard, where he conducted three concerts and took four rehearsals with the Boston Symphony Orchestra within a week. However, it was when he went to Washington that he vomited up two pints of blood, being treated by blood transfusion and sedation.[88] By the end of 1932 he was ill again, and on Boxing Day was admitted to a nursing home for a long convalescence, which enabled him to settle, composing the *Lyric Movement* for viola and orchestra and the *Brook Green Suite* for strings. Illness and composition were becoming bedfellows.

At the end of the following year Holst was admitted to a nursing home in Ealing, and Imogen recorded that for six to eight weeks he could do little more than read and take a bland milky diet.[89] There followed the critical advice of a surgeon. By now the diagnosis was duodenal ulcer. He was given the options of two different operations.[90] The first was a 'minor operation' from which success would be 'likely', but after which there would be 'life-long restrictions'. The second was a 'major operation', a serious one, but if it was successful there would be 'no future restrictions'. Holst chose the latter, which was carried out on 23 May 1934, although it was postponed by two and a half weeks because he was anaemic.[91] The hospital said it was 'a success'.[92] The only setback was Holst's death two days later. The strain on his heart, after all, proved to be too much.[93] So what are we to make of all this? Here we are well served by the balance of probabilities test. Today a course of Losec capsules or the like, or alternatively antibiotics to kill the germ (*Campylobacter pylori*) by which duodenal ulcers are often caused, would be cure enough. Yet until the late twentieth century surgery was offered for stubborn cases, of which there were many. The lesser operation offered is likely to have been one of cutting the vagus nerves to the stomach, thereby reducing stimulus to excessive gastric acid secretions which caused painful ulceration. That operation should be accompanied by a procedure called pyloroplasty, to facilitate drainage of material out of the stomach, as the channel from stomach to duodenum is often scarred by chronic ulceration. That adjunct in 1934 was not necessarily offered, especially as Holst was warned that there might always be restrictions thereafter. So it seems probable that instead he was treated by a partial gastrectomy (removal of the final third of the stomach), a procedure pioneered by Brahms's great friend Theodor Billroth, but, even in the most expert hands and notwithstanding the unfortunate supervention of death, it was certainly not without long-term post-operative complications of some notoriety.

We can only speculate, in the absence of a post mortem report, as to why Holst died two days later. In November 2013 there were no specific medical records in the Holst archive, although the death certificate gives his cause of death as: '1. Duodenal Ulcer (operation 23.5.34), 2. Myocardial Arterial Degeneration' (aka coronary artery disease). It was signed by Dr A. W. Hobbs.[94] There is nothing in his long-term medical history initially with all that cycling and walking to suggest that he had ischaemic heart disease with angina or serious irregularity of the heart rate. Adrian Boult wrote of his walking from Cheltenham to London.[95] However, remarks are recorded in the family correspondence, during the mid- to late 1920s and early 1930s, which suggest that he may have had a touch of heart failure. Our problem in analysing these possibilities is the liberal use of words such as 'strain' mixed up with diagnoses that he was 'doing too much', from which recovery was then sought by strenuous activities.

If he underwent surgery whilst already anaemic from blood loss due to the ulcer, as Imogen implied, then a major operation such as partial gastrectomy, with possible silent post-operative blood loss, may have precipitated a heart attack or failure and consequent death; this could occur even in a healthy individual,. On the day of surgery Isobel Holst wrote to Mrs Herbert Jones, saying that the operation had taken three hours (an unusually long time!) and been so great 'a shock to his system' that he would be unable to work much for the rest of 1934.[96] Alternatively and improbably, if pre-operatively he had been lying around in nursing homes 'confined to bed' on doctor's orders, then he might have developed a deep venous thrombosis and, after the further trigger of major surgery, died of a pulmonary embolus. Today an autopsy would be ordained by law, and the coroner would want to know why an individual perished two days after an elective operation.

His neuritis is also difficult to diagnose. Compression of the three main nerves to the arm are, in the case of the median and ulnar nerves, usually easy to diagnose and treat. Neuropathy of the radial nerve is a rare and nebulous condition, discussed more fully in the section on Schumann (Chapter 6). These may all have been described then as neuritis. To hazard an informed guess, it is more likely that Holst, like Imogen or Clara Schumann,[97] suffered from fibromyalgia, colloquially known these days as fibrositis, rather than neuritis. Finally, conditions of the shoulder itself can cause severe pain, not least in the hand. There can be great relief of shoulder to hand pain, as it is known, by successful surgery to the shoulder, but typically symptoms do not arise much before middle age. Holst's problem was career-threatening, as far as the piano was concerned, by his early to mid-twenties. This is a topic difficult to analyse because psychological factors undoubtedly obtrude and Holst was a tense, fraught man, described in Arthur Bliss's obituary as both solitary and a visionary.[98]

THE SAD TALE OF
✠ GEORGE GERSHWIN ✠
(1898–1937)

Death can be just, it can be kind, but it had no business taking our George
Ira Gershwin, 1937

Here is a case history which, because it fell within the twentieth century, illustrates a paradox in judging the probity of medical treatment. This is the sad case of George Gershwin, who died in 1937, aged thirty-eight, after surgery for a brain tumour. There are excellent detailed accounts of his tragic decline and fall, with a more intimate analysis of the medical records than is usually encountered with many other composers.[99]

By the early 1930s George Gershwin, the son of Russian Jewish émigrés, had become fabulously successful. During the period from 1934 to 1935 he had been overworking, but he was an energetic young man at both work and play. He complained that he felt listless, and lost his enthusiasm for social gaiety. Many put this down to his unrequited love for Paulette Goddard, who married Charlie Chaplin in 1935,[100] after which Gershwin went to a medically qualified psychoanalyst, Dr Gregory Zilboorg. Despite his punishing schedule, Gershwin attended analysis five times a week. Whether this presaged the start of organic disease is conjectural.

Silverstein would have us look back much further.[101] Gershwin described various stomach and bowel symptoms going back to 1922,[102] which were diagnosed as 'composer's stomach', another fiction. Many people experience such symptoms en passant. One needs retrospective focus, and perhaps that should be upon the word 'nausea', for it can forewarn of any disease causing pressure inside the skull, of which a brain tumour is the most notorious, especially if accompanied by a rising sensation in the upper abdomen and followed by drowsiness.[103] Clearly, very few patients experiencing nausea have a brain tumour, which is why clinical judgement is so important. In preparing his excellent article, Silverstein, a New York neurologist, spoke to Gershwin's sister and to Kay Swift, a paramour of George's in the 1930s.[104] Neither could recall his having complained of nausea before 1937; it was perhaps a spurious recollection, as he been talking of his stomach to doctors since the 1920s.[105]

Whilst playing his own Piano Concerto in F with the Los Angeles Symphony Orchestra on 11 February 1937, Gershwin blacked out, remaining upright on the piano stool for an estimated ten seconds, although the conductor was able to cover up the musical hiatus.[106] This was not a full epileptic seizure in that he did not fall off the stool, bite his tongue, wet himself or thrash around. Significantly, Gershwin observed later that, immediately before the attack, he experienced a nasty smell, like burning rubber,[107] something he also noticed even before this episode and again subsequently. That symptom, known as an epileptic aura, was to precede more 'fits' in the following months. He also complained of increasingly severe morning headaches and lethargy, symptoms dismissed by doctors, some of whom were friends, as neurotic,[108] although they were known by then to be typical amongst the symptoms of a developing brain tumour.

In her biography *The Memory of All That*, Peyser quotes the musician Mitch Miller as having said that Gershwin, whom Miller knew well, told him in 1934 that he was troubled by smelling the odour of burning garbage when clearly there was no garbage present.[109] Miller previously dated these smells to a day in 1934, which is well established with Gershwin boarding a train at Detroit with the Reisman Orchestra and mentioning it then.[110] Miller, when he met Silverstein in 1998,[111] was clear that Gershwin complained of 'severe headaches' in March 1936. By June 1937 the head-aches had worsened and he was admitted to hospital in Los Angeles on 23 June, when a blood test excluded syphilis and where he refused a lumbar puncture(LP), a procedure where a slim needle is passed into the fluid-containing sleeve (meninges) which protects the spinal cord within the spine. Laboratory analysis of this cerebrospinal fluid (CSF) is helpful in diagnosing various conditions. Had the procedure been carried out, it might have killed him within minutes, contrary to the view expressed by Greenberg.[112] Lumbar puncture in a patient whose brain is under pressure within the skull, as by then Gershwin's would have been, causes a sudden drop in pressure lower down in the spinal fluid. This can cause part of the brain to be pushed out of the skull into the upper neck, a process known as 'coning' which can stop the vital centres of breathing and heart control at the base of the brain, causing rapid death.[113]

At the hospital Gershwin complained of severe frontal headache and listlessness. He mentioned the bad smells and was found to be somewhat malcoordinated. His performance at the keyboard had recently become erratic. In spite of all this, he was discharged on 26 June with a note saying that it was 'most likely hysteria'.[114] Significantly, the backs of both eyes were examined with an ophthalmoscope and *said* to be normal. Subsequent events cast doubt upon that point. Also, there had been two odd episodes. In one he tried to push his chauffeur out of the car,[115] and on another occasion he squashed up some chocolates and wiped the resultant mess over his body and clothes.[116] Shortly thereafter, he deteriorated further. On 9 July 1937, Ira called and found his brother unrousable. Gershwin was quickly readmitted to hospital in Los Angeles, under the care of a neurosurgeon, Dr Carl Rand, who now found swelling at the back of the eyes (papilloedema) with an ophthalmoscope.[117] That is an ominous sign, indicating raised pressure within the brain. Other signs were elicited on examination to reinforce that conclusion. Such features were recorded previously as having been normal. A lumbar puncture was performed at which increased pressure was discovered, raising the question of whether it caused the brain to herniate (cone), as described above, thus hastening the inevitable end, a point to which we will return.[118]

Meanwhile, Gershwin's friend Emil Mosbacher contacted Professor Harvey Cushing on the east coast.[119] Cushing was the founding father of modern neurosurgery, but by then was retired. Accordingly, he recommended Dr Walter Dandy, who pioneered an X-ray technique known as pneumo-encephalography, whereby air is put into the cavities of the brain (ventriculogram) to see if it will outline a tumour.[120] Then an incredible scenario developed.[121] Walter Dandy was sailing in Chesapeake Bay, where he was 'ambushed' by the coastguards and taken by police escort to Newark airport in New Jersey, with a view to flying across to Los Angeles. At the airport, Dandy spoke by telephone to another eminent brain surgeon, Dr Howard Nafziger, who had sensibly been called in by Rand. He believed that the situation was immediately and urgently life-threatening. Hence, without waiting for Dandy, Nafziger carried out the ventriculogram, which revealed a tumour in the right temporal lobe of the brain.[122] Accordingly, a flap of bone was lifted from Gershwin's skull, and a large cystic tumour was discovered and decompressed. George Gershwin never regained consciousness, and died on 11 July. The pathology of the tumour within the cyst was a malignant glioblastoma, a particularly aggressive tumour.[123]

This was the worst of circumstances and one for which the prognosis was truly appalling. No blame should attach to Dandy, Rand or Nafziger for the tragedy. Tragedy it was because, with Gershwin, the USA lost its first composer of worldwide fame. Six months before his death, Gershwin told his sister Frances that he had so much more music in him, symphonies, concertos, operas … perhaps he sensed what was to overtake him. He had already expressed his dislike of Hollywood and told Frances that, once he was financially secure, he would 'devote my time to compose serious music'. Tragically, he ended by saying, 'I feel that I haven't scratched the surface.'[124] He was starting to write a string quartet.

Two conclusions are clear. Firstly, the famous composer may have been a little neurotic in his personality; many creative people can be. It is the clinician's duty to exercise clinical judgement and caution and never to moralise too much about patients' peculiarities. The symptoms observed or reported should have alerted Gershwin's doctors from an earlier stage to the likelihood of a brain tumour. This was potentially a point of some importance. If Gershwin had proved to have a more benign type of tumour such as a meningioma, then this delay might have militated against a full recovery after its belated removal. As it is, if Gershwin had come under Rand's, Nafziger's or Dandy's care months, or even a year or two, earlier, his death might not have been so dramatic but, with the type of tumour discovered, he was unlikely to have lived much beyond 1938. Moreover, the price to pay for palliative surgery in cases such as this sadly can be devastating in terms of disabilities after surgical intervention. One sometimes wonders about the quality of such prolongation of life. The brutal likelihood is that Gershwin's abilities as a composer, or as a concert pianist, would have evaporated. Thus we have the paradox that the doctor who did the right thing as a result experienced a profound, and possibly for him embarrassing, clinical failure. That was not Dr Nafziger's fault. Even with today's most sophisticated medical treatment, the prognosis has improved little from Gershwin's time.

The last word belongs to the compassionate Dr Walter Dandy, who, in his letter to Gershwin's doctor, said, 'I do not see what more could have been done to help Mr Gershwin. It was just one of those fulminating tumours.' He went on to suggest that his sudden death had been for the best. Dandy concluded, 'For a man as brilliant as he, with a recurring tumour, it would have been terrible; it would have been a slow death.'[125]

THE MYSTERIOUS CASE OF
✣ MAURICE RAVEL ✣
(1875–1937)

I still have so much music in my head … I haven't said anything yet, and
I still have so much to say.

Maurice Ravel, 1937

Some might criticise the medical or at least surgical care of Maurice Ravel,
a man who ended up in the hands of another famous brain surgeon. It
is revealing to review the last few years of his life, and for several reasons:

1   It may be that the record should be clarified, remembering that in
    English law we can judge treatment in 1937 only by the standards
    upheld then.
2   Here, in contrast to many other composers, is a case to which there
    was a relatively modern medical approach.
3   This is the most important of all our cases in being able to assess in
    sad detail the impact of brain impairment on the neural mechanisms
    of a man hearing music in his head and being unable to commit it to
    paper, and thus to the outside world. As Ravel complained, by 1933
    his mind was 'becoming clouded by fog'.

From the delightful pages of Roger Nichols's biography, we encounter a
small, wiry, witty man, who was not always very sociable.[126] His sparse
frame initially kept him out of the Great War, although he did later serve
at Verdun as a lorry driver.[127] He also underwent surgery for a hernia in
1916.[128] Ravel appeared to have few intimates, male or female, beyond his
mother and brother Edouard, although he had many loyal friends. Nichols
regards a period as long as nine or ten years as being the final chapter,
during which Ravel deteriorated, ultimately becoming locked-in musically. Eric Baeck, a Belgian neurologist, is a pre-eminent Ravel medical
scholar who believes that the period of serious brain degeneration was no
more than four or five years.[129] Ravel complained of insomnia, fatigue and
a decreased aptitude for composition intermittently for a longer period.[130]
Of course, we all have problems of lassitude with a disinclination to work,
and Maurice Ravel was a demanding taskmaster of himself, once saying,
'My object is technical perfection. I strive increasingly to this end.'[131]
A curious reference is that on 11 November 1918 Ravel had surgery for
'tubercular ganglions of the right lung'.[132] Just what 'tubercular ganglions'

were is elusive. Possibly significant is that two months later he went to Megève to walk in the mountains and ski, which seems improbable if surgery to a lung had occurred two months earlier. A medical guess is that lymph nodes in the neck were removed and examined for evidence of TB. Anyway, there is no follow-up on this medical item, whose importance presumably evaporated.

Henson places the onset of 'Ravel's pre-senile dementia' in 1927.[133] Ravel's friend Hélène Jourdan-Morhange called Dr Vallery-Radot to see him. He looked after Ravel for several years, but now Hélène said he was always making blunders and 'became so lost before his music'.[134] A year's rest was prescribed. Then in 1928 Madeleine Grey reported that, whilst playing his *Sonatine* in Madrid, he jumped from the first movement to the coda of the finale,[135] which justifies Nichols's view. Alternatively, it might just have been because he was distracted, even annoyed, by the noisy audience. Henson comments that the period 1928–31 is not well documented, although the two piano concertos came to fruition and *Bolero* had its premiere then.[136] He was being treated by prolonged total rest at this time.[137]

Regarding that most famous and possibly vexatious of pieces, many have attached medical importance to *Bolero*. Kerner reflected that the monotony of *Bolero* was indicative of Niemann-Pick disease (aka Pick's, a form of pre-senile dementia), to which we will shortly return.[138] In 1930, Ravel criticised Toscanini for playing *Bolero* much faster than he, Ravel, meant it to be played, emphasising that he wanted there to be the same monotonous tempo throughout.[139] It was, he said, 'experimental: orchestral tissue without music'.[140] Ravel seems to have been clear in his directions for his most controversial composition. It remains a moot point whether we should let the music explain the underlying disease, or the converse. The Ravel scholar Roy Howat has generously shared his suggested explanation for *Bolero*.[141] For many years Ravel suffered from insomnia. Then in the 1920s came his American tour, with long distances spent in overnight sleeping cars. Clickety-clack, clickety-clack went the train as it lulled the composer gratefully to sleep. Whether acknowledgement of soothing train noise was a conscious or unconscious act remains enigmatic, but it is plausible. There is no doubt as to the repetitive nature of *Bolero*. But the same may be said of much music by American minimalists of the late twentieth century, such as Philip Glass, Steve Reich and John Adams, whose mental health is not questioned. Some authorities regard *Bolero* as an example of perseveration,[142] a feature typical in atrophy of the frontal and temporal brain lobes. Just before he died Ravel laughed about *Bolero*: 'What a joke I played on the musical world.'[143]

In March 1929 Ravel met Paul Wittgenstein in Vienna. He was of that great family and had become a famous pianist. By now he was also a right-arm amputee from the Great War.[144] Wittgenstein commissioned a Piano Concerto for the Left Hand from Ravel, who also embarked upon the two-handed G major Concerto, and the two were composed roughly in parallel. Nichols reflects that in 1930 Ravel was composing more and sleeping less, energetically contrary to some of the earlier observations. This is reasonable evidence that, at that time, he was neither ill nor depressed, but that his mood was cyclothymic. Generally neurological illness, in common with depression, ebbs and flows. Eventually, in January 1932, both concertos were premiered. Contractually, Wittgenstein played the Left Hand Concerto, and Ravel's friend Marguerite Long the G major. It has been asked why Ravel himself did not play the G major Concerto. There had been disputes,[145] but was it his health? The more probable and pragmatic reason is that Mme Long was a better pianist.

Henson describes variable decline in Ravel's health during 1932.[146] On 28 August 1932 he attended a festival of his own music at San Sebastian. Signs of lassitude and amnesia were both prevalent and awkward. He spoke of amnesia and 'senile decay',[147] while others spoke of inappropriate behaviour (often an early sign of brain pathology, particularly in the frontal lobes of the brain). It is difficult today to judge forgetfulness, even if its exhibitor describes 'amnesia' as Ravel did.[148] Absent-mindedness has been a metaphor over centuries for clever people.

On 8 October 1932, Ravel was in a taxi which was involved in an accident. He sustained cuts to his face and probably suffered bruising of the right lung with possible bleeding, although he told Falla that it was not very serious.[149] Whether he briefly lost consciousness remains uncertain. Some have suggested that the accident caused a 'mild to moderate head injury'.[150] He took three months to recover, experiencing insomnia and a supressed appetite, as he had much earlier. Then he was invited to write music for a film about Don Quixote, with the improbable cast of Chaliapin as the Don and George Robey as Sancho Panza. He agreed and then appeared to default. Later he did compose three songs upon the Quixote theme, finishing them in April 1933. Sadly, they were to be his swan-songs and, some might say significantly, all he ever composed after the accident. Otte and colleagues emphasise that the decline in his abilities came after the taxi accident, despite the head injury appearing to be minor.[151] It is said that a minor injury such as this can accelerate deterioration of pre-existing brain disease.[152] The point is interesting, but the taxi episode seems to be but one benchmark along a longer and vacillating clinical course. Otte's clinical theme is that we may underestimate the severity of apparently minor head injuries, with Ravel a famous example. It is a view popular today with personal injury lawyers.

In June 1932 Ravel had to be rescued from the sea. Although he was normally a good swimmer, there was incoordination between his arms and legs; he said he could no longer swim.[153] This was also the time of his skimming a pebble into a lady's face, rather than across the water as he intended.[154] He unsuccessfully attempted composition by using his student Manuel Rosenthal as an amanuensis.[155] In 1934 he said that he felt hazy and that he went out and about less, although ideas floated in and out of his head, with nothing transpiring; he intermittently attempted to compose an opera about Joan of Arc, a project in process since 1927, which never came to fruition. In November 1933 he conducted for the last time, with Marguerite Long playing the G major Concerto.[156] He said of *St Joan*: 'It's there in my head, I can hear it but I will never write it down. It's the end. I can't write my music down anymore.'[157] With that, he went to a clinic in Switzerland where little more than rest and pampering were the regimen. By then he was experiencing severe difficulty in writing letters.

Ravel and Alajouanine

Ravel consulted the great French neurologist Professor Alajouanine in 1936. It is a sad account of the impaired musical mind.[158] One of the touching aspects is that Ravel appears to have had good insight into his own predicament. He had always been a somewhat self-deprecatory man anyway. Furthermore he was worried, if not scared, because his father, in 1908, had developed a dementing cerebral atrophy. It is worth recounting Alajouanine's report regarding his dealings with Ravel.[159] Here are the patient and his disease, with the impaired musical genius attached to both, in the clinical laboratory. Alajouanine worked within a framework of sensitivity to Ravel, the wounded bird he perhaps hoped to set free. He explained expressive aphasia, which is knowing what you want to say without being able to articulate the words, whilst realising that Ravel described perfectly its musical counterpart, in which he had tunes in his head but was incapable of musical notation (amusia). Apraxia is similar in motor function. Ravel wanted to light a cigarette; he knew how, but somehow could not always coordinate a meeting between cigarette and lighter.[160]

Of great interest were the sessions that Alajouanine and Ravel had with two first-class pianists, one of whom was also a neurologist. They used *Le tombeau de Couperin* and *Ma mère l'oye*. Ravel's tune recognition was swift and accurate, his ability to name notes poor, and to read them worse, whilst his ability to reproduce notes at the piano himself was mixed.[161] However, when either of the two pianists made slight deliberate mistakes, by playing the wrong note or omitting one, and later by altering the rhythm, Ravel pounced upon this error at once. This ability was still preserved in June 1937, when he identified a slight change of metre whilst Madeleine Grey was singing one of the *Don Quixote* songs with Francis Poulenc as pianist.[162] Given a one- or two-note prompt, he could sing quite well to order. He performed better with his own music than with that of others. For those disposed to localising the disease in Ravel's brain, it is interesting that he could play *Ma mère l'oye* with his right hand much better than with his left, although he could play scales in major and minor keys quite well with both. Alajouanine summarised that Ravel had aphasia, apraxia and alexia (inability to write down a thought), affecting his reading or use of musical notation as well as piano playing, whereas his memory, musical recognition and aesthetic judgement remained well preserved.

Aphasia or dysphasia sadly is quite common after head injuries or strokes; fortunately most patients so affected are neither amusic nor dysmusic.[163] There are even people who can sing, but not say, their name and address. This is a cornerstone of recent interest in music therapy. Also it suggests a separation of words from music within the brain. Curiously the opposite is often not the case, with 75% of people with amusia also being aphasic. Alajouanine believed that Ravel's diagnosis belonged to a group of cerebral atrophies distinct from Pick's disease. Functional MRI scans will soon differentiate this area.

A Neurological Diagnosis

Although much less frequent than Alzheimer's, a diagnosis advanced by Dalessio,[164] Pick's disease is the second commonest cause of pre-senile dementia in patients under the age of sixty-five. Ravel died when he was sixty-two. Ravel's detailed memory for little pathways in the forest of Rambouillet late in his illness is very much against a diagnosis of Alzheimer's,[165] a late feature of which is a failure to empathise with or even recognise friends and family. For all Ravel's reserved manner, this was not clinically evident even at the very end. Likewise, the manuscripts of the two piano concertos are beautifully handwritten.

Baeck has researched Ravel's neurological illness in detail.[166] He also analysed alleged stylistic anomalies in the two concertos and found them similar to ones found in *La valse, Le tombeau de Couperin* and *Ma mère l'Oye*, which were composed much earlier.[167] Baeck then proposed a diagnosis of cortico-basal degeneration (CBD).[168] This was rejected by Amaducci et al., who claimed that Ravel showed no signs of incoordination, a characteristic of CBD.[169] Problems with lighting cigarettes, throwing pebbles or even swimming may all be regarded as incoordination. Another article pointed to the absence of features of Parkinson's disease, sometimes a feature of CBD.[170]

After 2004 Baeck favoured a diagnosis of a form of Pick's disease, known in the 1920s as fronto-temporal degeneration.[171] It is the exhibition of compulsive rituals and perseveration in Pick's disease that has intrigued musicologists,[172] because, firstly, of *Bolero* with its apparent use of monotonous repetition and, secondly, of patterns in the Left Hand Concerto. Baeck commented that there are no reasons, be they chronological, neurocognitive or musical, to argue that the concerto was influenced by cerebral disease.[173] Wittgenstein's absence of a right hand was the problem. On a similar note, Amaducci and Marins argued that the rhythmic and harmonic complexities in *Bolero* were cleverly and deliberately pieced together and not indicative of brain disease.[174] As Baeck pointed out, its structures are very deliberate,[175] just as Ravel said he meant them to be. He also argued that if the alleged stylistic idiosyncrasies in *Bolero* were neurologically determined, then why are they not increasingly apparent in his subsequent compositions? This does not contradict Baeck's diagnosis of Pick's; it merely reaffirms that neither *Bolero* nor the Left Hand Concerto was the product of a mind affected by it. He also described the G major Concerto as a magisterial structural cohesion.[176]

It is easy to regard Ravel's death as the disease's end point. But, as we will see in a moment, death was sudden and secondary to surgery. He might otherwise have lived miserably with that disease for another ten years or more, ultimately declining in an asylum, when later features of Pick's such as aggression or sexual disinhibition might have prevailed. Suggestions that he was bisexual or asexual, possibly impotent,[177] or Robert Craft's view that, as a person, Ravel 'failed to evolve' are speculative and, in Craft's case, possibly specious.[178] Many years ago Howat visited the village where Ravel lived.[179] There were still old people there who remembered a man who was kindly, civil and discreet, particularly when saying early morning adieus to lady visitors. But that is possibly counter-speculation.

The Last Year, Surgery and Death

By 1937 Ravel had seriously deteriorated. On 29 October 1937 he signed his last (and dictated) letter, which was to the conductor Ernest Ansermet, although he had coached his friend Jacques Février to play the Left Hand Concerto in preparation for a concert to be conducted by Charles Munch.[180] In November 1937 he attended his last concert, a performance of *Daphnis et Chloé*, emerging at the end in tears and stammering that he still had so much music in his head, so much more to say.[181] Musically, this had become a locked-in syndrome. Ravel then consulted Professor Clovis Vincent, a neurosurgeon in Paris, having previously been advised against surgery by surgeons in several countries.[182] Vincent proffered the contrary view, and by then Ravel was possibly clutching at straws, although it is intriguing that Jourdan-Morhange declared Vincent to have disregarded the taxi accident in October 1932 as part of Ravel's aetiology.[183] Baeck reports that case records are now missing or unclear,[184] although it is touching to read of Ravel's discussion as to the indications for surgery and particularly the distress shown when, preparatory to the operation, his head was shaved of what been a fine head of silvery hair, a fact mentioned by Marguerite Long who claimed that Ravel had not wanted to undergo surgery, saying, 'He preferred the worst of declines to confronting death.'[185] Equivocation, being upon the horns of a dilemma, is both natural and quite common amongst those confronting imminent, risky surgery. Vincent's main indication for operating may have been to exclude a brain tumour.[186] There was probably another reason. Vincent believed that Ravel had a large head. My own impression, sustained by biographical detail, is that his head was fine, and it was just that he had a very small body. Vincent attributed the head size to hydrocephalus (a fluid blockage in the brain, causing 'water on the brain'). Evidently he contemplated a surgical solution to that problem, should it be progressive.[187]

Here it is worth reflecting that Moniz, a Portuguese surgeon, in 1927 first used the technique of injecting blood vessels to the brain with a dye in order to outline pathology such as tumours on an X-ray (cerebral angiography).[188] We saw with Gershwin that, in America, Dandy pioneered achieving a similar end by injecting air to outline the ventricles (chambers) within the brain,[189] and that was in use in 1937, as was taking electrical tracings or 'brain waves' known as an electro-encephalogram (EEG).[190] There is no evidence of angiography or EEG being used, and it is unclear whether ventriculograms were undertaken, although Baeck believes they were.[191] The argument goes that, without one, how could

Professor Vincent believe, as he did, that there was an enlargement of the ventricles within the brain causing hydrocephalus?

So opening Ravel's head (craniotomy) was planned firstly as an investigation, and possibly to then become a treatment. When the right frontal side of his head was opened (craniotomy) under local anaesthetic on 17 December 1937, not much was found or done.[192] In particular, no tumour or old haemorrhage was identified. Following the operation, he asked for his brother and old housekeeper. Later, he sank into a coma. On 28 December 1937, Ravel died peacefully. There was no autopsy. Today in England and Wales an autopsy would be ordered by the coroner in any case where death occurs up to thirty days after surgery, whether the relatives want it or not. This was 1937, and the most likely cause of death was that he experienced raised pressure in the brain secondary to haemorrhage after surgery, causing a blood clot,[193] or just post-operative brain swelling. Such a blood clot could have been easily surgically evacuated by removing the stitches and lifting out the flap of bone raised at the first operation. Any such haematoma would then have been removed, relieving the ultimately fatal pressure upon Ravel's already compromised brain. Whereas such clots are easier to diagnose today with scans, in Ravel's case that should not have been especially challenging in 1937.

By today's standards a more precise diagnosis should have preceded or prevented surgery, and if surgery was to be undertaken then a much more proactive programme of aftercare would be imperative. By the standards of the time we can probably exonerate Professor Clovis Vincent. Above all else, unless there had been a benign tumour, the chances of surgery restoring Ravel to anything like his former creative self were very slim anyway. The case history is not suggestive of a slowly growing tumour, nor of a post-head-injury syndrome, although it would have been right to consider both pre-operatively. A last word here: if there had been a haematoma since the taxi accident because of the bump to Ravel's head, then that too would have been discovered at surgery, and clearly it was not. There is a similarity with the case of George Gershwin. The only two available diagnoses, whose elimination might have enabled Ravel to regain some of his pre-eminence, were excluded by Professor Vincent's otherwise questionable operation. On reading accounts surrounding his surgery, it is unclear how much of the informed consent for surgery was given by Maurice Ravel and how much by his brother Edouard. We do know that, like any other rational being, he was terrified pre-operatively and said, 'They are going to cut my head off.'[194] Just before surgery, seeing a mirror reflection of his head enveloped in towels, he laughed when he was told that he resembled Lawrence of Arabia.[195] That is evidence of a witty intellect that remained intact, if impaired.

Perhaps Ravel would have wanted us to conclude his story on an upbeat note. Recently, Seeley and colleagues have described a scientist, Anne Adams, who suffered from degenerative brain disease.[196] It was noticed that, a decade before language deficits developed, she became driven to paint and did so in a garish 'expressive, transmodal style'. A favourite subject was her painting of Ravel's *Bolero*. As she worsened, becoming almost mute, her style changed, becoming much more realistically photographic and less disturbed or disturbing. Her sequential brain scan images revealed progressive degenerative changes in the left lower fronto-temporal areas of the brain (the seat of language function), concurrent with an increase in grey matter in the rear, right-sided occipital brain cortex, which is the seat of visual function. The inference was that the loss of language in Dr Adams's case was offset by an enhanced visual creativity. This rests comfortably with Miller's work on enhanced artistic creativity with temporal lobe degeneration.[197] This should not deflect us from accepting the nature of Ravel's locked-in creativity, with music unable to get out. This seems worse than the inner world from which extraneous distraction is excluded, which becomes the lot of the deaf composer.[198]

There is one small footnote which cannot be omitted, particularly as we are about to leave the hazy world of Ravel for that tortured nightmare which was the concluding passage of Smetana's musical life, namely syphilis. Nichols reported that, in 1952, a nurse who had looked after Ravel in his final illness recalled that she had seen a report concerning the Wassermann blood test (WR) for syphilis in Ravel's case, and that it had been positive.[199] Nichols's source was the memoirs of the singer Madeleine Grey.[200] Once more, such information should be analysed forensically. Amaducci, Grassi and Boller stated that a blood test was performed and showed no evidence of syphilis,[201] a view recorded by Dalessio.[202] It is supposed that these views derive from the unpublished MD thesis by Mercier. Either way, we should ask what level of experience and training the nurse had. Quite simply, was she competent to read and interpret the blood test result? Even today, trained doctors can have occasional difficulty in understanding changes in reference standards and terminology used in reporting laboratory results. Perhaps, after fifteen years, the nurse remembered seeing a laboratory report of a WR test, which is vitally different from seeing that one was positive. It should also be asked what proportion of WR tests in the mid-1930s gave a false positive result. We know that as many as 7% did in the USA. As this test would have been done (if indeed it was done) in preparation for Ravel's brain surgery, then it raises the even more difficult question – was Professor Vincent aware of this laboratory report and, if not, why not? If he had been aware of it and it was positive, then why was he surgically exploring Ravel's brain, having by then found a diagnosis? To counterbalance this apparent discord, one can conclude upon a balance of probabilities that the picture of Ravel described by many, including Alajouanine, was strikingly not that of third-stage neurosyphilis. Furthermore, on a balance of probabilities, Professor Vincent would have known of the WR result, had it been taken, and he would not have operated had it been positive. Syphilis is extremely unlikely to be any part of Ravel's medical history.

In a recent exchange, Nichols has emphasised his belief that further research may ultimately bring us much closer to a diagnosis.[203] He subscribes to an Italian view from a recent literature review that 'comorbidities' may ultimately prove to be the cause of Ravel's possibly multifactorial disease.[204] I believe that the water is deeply muddied by a host of erudite neuro-psychological debate, much of which advances only modestly from Alajouanine in 1948. The suggestion of a genetic mutation in brain chemistry is interesting.[205] It is an attempt to define scientifically the accurate identity of Ravel's pre-senile dementia, about which broad diagnosis there should be little doubt anyway. It has recently been suggested that Ravel's right craniotomy may have missed a small blood clot (subdural haematoma) caused by the taxi accident.[206] That is implausible because such a collection of old blood would have caused the brain to shift from right to left, and should have been evident at the craniotomy. It would have been evident on the ventriculogram X-ray if Vincent had done one prior to surgery. If it was so small a clot as to cause no shift in the brain, or to be missed at surgery, then its clinical significance is open to debate. On a balance of probabilities we can confidently discard this theory too. What cannot be denied is that Ravel's death was the result of surgery.

With respect to Nichols's excellent book, surely there were enough composers who allegedly had the French pox without more being recruited. I felt indignant that this nurse may have disclosed strictly confidential, sensitive information, if it was true, let alone untrue, only fifteen years after Ravel's death. Curiously, it is comfortable to realise that poor old Donizetti caught the pox about a hundred years earlier, and our engagement with that can be much more jocund than in the case of Ravel, who died within the lifetimes of some people reading these pages. So where does speculative analysis of clinical records merge into a historical free-for-all, not least amongst those prone to write about medical ailments? Winston Churchill's personal doctor, Lord Moran, was not slow in going into print, and there are many other examples. Somehow the lapse of a hundred years seems much more respectful than fifteen, and surely Ravel deserves better.

Tauopathies are part of Cavallera's review.[207] This is a topical term, as Alzheimer's is the best-known and most researched of that group of disorders. This seems to be a more profitable line for future research than speculation about chronic endocrine and thus sexual dysfunction. There is little doubt that pre-senile dementias will become more accurately described, and this is one of medicine's current growth areas. Add to that the analyses of experts such as Baeck, and a more accurate neurological map of music and the brain could usefully emerge.

Postscript

There are also composers dealt with in other chapters whose treatment, by the standards of their own times, might be questioned. These include Mozart, Beethoven, Rossini, Shostakovich and especially Schumann and Elgar.

Chapter 4

Syphilis

Beware the dreaded spirochaete

Anon.

Introduction

THE APHORISM 'Beware the dreaded spirochaete' was wise. A spirochaete (*Treponema pallidum*) causes syphilis, an infection which may
manifest itself in many forms. Sir Jonathan Hutchinson, the leading nineteenth-century specialist, described syphilis as 'the great imitator', hence
the caution in judging case histories preceding the standard blood test.
That test (the WR) was an antibody test introduced by Wassermann in
1905, immortalising his name.[1] There can be both false positives and neg-
atives. There are more recent blood tests (e.g. VDRL), which are beyond
the scope of this book.

Few diseases have been implicated more often with past composers,
reflecting partly the overall incidence and ubiquity of the condition, but
also the enthusiasm and sometimes carelessness with which it has been
over-diagnosed retrospectively. The lists below show composers who were
definitely syphilitic and those alleged by some to have possibly been so.

Known Syphilitics

Schubert
Donizetti
Smetana
Delius
Wolf
Chabrier

Some Alleged Syphilitics

Vivaldi
Mozart
Beethoven
Schumann
Tchaikovsky
Duparc
Ravel
Sibelius
Gershwin
Britten

Syphilis is so important in musicology that a short digression into the history of this disease and its clinical pathology follows.

A Short History of Syphilis

A night in the arms of Venus leads to a lifetime on Mercury

Anon.

Traditionally, syphilis first appeared when the French army invaded Naples in 1494.[2] This may explain its soubriquet, the French pox; it is known in France as the Italian pox. The age-old question is whether Columbus's expedition took the disease to the Americas or whether his crew brought it to Europe. Waivers described a physician in Barcelona, Dr Ruiz Diaz de Isla, who had seen Vincente Pinzon, the captain of Columbus's second ship, the *Niña*, avowing that he had syphilis, curiously a disease supposedly unrecognised previously in Europe.[3] So how did he recognise it?

Rothschild gives a definitive account of the history of syphilis.[4] From a medical, archaeological and anthropological viewpoint, syphilis is easier than many other diseases to study retrospectively because it frequently affects the skeleton. Much is known about this disease from the Oslo study of patients with untreated syphilis over several decades.[5] In 1999, the World Health Organization estimated there to be 12 million cases of syphilis worldwide. It remains a major problem, with dangers in the West of complacency.[6] Re-emergent syphilis today is often partnered by the HIV/AIDS virus.

Treatment before Penicillin

The earliest proponent for treating syphilis with mercury was Paracelsus (1493–1541).[7] Its attraction, apart from mystical properties, was that, as a powerful diuretic, it made the urine 'flush out the badness'. It also caused excessive salivation, sometimes foul-tasting. Indeed, dosage of mercury was titrated against the volume of saliva. This and the appearance of a blue line on the gums were considered as points at which treatment should stop. In many cases teeth fell out, joining disabling tremors (hatters' shakes), inflammation of the lungs and ultimately kidney failure as awful complications of treatment with mercury. O'Shea concludes that mercury was probably beneficial only if ingested or applied topically in the first stage of syphilis.[8] In 1906 Salvarsan, an arsenical medicine, was introduced because it might have been less toxic and more effective than mercury. The Oslo study cast doubt upon the efficacy of any treatment for syphilis prior to penicillin's introduction, with one probable exception.[9] In 1927, Julius Wagner-Jauregg won the Nobel Prize for medicine.[10] He had noted that the features of syphilis could regress if the patient had suffered a high fever. Thus he deliberately induced malaria in syphilitic sufferers on the basis that he then had a good remedy, with quinine, for malaria, whose fevers had by now 'treated' the syphilis. In 1942 penicillin overtook all previous remedies, and it is still used today. But doctors are stubborn and some were still using toxic mercurial drugs during the 1950s.

Features of Syphilis

There are four principal clinical manifestations:

1 Primary syphilis occurs nine to ninety days after contact and at the points of contact. Painless open sores known as chancres appear, usually in the anogenital region, regressing after three to six weeks. The transmission of syphilis is almost entirely due to sexual contact, including kissing. For medical workers, inoculation or contamination from mucous membranes can transmit the disease.

2 Secondary syphilis occurs, but not in all patients, six to ten weeks after the primary manifestation, and is typified by rashes on the skin and wart-like lesions (condylomata lata) around the perianal mucous membranes. Rarely arthritis, hepatitis and neuritis of the

optic (sight) or acoustic (hearing) nerves occur. Kidney disease and periostitis (painful inflammation of the bone) may follow.

3 Latent syphilis is a stage in which there are no symptoms and little external evidence of the latent disease apart from a positive WR test. Hayden alternatively describes lengthy periods of prolonged suffering between the first and third stages, which she terms 'hidden syphilis'.[11] Today, complaints similar to those of a gastric ulcer are rare symptoms, with the risk of missing the diagnosis.

4 Tertiary syphilis occurs in 10–30% of those initially infected and remaining untreated or undiagnosed, and on average three to fifteen years after the initial inoculum. Hayden believes this figure to be a gross underestimation.[12] There are three types of tertiary syphilis which may overlap:

a Gummata, ugly lumps, may occur internally, for example in the bone, or externally, for example on the face.

b Cardiovascular syphilis can both damage the aortic heart valve and cause aneurysm.

c Neurosyphilis includes the most awful features of the disease, which can manifest themselves in three ways:

i Meningo-vascular neurosyphilis affects the membranes around the brain (meninges) and is rare, with a long course, including chronic headache, ultimately declining into dementia and coma. Patients may become blind or deaf.

The two most dreaded results of the spirochaete at its worst are:

ii **Tabes dorsalis,** where there are severe lightning pains, usually in the legs. These may be associated with disorders of sensation, especially position sense. Incontinence of urine, or even double incontinence, usually associated with male impotence, may occur. Paralysis of limbs usually follows. Whilst the subject remains mentally intact, the gait becomes high-stepping and increasingly chaotic, before a wheelchair is ultimately called for upon a permanent basis. Cranial nerves may also be destroyed at this stage, with blindness or deafness.

iii The alternative to these gruesome sufferings is **general paralysis of the insane (GPI)**, from which most occupants of mental asylums in pre-penicillin Europe and North America suffered. A residuum of syphilitic patients continued into the 1970s. Firstly, the patient's family will often notice intellectual and personal deterioration, with manic and megalomanic delusions. Speech deteriorates and half of the patients become epileptic.

This is a truly terrible disease, and it is little wonder that it aroused such fear and repulsion. Some of the great musical minds which have given us peace, tenderness and leaps of joy were suffering from syphilis, a fact worth remembering when we enjoy the Vltava's mellifluous passage through Smetana's Prague.

✢ FRANZ SCHUBERT ✢
(1797–1828)

The art of music here entombed a rich possession, but even fairer hopes.

Franz Grillparzer, 1828

On 21 March 1839 at the Leipzig Gewandhaus the thirty-year-old Felix Mendelssohn conducted the first complete performance of Schubert's 'Great' C major Symphony, the Ninth. The scores had been discovered amongst papers at the house of Schubert's brother Ferdinand by Robert Schumann on New Year's Day 1837, eight years after Schubert's death. This rather tragic trio of young composers highlights that image of early demise amongst romantic artists. Schubert's death, at the age of thirty-one, raises three broad questions today. Of what did he suffer for his last five or six years, and what caused his death? Thirdly, Grillparzer's poetic words pose the tantalising question as to what music we might have been left, had he lived longer. The Schubert scholar Brian Newbould believes that the fusion of Classic and Romantic style and technique evident in the Eighth and Ninth Symphonies would have matured with subsequent symphonies.[13] Newbould completed the 'Unfinished', as well as the Seventh Symphony and the embryonic Tenth. He believes that Schubert sketched out three, possibly four, movements of the 'Unfinished' before then writing an incomplete orchestral score.[14] It was suggested that Schubert stopped composing the Eighth as there developed in his mind an association between it and the sexual act which, at the time of composition, had caused syphilis.[15] Newbould's pragmatic view, that art and reality were not so irrevocably intertwined as to prevent him completing the symphony, seems more probable, not least because the dates of acquiring syphilis and working on the 'Unfinished' don't coincide very well.[16] An overview of the Deutsch classification of nearly a thousand compositions reveals that this swift composer left a number of works incomplete throughout his career,[17] sometimes for commercial reasons, as he turned to potentially more rewarding projects. Now we have two keys to his life and work: the diagnosis of syphilis in his mid-twenties and an immense canon of composition by the age of thirty-one. Are they irrevocably linked?

How sound is the diagnosis of syphilis? The earliest 'allusion' to it was in a letter Schubert wrote in 1823 saying, 'My state of health prevents me from leaving the house.'[18] In 1907 Deutsch quoted statements from three of Schubert's friends (Kenner 1858, von Chézy 1863, Schober 1868), which leave us with little doubt that it was their belief. Schober wrote that Schubert 'frequented taverns and composed some of his best songs in them, just as he did in hospital, where he found himself as a result of excessively indulgent sensory living and its consequences'.[19] Clearly, that is retrospective judgement. Similarly, Kenner declared that 'The craving for pleasure dragged his soul down to the slough of moral degradation.'[20] McKay reported Schubert's increasing mood swings, often inflamed by alcohol, by 1824.[21]

Eric Sams has constructed a case where, not just on a balance of probabilities but almost beyond all reasonable doubt, Schubert had syphilis.[22] He wrote with the medical assistance of Dr R. A. Henson and by erecting a scaffold of the generally recognised features and timescale of syphilis. Upon that framework he hung recorded features like alopecia, and events such as Schubert having been housebound or hospitalised. A good pattern of convergence thereby emerged; syphilis fitted the known facts and their timing. Above all, Sams summarised from medical textbooks six symptoms which are typical of syphilis, namely iritis (an inflammation within the eye), headache, facial rash, alopecia, bone pain and vocal disorder. For all six there is corroborative evidence with Schubert. It could be argued that iritis is assumed because Schubert complained of eye pain which, like headaches, might have been due to working in poor light with inappropriate spectacles, but it is the combination of symptoms which is convincing.

Importance has been attached to remarks in the diary of Schubert's associate Eduard von Bauernfeld that 'Schubert is ailing; he needs young peacocks like Benvenuto Cellini.'[23] That renaissance figure openly professed his own syphilitic diagnosis, advocating its treatment by eating young peacocks, which he claimed had cured him.[24] It was clearly argued that needing young peacocks therefore implied that Schubert was syphilitic. Maynard Solomon went further, believing both Cellini and Schubert to have been gay,[25] although Cellini claimed to have contracted syphilis from a woman. Solomon's view was also based not only on Schubert being unmarried, but on the belief that his need for young peacocks was a metaphor for needing flamboyantly dressed, effeminate young men.[26] From all we know, Schubert would surely have loved to have been married. In 1827 friends suggested that he might marry Gusti Grünwedel, a girl said to be fond of him. He immediately stormed out, visiting St Peter's church and returning half an hour later to say that no happiness was granted to him on earth.[27] An obvious explanation for such self-imposed celibacy is syphilis. Moreover, Schubert's social circle was conspicuously heterosexual, and his close friend Schober was a notorious womaniser. And why do gay men have to be flamboyantly dressed or effeminate? Even if Schubert did need male company, then how normal that would be. Most men do. Rita Steblin's dissection of Solomon's hypotheses, based as it is upon meticulous citation of diaries and correspondence, is a paragon of resisting the salacious by applying the objectively studious.[28] Such rigour might also be applied to McKay's tentative suggestion that he smoked opium, the evidence for which seems tenuous, as she seems to concede.[29]

Sams placed the probable onset of Schubert's syphilis in early 1823,[30] which enables us to study the effect upon both the quantity and the nature of his compositions, and upon his mood and habitude. With nearly a thousand works composed by the time he died, we marvel not just at his industry, but at the speed and ease with which he worked. From his own writings his awful realisation of the personal catastrophe which had overtaken him is clear. His poem 'My Prayer' was written in 1823, allegedly whilst in hospital, and reveals not only his physical debilitation but his mental torment, as he says:[31]

> See abased in dust and mire
> Scorched by agonising fire
> In torture I go my way
> Nearing doom's destructive day

Notwithstanding contrivance in translation, there in a stanza is his self-realisation, with a determination to continue composing. Schubert did not actually expect too much from life. He had written, 'I have come into this world for no purpose but to compose.'[32] Despite frequent periods of illness, Schubert's indispositions were insufficient to stop him composing until nearly the end. Whereas John Reed applauded the continuing production line of composition in Schubert's final year, he pointed to more inconsistency in quality than in earlier years.[33] As Schober had recorded, he composed in pubs and in hospital. Nevertheless, a sense of despair, with the very probable realisation of his syphilis, is also well recorded. In late 1823 he had written to Schober that he doubted if he would ever be well again.[34]

Realising that, despite his health's vicissitudes, Schubert continued composing just as freely and quickly, one asks whether the nature of the music itself then changed. It is convenient to regard the 'Unfinished' (October–November 1822) and *Schwanengesang* (completed August 1828) as the 'bookends' between which much of the great music from this increasingly sick man reposes. *Die schöne Müllerin* was composed in late 1823, soon after Schubert's realisation of his syphilis. Newbould regards the cycle as progressing from initial promise through disillusion to tragedy and also asks whether Schubert, who knew his days were numbered, composed more urgently than he might otherwise have done. Newbould probably answers his own question, in that Schubert had always been astonishingly productive. We conclude that the quantitative output of music did not change much, but the question remains as to whether his music became sadder after the 1822/23 waterline. It is easy to regard the first five symphonies as the sunny ones, before the sadness and perhaps resignation of the 'Unfinished'. Then, during the summer of 1825, when his health improved albeit temporarily, he composed his Ninth Symphony, sometimes nicknamed 'Sommerreise', which he revised shortly before his death in 1828. It is the exuberant, bustling pace which first strikes many listeners and sometimes taxes performers. What is stranger, in considering the impact of illness on composition, is to compare the charming Octet, composed in February 1824, with the 'Death and the Maiden' String Quartet from the next month. The miracle is the speed of composition with both, but it is from the daily details that an explanation for their dramatic difference emerges. In early 1824, Schubert's hair had grown back. He was on a new treatment, and Schwind told Schober in March 1824 that Schubert felt better.[35] It was to be short-lived, for at the end of March he wrote to Kupelweiser, 'When I go to sleep I hope never to wake again.'[36] 'Death and the Maiden' now comes as no surprise.

It seems reasonable to believe that, had Schubert lived to be sixty or seventy, he might not have composed *Winterreise* (February–October 1827) or the fateful String Quintet in C, which he did only weeks before his death. Nevertheless, his friend Spaun believed that it was *Winterreise* which made him gloomy, and not that this sad music was a product of his mood, if only in the first half of the cycle.[37] McKay does not regard him as having been depressed during its composition. The effect of illness and mood upon composition is most vividly made in contrasting the cheerful 'Trout' Quintet, written in the autumn of 1819, with that final String Quintet. No contrast could be more stark. Probably a healthy Schubert in autumn 1828 would have composed something very different. Instead, by then he was complaining further of headaches, sometimes associated with nausea, and dizziness. Sams conjectured that this might have been due to mercury toxicity,[38] although notable in Schubert's medical history is the absence of reference to other mercury overdose features, which were well known then. Perhaps this is where Rold's scepticism as to the diagnosis of syphilis may arise.[39]

Perhaps the key to Schubert's whole approach comes before these incomparable later works. We return to the end of 1823, remembering that Schubert's operas were never successful. In December his rapidly composed music for an almost unknown play, *Rosamunde*, was another theatrical failure but, soon thereafter, with spirits undaunted, came the

Octet and then the more portentous A minor String Quartet. Our conclusion surely must be that, feeling well or wretched, happy or despairing,
he just relentlessly continued composing.

And so to the end, as we address the final mystery – what killed him?
After his return on 20 September 1827 from a particularly happy holiday
in Graz, his health varied. Nevertheless, his travelling companion, Jenger,
reported that in the summer of 1828 Schubert was working diligently on
a new mass (D950), No. 6 in E flat, and on an incomplete symphony
(D936A).[40] In *Schubert: The Final Years*, Reed gives a detailed chronology
of the still productive final months from April until November 1828.[41] That
summer Dr Rinna recommended that Schubert move out of Vienna to stay
with his brother Ferdinand. Sadly, the lodgings were both damp and insanitary, far from the ideal of fresh air and exercise. To this accommodation
McKay traces the beginning of the end. Schubert composed only one song
that August, although by early October he was well enough for a three-day
walking trip with Ferdinand and two friends to pay their obsequies at
Haydn's grave in Eisenstadt.[42] On his return he became unwell again.

As an aside, Reed asks why Schubert diverted his attentions to liturgical
composition in his last year.[43] Was it a premonition of death's imminence?
Reed believes not, reminding us that the church was a good paymaster
and argued, as others have done,[44] that Schubert was not a conventionally
religious man, although he says church music was in his blood.[45] Perhaps
there is a deeper spirituality in the unsurpassed String Quintet than in
Hymnus an den Heiligen Geist (May 1828), the Mass in E flat (July 1828)
or the offertorium *Intende voci* D963, composed a few weeks before the
end. Shortly before Schubert died he met a friend to whom he said,
'Sometimes it seems to me as though I am no longer of this world',[46]
a saying which remains enigmatic. Amongst these essays into religion,
however motivated, Schubert that summer had continued to enjoy parties
and visits to his favourite inns, despite complaining of weakness, lassitude, nausea and headaches. They may have been early manifestations of
meningo-vascular syphilis, as implied by Sams and Rold.[47] Significantly,
Schubert had suffered nausea, sickness and diarrhoea in 1826 and again in
1827, when typhoid had been endemic. Some believe typhoid may have
caused Schubert's death.[48]

It was with total bathos that the composer of the 'Trout' Quintet succumbed to what may have been a fatal fish supper. On 31 October 1828,
Schubert ordered fish in the restaurant 'The Red Cross'.[49] After eating a
little he complained of nausea and immediately vomited: probably a case
of acute gastroenteritis. On this and earlier occasions, Schubert said he

felt as if he had been poisoned.[50] There is no evidence that he had. Four days later, he attended a requiem composed by his brother and took a three-hour walk. On 12 November he wrote to his friend Schober, saying that he had been vomiting and unable to keep anything down for eleven days, and that now he could only totter about in his room.[51] He then cancelled his second lesson in counterpoint with Simon Sechter. Baron Schönstein's record of a bibulous dinner party on 8 or 9 November, at which Schubert imbibed freely,[52] is, on balance, totally inconsistent with all the other accounts given for Schubert's last two weeks. It is probably best regarded as an inaccurate recollection. Two physicians attended and declared him to be suffering from 'Bauchtyphus'. It is extremely unlikely to have been what is now known as typhus. In his article of 1947, 'Schubert's Last Illness', Walker explained that the term 'Bauchtyphus' would then have included typhoid fever.[53] How poignant it is that his last professional task had been to correct proofs of the second volume of *Winterreise*, whose final song, 'The Hurdy-Gurdy Man', is such a harbinger of gloom.

Dr Vering, who specialised in syphilis, was one of the physicians who attended on 16 November. Schubert's brother and half-sister were loving in their care. By 17 November he was delirious, and it is popularly supposed that, in a lucid interval, he spoke of his idol, Beethoven.[54] On the 18th in the afternoon he allegedly turned from his doctor, saying, 'Here, here is my end', after which he passed away the next day. The actual cause of death given by the two attending physicians was 'Nervenfieber', a blanket term given then to many causes of death, whilst avoiding registration of syphilis and thereby sparing his family's feelings.[55] One possibility was typhoid, of which there were several features, although a rose red rash and diarrhoea, both typical, were not recorded. Also, Schubert's delirium during his last two days is described, but not high fever. There we should not tarry; clinical thermometers were not used in 1828. The conspicuous absence of diarrhoea in the contemporary accounts could improbably be explained by a failure to mention it out of delicate considerations.

The certainties are that Schubert had a final illness whose most conspicuous feature was persistent vomiting. This would lead to a dangerous degree of dehydration and a disturbance in the balance of the salts (electrolytes) in his blood. How strange it is that experts explaining his death have not incriminated fluid depletion with electrolyte imbalance, which was inevitable in Schubert's case within two or three days, despite postulating alcohol excess, malnutrition[56] and immune suppression,[57] as well as mercury poisoning.[58] Even scurvy is considered,[59] and yet such depletion of water and salts causes lassitude, weakness and delirium, leading ultimately to coma and death. Whether the causative germ was that for typhoid remains hypothetical and unimportant. Today people die from clostridial or coliform infections, despite antibiotics. Back in Schubert's time – who can tell? So stick to what we know. Today he would have been supported by intravenous infusion (IV) of a solution with appropriate dosage of salts such as sodium. This great medical advance was not available until the early part of the twentieth century, when it was developed by a pathologist, Justine Johnstone, and her husband, Walter Wanger.

Dr Vering proclaimed Schubert's case to be 'hopeless' and attributed this to an 'advanced disintegration of the blood'.[60] Although one doubts whether red blood corpuscles were studied down a microscope, Sams observed in his overview that such disintegration may be a feature in tertiary syphilis.[61] Sams also quoted Kerner, who had written of narrowing or blockage of a cerebral artery (main artery to the brain) progressing to a stroke. Such changes may occur rarely in meningo-vascular syphilis but, as Rold elucidates, none of the well-recorded clinical features at the time accord either with a stroke or with the classic features of tertiary neurosyphilis, nor with those of mercury treatment, which were well known in Schubert's time.[62] Rold also points to the oddity of Sams apparently ignoring Schubert's final gastrointestinal symptoms in his analysis.

Chronic syphilis may reduce a resistance to other forms of infection,[63] and, upon a balance of probabilities, that is the limit of its culpability in Schubert's death. The contemporary accounts of those final, fateful three weeks in Schubert's life have little resonance with the various hideous manifestations of tertiary syphilis. Schubert continued composing until the fish supper on 31 October, whereafter silence prevailed. That is the clinical story of a sudden, presumably infectious, illness and not the culmination of chronic syphilis, which Kerner, quoted by Sams, believed was the cause of death.[64]

For those who believe in the pre-ordained, Schubert's story is a sad tale, and his end was marked by a human virtue seldom ascribed to him, as it has been to Beethoven. 'Courage', the twenty-second song in *Winterreise*, tells us in the words of Wilhelm Müller so much about the brave Schubert:

> Merrily off into the world
> Spite all wind and weather
> If we can't have gods on earth
> We are gods ourselves.

Schubert was surely a god amongst composers.

✢ BEDŘICH SMETANA ✢
(1824–1884)

Má Vlast

Smetana showed early promise, especially as a pianist and teacher. He married one of his students, Katerina Kolorova. After the failure of his music school in Prague in 1848, and amidst other setbacks, he tried his luck in Gothenburg as a music teacher and composer.[65] Between 1854 and 1856 three of his four daughters died. He dedicated the G minor Piano Trio to the memory of his eldest child, who had succumbed to scarlet fever.[66] By then Katerina was also a sick woman. Smetana decided to take her away from the cold of Scandinavia. Whilst returning to Bohemia during 1859 Katerina died of TB in Dresden.[67] Within a few months Smetana married his brother's sister-in-law Bettina Ferdinandova.[68] It was to be a frenetic but loveless marriage.

In 1862 he conducted two of his symphonic poems and played Beethoven's Third Piano Concerto to a nearly empty hall in Prague. That same year he started to study and use the Czech language, having hitherto lived, worked and corresponded in German. He had been criticised in this nascent era of Czech nationalism for being too German. His opera *The Brandenburgers in Bohemia*, which was premiered in 1863, received a mixed reception, but so did *The Bartered Bride* in 1866, with warm audience applause but indifferent critics.[69]

Details of his medical history and diaries were studied by Feldman, a German ENT surgeon.[70] These reveal how Smetana was overtaken by his disease and yet somehow strove on and in many ways triumphed, with the bittersweet paradox that ultimately his music became a success, but only when he himself could no longer hear it. In April 1874 he recorded in his diary that he had 'a purulent ulcer', which lasted for eighteen days, and then developed a sore throat followed by a rash.[71] Where the ulcer was remains unknown. Today there can be little doubt that the cause was syphilis, although until 1907 there was no reliable diagnostic test for syphilis.

On 28 July 1874, Smetana recorded, 'My ears are blocked and at the same time my head seems to swim and I feel giddy.'[72] He consulted Professor Zoufal, an otologist, who diagnosed catarrh, for which he recommended deep breathing.[73] Smetana then entered an understandably nervous phase, temporarily giving up composition. In September he warned his employers, 'I may lose my hearing', saying that the buzzing in his ears was like being by a huge waterfall.[74] By 20 October 1874 he was almost completely deaf. The onset of deafness in syphilis may be rapid, in Smetana's case taking two to three months from onset to total deafness.[75] Then we reach the crucial moment, for what did he do: despair, retire or contemplate suicide? No, instead he continued with *Má Vlast*, of which *Vltava* was composed between 20 November and 8 December 1874.[76] He did contemplate suicide later. Better medical opinion would have been unlikely to lead to more efficacious treatment, for none was available then. Meanwhile he stoically learned to lip-read and continued to play the piano.[77]

In spite of these hideous impedimenta, and constant difficulties over payment, he went to the opera saying he could follow the music from the conductor's baton. Then he found that if he read or wrote music for over an hour, he got awful noises in his head, observing that he could have accepted the total silence of deafness if it had not been for the noises. In 1876 whilst suffering from severe tinnitus (ringing in the ears), he completed the First String Quartet, known as 'From My Life', in which the high E note in the final movement illustrates the piercing whistling in his head by which he was haunted.[78] It is astonishing that he could compose at all, especially as he became depressed and quarrelled with Bettina.[79] On his fifty-second birthday he confided to his diary, 'If my illness is incurable then I would prefer to be delivered from this miserable existence.'[80] He said later that he was kept alive by his family and by his need to continue working 'for my people and my country', and so his opera *The Kiss* was 'another triumph' in November 1876.[81]

He completed a seventh opera, *The Secret*, during 1878, in just eight months. The Theatre Association paid him for just one benefit night.[82] Surprisingly, he still performed in Prague, where he had been a splendid pianist. On one occasion, by now totally deaf, whilst playing he suddenly shouted 'pianissimo' to the consternation of fellow soloists and listeners alike.[83] He completed *Má Vlast* with the symphonic poems *Tábor* and *Blaník* in 1878–79. In 1879 he wrote to a friend, Jan Neruda, saying, 'I'm terrified I'll go mad.'[84] By the early 1880s people had started to shun him, and he was angered that others altered his work. His inappropriate behaviour was increasingly recorded.

In 1882 he was still at work completing his last opera, *The Devil's Wall*, started three years earlier.[85] This was in spite of constant pounding and hissing in his head. The premiere was chaotic. He said he was always cold and that he felt stunned and drowsy.[86] During the autumn of 1882 he started to lose both his memory and his power of speech,[87] and his reason sometimes deserted him in early 1883 when he may have suffered a stroke.[88] His last significant composition was the Second String Quartet, in which he re-used some earlier music. He said, 'No-one knows how musical ideas run away from a deaf person.'[89] The quartet is said to have reflected both his deafness and his by now failing memory, although Arnold Schoenberg said it was a work ahead of its time.[90] His total canon after becoming totally deaf included three operas, five-sixths of *Má Vlast*, two quartets and various piano pieces, including the sequences *Dreams* and *Czech Dances*. Also there were pieces for violin and piano, songs and nine choral works.

Some inner creative force still drove him on to attempt writing an opera based on Shakespeare's *Twelfth Night*, which he had started in 1874, grown tired of and then taken up again.[91] Smetana still wrote down fragments of *Viola* at a time when he started to hallucinate and then failed to recognise family and friends. Large comments that *Prague Carnival*, also resurrected in June 1883, 'is a work of highly skilled and imaginative craftsmanship', although there were errors.[92] Smetana became intermittently violent and impossible to manage at home, from which he tried to escape. On 23 April 1884 he was taken to the Prague lunatic asylum,[93] much to the distress of his surviving daughter Zofie. By now he was shouting, struggling, dribbling, weak and emaciated. Three weeks later his torment was relieved by an inevitable death, probably from pneumonia.[94]

Almost undoubtedly the cause of all these sufferings was syphilis, although the death certificate gave senile dementia as the cause of death. Despite that certificate, his family believed that Smetana died of syphilis.[95] The day after his death, Professor Hlava undertook an autopsy. Dr Ernst Levin, an Edinburgh neurologist, translated his report, which appears as an appendix in Clapham's biography.[96] Hlava reported syphilitic features, including atrophy of the auditory nerves. More recently, Professor Emanuel Vlček obtained samples of muscle by exhumation,[97] concluding that the diagnosis was syphilis. Debate intensified when Dr Jiří Ramba questioned the validity of such scientific analysis upon human tissues with more than a century's opportunity to decay.[98] The fact is that the well-recorded clinical course in Smetana's case would leave most clinicians with little doubt that he had died of tertiary syphilis, manifest as general paralysis of the insane.

The striking conclusion to draw from this sad story is admiration of Smetana for his courage and musical genius. Deprived of the most vital of musical sensations, he productively soldiered on. Then his higher brain functions in turn became 'switched off'. By this stage something indomitable was still driving him to write just one more opera. A supreme triumph of the spirit over impending madness was the Second String Quartet. Could a greater triumph have arisen from such distress and disorder?

✣ FREDERICK DELIUS ✣
(1862–1934)

To the end I never lost my awe of him; there was a presence about him always.

Eric Fenby, 1936

This Yorkshireman, born of a prosperous German family, lived for his productive years and those of his physical disintegration at Grez-sur-Loing in France.[99] As a young man, when he was supposed to be growing oranges, Delius was moved by the music of the Afro-American community in Florida and learned much from their harmonies. He then went to Leipzig, where he learned composition and befriended Grieg and Grainger. After Leipzig he moved to Paris, where he led a colourful, sociable and Bohemian life with painters including Munch and Gauguin. It is generally believed that during 1895 in Paris he contracted the French pox:[100] as Balfour Gardiner put it, 'the malady he caught in the pursuit of pleasure'. It became latent and in 1896 he met the painter Jelka Rosen, the granddaughter of Beethoven's pupil Moscheles. They married in 1903, but remained childless, and Delius unfaithful.

We know that he had been in reasonable health, even dragging Thomas Beecham up Norwegian mountains in 1908, when Delius was unimpressed with the conductor's fitness.[101] Beecham recounted how later that year Delius had complained of headaches, backache and experienced a severe bilious attack.[102] He looked haggard in 1911 when he visited various spas, experiencing some relief, and still enjoyed walking.[103] His compositions at this time, such as *Summer Night on the River* (1911) or *On Hearing the First Cuckoo in Spring* (1912), reveal no clue of his impending medical catastrophe.

Eric Fenby later reflected that Delius was deeply seared by the wastage of youth in the Great War's carnage.[104] His response had been composition of the pantheistic Requiem. In 1917 he and Jelka had to leave France, after concealing their best paintings and wine.[105] In England he had composed the more classical Violin and Cello Concerto, as well as the Violin Concerto, Cello Concerto and String Quartet. At the war's end they returned to France, and in 1918 a tour of spas seeking 'the cure' recommenced, continuing intermittently well into the 1920s.

Delius started to lose the use of his hands during 1921 although, when at his Norwegian chalet in July and August, he could still walk clumsily with two sticks,[106] having presumably still retained some manual strength. In 1920 composition of the incidental music for James Elroy-Flecker's play *Hassan* started and was dependent upon Percy Grainger's cheerfully energetic help. With Grainger, Delius could still be mischievous, but with Jelka, as the 1920s unfolded, he was intermittently a complete misery. As his paralysis and then eyesight deteriorated, Jelka was poor at taking down musical dictation, especially after Delius became totally blind early in 1925, by which time he was using a bath chair. And yet the first quarter of the twentieth century was Delius's richest passage of composition; Jefferson describes his patience and fortitude, despite great pain.[107] Perhaps the fate of the world influenced his composition more than the inexorable disease overtaking him. By 1928 the paralysis was almost complete. His music, by then unique and underivative, was a superb example of courageous determination overcoming pain and disability. Delius's stylistic development, as Payne elucidates, came from within this very self-contained and self-centred man.[108] Not only this, but for all its loveliness, the music remains impersonal and free of the 'self' of an essentially selfish man. In time, as he was felled from mountain top to invalid carriage, that same self-containment gave him the inner strength to sustain composition through infirmity. It is also a measure of Jelka's devotion and guidance that this man, otherwise so independent, even disdainful of the company and opinion of others, still recognised his need of them. Sacrifice of her own independence and creativity preserved his within its own paralysed body.

During 1928 Delius's plight came to the ears of a fellow Yorkshireman, Eric Fenby.[109] There was then born a creative whole, where two minds met and worked to one purpose, even if their workplace was sometimes uncongenial. Special people may collaborate with a meeting of minds, sometimes in friendship and sometimes not, creating a fusion of two into one final product. With Delius and Fenby, there was only ever one product from initial conception to first performance. Perhaps Foss unintentionally explained the reason why this union was possible at all, observing that Delius 'thought the sounds first and then sought means for producing these particular sounds'.[110] Initially the collaboration was disastrous, with Fenby unable to follow Delius's monotone or even to keep up with his dictation. That Fenby did not give up after Delius's initial bullying was largely due to Jelka's kindly and firm support.[111] Inititally, both men must have been tentative, and probably nervous, one becoming domineering, the other timorous. In his film *A Song of Summer*, Ken Russell directed his Delius and Fenby, once the ice had been broken, not so much as master and boy but as adjoined musical minds.[112] Whilst dictating his orchestral piece *A Song of Summer* to Fenby, Delius bade him to imagine they were sitting on the cliffs in the heather looking out to sea. Fenby later commented that in fact the process was far more nerve-wracking than that.

As Grainger had been before, Fenby increasingly and modestly became adviser and collaborator. Russell's film helps us to understand the relationship and the music that emerged and how it came together, as well as the impact of disease upon the composer and composition.[113] Fenby was young, eager and anxious to help, above all probably selfless, even though much later he described Delius as 'a selfish, miserable, syphilitic old bastard'. On a bad day, he must have been just that. To many his situation seemed pitiful. However, the composer's sister Clare said that he was 'so full of fun' and that 'sympathy would be wasted on him'.[114] When Neville Cardus met Delius in 1929 at the Delius Festival he commented, 'There was nothing pitiable about him – face strong and disdainful, every line graven on it by intrepid living', whilst regarding his music as 'recollecting emotion in tranquillity'.[115] Delius was clearly a wounded giant, acutely aware of his own dreadful mortality. He had been sociable, amorous and personable as a young man in the USA and Paris but, even before syphilis exacted its frightful toll, became increasingly solitary, probably by preference rather than because of disease. Undoubtedly he was selfish, but how could he have been otherwise? He was by now totally dependent on Jelka, Fenby and his male nurses.

It is hard to conceive of this once handsome, lively man, with aquiline features and of an independent inclination, lying in a bath chair unable to see, unable to walk, unable very probably to care for basic bodily tasks and unable to write, being less restricted than Ravel. Both of them could hear the music in their heads, but thereafter their paths diverged. Delius's power of speech and song remained intact, for he was also able to dictate musical notation. Here was an issue of capturing raw, unbridled creativity, but in real time, something which was impossible for Ravel, who could think of the tune, because that part of his brain was both able to conceive and conceptualise musical form (see Chapter 3). However, Ravel was unable to exercise the only means by which conceived music can be outwardly expressed: by playing it, singing it, writing the constituent notes down or literally dictating the piece note by note, as Delius did with Fenby. The expressive part of Ravel's brain was so much switched off that music could not be exteriorised. In contrast, the haggard figure of the blind Delius was still able to get his music out, albeit thanks to Fenby. Clearly, it was a laborious process, but they managed at a price. Ravel as a creative musician was locked in and stopped in his tracks. By contrast Delius, although greatly disabled, was able to continue triumphantly with the help of others, at least fourteen compositions arising from the Delius–Fenby collaboration. After *Irmelin* and *Fantastic Dance* in 1931, there was no more significant composition. Yet there is no evidence of intellectual decline or even resignation in Delius's last eighteen months. This is exemplified by Elgar's visit to Delius at Grez-sur-Loing in 1933, when he had gone to Paris to conduct his Violin Concerto with the young Yehudi Menuhin. Acting upon a whim, Elgar had written tentatively to Delius, suggesting that he might visit him before returning to England. Delius replied promptly: 'In spite of my infirmities, I manage to get something out of life and I should love to see you.'[116] One learns so much about Delius, his intellect and his attitudes in 1933 from that one brief note. Moreover, the two men continued to correspond until their deaths in 1934.[117]

Elgar published his impressions of the visit and of Delius in the *Daily Telegraph*.[118] It is a charming, vivid account. One can almost hear the cicadas chirping in the garden as the two grand old men sipped champagne and discussed music, Charles Dickens and the merits of air flight, which Elgar suggested was rather like Delius's music. Clinically the account is important, because Elgar was amused that every time Delius had a good idea or made a decision, he confirmed this by raising his left hand. Here we learn that paralysis of the arm was incomplete. Even more significantly, on taking his leave, Delius clasped Elgar's hands with his own as a return visit by Mr and Mrs Delius to Elgar in England was mooted. Delius was probably energised by the prospect of the visit and on his best behaviour, but Elgar's image of Delius is far from the ultimate, impossible, tortured wreck of Ken Russell's film. Furthermore, we have abundant evidence that Delius's intellectual, aesthetic and conversational faculties were unimpaired and that his spirit was undimmed, which was the measure of the man. That he had tertiary syphilis, typically of the tabes dorsalis type, is beyond all reasonable doubt. It is good to learn that he was still capable of enjoying a convivial glass of champagne with a colleague whose mind was met with much of Delius's wry, charming speed of thought. Fenby tells us, 'There was nothing of the sickly, morbid, blind composer, as known by popular fiction, but a man with a heart like a lion and a spirit that was as untameable as it was stern';[119] he was a man who 'still got something out of life'. For all his own misfortunes, Delius saw many of life's sadnesses, but was so detached that he did not participate in them. Despite mood swings which were sudden and upsetting, he never complained much about his own disability.

In the early summer of 1934, Eric Fenby left Grez, sensing that he had done all he could and went to London to assist with some publishing matters. He was swiftly recalled. The idyll created and sustained by Jelka and Frederick Delius, in spite of everything, was suddenly doubly stricken. She had undergone emergency major surgery at Fontainebleau for what proved to be incurable cancer.[120] He, in turn, had been greatly distressed by these circumstances at a time when his tabes dorsalis was relapsing, with severe shooting pains.[121] He died on 10 June 1934, both painfully and quickly,[122] and was buried not in the garden at Grez, on account of French law, but at Limpsfield in Surrey near his mother, with a funeral where the music had been arranged and the oration given by that great Delian Sir Thomas Beecham. Jelka was soon to lie permanently beside him, thus ending a remarkably sustained period of musical composition through the ravages of a long-term, then incurable disease.

Mind or Matter: Elgar and Delius

To compare Elgar and Delius musically is at first sight a departure from this book's thesis. It is only when contemplating them with a medical slant that the comparison becomes relevant. They who met in a spirit of friendship only during the last year of both their lives were contrapuntal mirror images. At least some of the musical expression from two exceptionally instinctive men came from their personalities and their afflictions. Elgar was an active man, shrouded by a moody, insecure, restless temperament. Delius was a ruthlessly self-confident loner, with a mind long trapped in a grossly failing body. Without that steely reserve and Jelka, how else could Delius have been able to tell Elgar in 1933 that, for all his infirmities, he still got something out of life? It is here that the numerous contrasts between and within the two composers become intriguing. Elgar lived in a conspicuously Edwardian, genteel English manner. Delius eschewed England, living, despite his incapacity, in many ways contentedly in France. Elgar became greatly troubled by the England of which he became a baronet in 1931. He renounced his Catholicism, whereas Delius had always been an atheist.

After Alice died, Elgar, still a vigorous man, composed little more, whilst the blind and paralysed Delius was energised by his wish to exteriorise the music still in his head. With Fenby came *A Late Lark*, *A Song of Summer*, *Cynara* and the *Irmelin Prelude*, probably arising from Delius's unshakeable inner strength and self-conviction. Point and counterpoint: Delius had a tortured body and it was lovingly cared for. Elgar, after Alice's death, became something of a tortured soul, at times spiritually alone.[123] Delius, the supreme egoist, wrote lovely but impersonal music, even explaining to Fenby in 1928 that he was not bothered too much about being blind; he had seen enough to feed his fervent musical imagination. Elgar wrote his First Symphony with 'a great hope and charity for the future', later saying that Gerontius's heavenly journey was 'the best of me'. Such reflections could not have come from Delius, a much more settled person than Elgar. Delius never musically sought his own self or his own salvation, both of which caused Elgar the anguish we hear in the Violin and Cello Concertos. Yet both men had an intense love of nature and the countryside and, at heart, both probably were solitary. With Delius that is clear to us immediately; Elgar is more complicated, as we see a man possibly most contented when young by the River Teme in the Golden Valley. We meet Elgar in society with all its trappings, uncomfortable with it and lonely without it.

✠ HUGO WOLF ✠
(1860–1903)

If I were only Hugo Wolf

Hugo Wolf, c.1900

Early in his career Hugo Wolf shared an impecunious flat with Mahler in Vienna. Whilst there, an influential mentor was the would-be composer and rich dilettante Adalbert von Goldschmidt. Alma Mahler claimed that in about 1878 Goldschmidt took Wolf to a brothel to be sexually initiated.[124] It has subsequently been assumed that he contracted syphilis then, but Alma could be an unreliable witness. Walker quotes Springer, who in 1926 boldly stated that Wolf contracted syphilis when he was seventeen.[125] This may have been because at that time he began to eat and travel separately from his friends. Perhaps, knowing he was syphilitic, he wished to spare those who were good to him from cross-infection as he understood it.

From this time his story becomes distinctly cyclothymic with his famous love for a French beauty, Vally Franck,[126] and periods of intense composition interspersed with despondency, although a tendency to cyclothymia had preceded his contracting syphilis. When Vally returned to France, Wolf despaired, going on to reject advice from Brahms as well as to fall out with his father and friends. After that a musical silence for half a year may have been in response to his father's death. During the 1880s his cyclothymia worsened, being reflected in the bleakness of some of his songs. In the late 1880s, a zenith of creativity came when he set some of Eichendorff's poetry to music.[127] There followed the popular *Italian Serenade* as well as *Italian Songbook*.[128] Then in 1891 Wolf became lethargic and fell victim to feverish throat infections,[129] which may, with the benefit of hindsight, have been due to syphilis. Alternatively, perhaps it was only then that he caught syphilis, avoiding an obvious earlier moral conflict between knowing he was probably syphilitic and any physical token of his love for Vally Franck. In 1893 he talked of hanging himself.[130]

Walker describes 1891–94 as the 'Lean Years',[131] which is justified from Wolf's chronology of compositions. By personality Wolf seems always to have been temperamentally stubborn and capricious. During lunch in April 1897 with Mr and Mrs Engelbert Humperdinck, his behaviour was erratic and he suddenly absconded as he bade them farewell, possibly showing the beginning of insanity.[132] Clinically we should examine earlier events. In 1896 Wolf was taken to a neurologist, who found unreactive pupils (possibly Argyll Robertson pupils), a probable sign of syphilis, although he had sustained a significant eye injury due to flying cinders.[133] It was also in 1897 that he took up cycling and was constantly falling off – perhaps evidence of declining coordination.[134] Nevertheless, this was also a year of renewed vigour in which he secured the performance of his second opera, *Der Corregidor*, whereafter he started composing his last, *Manuel Venegas*.

Again, there were signs at the lunch table. On 19 September 1897 Wolf met his friend Hellmer, to whom he declared himself to be the new Director of the Vienna Opera.[135] The next day, meeting Hellmer's parents, he added that he had sacked Mahler.[136] Dr Gorhan of the Mödling Infirmary declared that Wolf should be placed in an asylum urgently.[137] Now we encounter an intimate association between developing madness and composition. At the infirmary friends later discovered the first fifty pages of *Manuel Venegas* in a good hand and without signs of incipient madness.[138] New music for the symphonic poem *Penthesilea*, originally started in 1883, and a first movement for the third *Italian Serenade* were also discovered. However, most of his final attempts at composition in the asylum, from which he plotted an escape, showed, if anything, that innate inner resolve to compose in spite of everything. By now he was writing to friends about grandiose schemes for composition and performance with future fame and fortune. Such delusional megalomania is typical of GPI. Nevertheless, on 29 April 1898, *Der Corregidor* was successfully produced in Strassburg.[139] A month later he threw himself into the Traunsee, where he was invigorated by cold water and decided to swim back. Now he was hospitalised permanently.[140]

People were kind to him, including the Emperor, and by early 1898 he was reconciled with another former love, Melanie Kochert, who, with Wolf's sister Käthie, cared for him until his death, shortly after which Melanie took her own life.[141] By 1899 there was incipient paralysis and his eyesight started to deteriorate. Once the twentieth century had begun, chest infections and convulsions ensued and his psyche sometimes seemed turned inside out; as he said, 'If I were only Hugo Wolf', believing the world was made of cardboard.[142]

On 22 February 1903, by now very wasted and demented, he died. There had been no significant composition since that in 1897 at the asylum. He had said, 'When I can compose no more you may throw me on a dung-hill.'[143] Instead, he holds a place of honour in the Vienna Central Cemetery close to Schubert and Beethoven. It is curious that biographers such as Newman and Walker hardly mention syphilis, of which Wolf surely died.

Newman's objectivity may be questioned because he permitted himself no such reticence with Beethoven, who was not syphilitic (see Chapter 11). A more fitting testimony is that of Sams and Youens, who regard Wolf's particular genius as writing song and word together, not just setting words to music.[144]

Gaetano Donizetti (1797–1848)

This creator of bel canto was born in Bergamo of penniless parents, dying there fifty years later.[145] Despite this start, his musical fecundity was astonishing, as was his application. He produced short pieces at one sitting, and in nineteen years composed fifty operas, as many as five in a year,[146] provoking the view that he spread his talents very thinly. There is a lithograph of him writing with both hands simultaneously.[147] His first real triumph was with *Anna Bolena* in 1830.

After marrying Virginia, a lawyer's daughter, in 1827, he went on to even greater success with *Lucia di Lammermoor* in 1835. Two years later Virginia, who had already lost two children, died after childbirth.[148] Donizetti perhaps never recovered from the loss of his adored wife. One stillborn child bore abnormalities consistent with parental syphilis, although Virginia is said to have died of post-puerperal sepsis (likely) or German measles (less so).[149] The following year he moved to Paris and, perhaps like Rossini, he hoped to make enough money to then retire. *Don Pasquale* in 1843 was the pinnacle of his success. By then he was contractually able to divide his time between Paris and Vienna, where he had become Kapellmeister and was befriended by Metternich. Donizetti started to deteriorate, at first losing his formidable powers of concentration in the early 1840s. Weinstock infers that his downward course started as early as 1835.[150] Headaches became worse and more frequent. By December 1844 he wrote, 'I am half destroyed, it's a miracle I'm still on my feet.'[151] He was both restless and depressed, and experienced severe headaches and 'fevers' as he declined during 1845.[152] His last completed opera, *Don Sebastien roi de Portugal*, was said to have failed because of its libretto being described as 'a funeral in five acts'.[153] Ashbrook praised the music, but drew attention to the erratic nature of Donizetti's rehearsals.[154] Its composition had been more laboured than that of any of the earlier fluent works. Incipient disease probably had more to do with his final flop than the libretto did. Nevertheless, in 1845 he was still driven on to compose the incomplete work *Gemma di Vergy*. However, 1845 was the year in which he first needed a minder because he indulged in depravity with many women, most likely including prostitutes,[155] from whom he had probably caught syphilis whilst a student.[156]

He consulted specialists in January 1846, including one in venereal disease, whereafter inevitable remedies such as leeches, footbaths and bleeding added to his miseries.[157] He was placed in a sanatorium disguised as a country house outside Paris, where he declined into a monosyllabic, drooling, dribbling vegetable-like state. After a period requiring restraint, he became somnolent, just grunting harmlessly. His nephew Andrea was keen to return Uncle Gaetano to Bergamo, where his illustrious career had begun. The French authorities had been reluctant to allow Donizetti to return home, fearing the journey would be too arduous for his now feeble condition. They even put a guard on his door.[158] Finally, on 19 September 1847, Andrea took him upon a seventeen-day journey back to Bergamo.[159] There he was lovingly attended by friends until his death on 8 April 1848.[160]

The autopsy was unequivocal in finding changes typically associated with tertiary syphilis,[161] which the Donizetti Society website disputes.[162] This counter-argument seems to be based on his having suffered from headaches, nausea and 'lightning indispositions' over many years for, in the society's view, the symptoms had an 'unrealistically long gestation'. Ashbrook depicts his physical and mental deterioration from at least 1843, as do Smart and Budden.[163] But a lengthy gestation may be typical of syphilis. The same source implied that his fervour of composition indicated a 'cerebral dysrhythmia quite beyond a normal span'. In a single word, a more probable explanation for such fervour is 'genius'. When asked which of his operas he favoured most, he immediately replied, 'A father always has a preference for a crippled child, and I have so many.'[164]

Emmanuel Chabrier (1841–1894)

Chabrier is best known for joyous pieces such as *Suite pastorale*. Ravel declared him to be his greatest influence.[165] Poulenc rated him with Debussy in the evolution of French music.[166] He became a full-time composer only in 1880, the year in which a 'nervous disorder', possibly the onset of syphilis, was first noted.[167] Despite his success with *España* in 1883, in quick succession his life disintegrated with the death of an infant child and later that of his wife. By 1891 composition was tailing off.[168] In 1892 he went bankrupt and became depressed: This may have been a harbinger of syphilis, for in 1893–94 he developed what sounds to have been a characteristic pattern of GPI. Thus, by the time his opera *Gwendoline* was at last premiered in 1893, he was beyond recognising it as his own.[169] There are sensible grounds for assuming the diagnosis of syphilis, and Howat reports that Roger Delage can even account for when Chabrier caught syphilis and from whom.[170]

Prescription for Syphilis

Syphilis is a subject with considerable resonance for us today, with public interest in celebrity and 'private life'. Donizetti, Delius, Smetana, Chabrier, Schubert and Wolf beyond reasonable doubt all had syphilis, which makes it all the more inexplicable that Hayden, in her book *Pox*, should omit the first four, despite obvious efforts to persuade us that Schumann (Chapter 6) and Beethoven (Chapter 11) were syphilitic.[171] Today, penicillin would almost certainly have relieved their sufferings. Syphilis cannot be absolutely excluded in Schumann's case, but is improbable. For composers to be seen in other chapters, including Mozart, Beethoven, Tchaikovsky, Gershwin, Ravel or Britten, it can be discounted. If this book, inevitably flawed too, can lead to some firm ground rules for published research into medical aspects of biography, then the effort will have been thrice rewarded. We are all the curators of reputation.

Chapter 5

Alcoholism

Drunkenness is a temporary suicide: the happiness that it brings is merely
negative, a momentary cessation of unhappiness
Bertrand Russell, *The Conquest of Happiness*, 1930

Introduction

JUST AS SYPHILIS has been over-diagnosed, we come to alcohol,
another perceived result of over-indulgence. Of Breitenfeld's seventy-seven 'substance abusers' amongst composers, the major culprit was
alcohol.[1] So we see reputations inaccurately disfigured in musical pathography. An even more vital question is whether alcohol fuels creativity.
Alcoholism is a disease and not a crime, although sadly either may lead to
the other. There are good basic definitions of alcoholism. Pragmatically,
the wisest one is possibly that the sufferer is a person who apprehends
that he or she has a problem but is incapable of doing anything about
it.[2] The World Health Organization categorises criteria,[3] but Kessell and
Walton stressed the importance of a diagnostic gradient;[4] this is difficult
with today's national obsession with tick-boxes. They also highlighted the
permanent physical damage that is a consequence of chronic alcoholism.
That the social drinker, who deliberately and enjoyably gets tipsy occasionally, is not an alcoholic has been a comfort for many of us. More
importantly, the excessive drinker is not necessarily an alcoholic, being
separated from the latter by the absence of an inexorable deterioration
over the years. The key is decline and dependence, and in 2001 there were
said to be 2.8 million dependent drinkers in the UK.[5]

With some alcoholics the condition initially is a pleasure; they are usually the self-indulgent type.[6] For most it is a condition from which the
patient would dearly love to be free. One day an inborn error of metabolism may be discovered with, hopefully, cures structured thereupon.
Reformed alcoholics have to remain teetotal because drinking any alcohol

may trigger their illness. Such self-discipline is admirable. Meanwhile, there are identifiable psychological, social and geographical factors pre-disposing to alcoholism. What is striking is the paucity of true alcoholics amongst composers. There is one simple reason for composers being so relatively free of this disease: established alcoholism is inconsistent with sustained, serious musical composition. That novelists and poets may have been apparently more susceptible is beyond the scope of this book. The following list includes composers to whom ascriptions of alcoholism, or alcohol abuse, have been made, in some cases frequently. Not everyone who is seductively recruited by alcohol remains its prisoner.

Alcohol and Composers

(a) Alleged but unsubstantiated alcoholics
    Handel
    Mozart
    Beethoven
    Schubert
    Schumann
    Wagner
    Brahms
    Bruckner
    Tchaikovsky
    Dvořák
    Debussy
    Elgar
    Shostakovich
    Britten

(b) Excessive drinkers
    Sibelius
    Liszt
    Warlock (Heseltine)

(c) Alcoholics
    Musorgsky
    Satie
    Lambert
    Arnold

(d) Possible alcoholics

M. Praetorius
W. F. Bach
J. C. Bach
Field
Nicolai
Delibes
Glinka
Scriabin
Glazunov

The list indicates that we should judge composers along a gradient of consumption. Group (a) reveals frequent misjudgements. Handel was a huge man with an enormous appetite for food and drink. There is little evidence for his being a habitual drunkard. Schubert, Brahms and Bruckner were well known for supporting the Viennese pub trade. Perhaps significantly all three were bachelors who ate out. Schubertiads were undoubtedly bibulous affairs and, by most accounts, very jolly ones – reasonable evidence for their author's not being an alcoholic, although he did sporadically drown his sorrows. Schumann was a heavy drinker, but that does not make him an alcoholic, and he should be judged in the context of his overriding manic-depressive psychosis. There is some evidence that alcohol hindered his composition. It was not a significant component of his grave mental illness. Britten's doctor told me that his patient was believed to be alcoholic by a distinguished cardiologist, largely on the basis of his being an 'artistic type' who enjoyed a stiff drink before dinner.[7] Britten's biography is hardly punctuated by accounts of his falling about drunk and incapable.

Shostakovich and Debussy, and even Elgar, were perhaps more solitary in their use of alcohol, possibly as a comfort during adversity. Dvořák was said on more than one occasion to have consumed 'more than his measure of beer'. We are not acquainted with what his 'measure' was. A weakness for having a few pints does not constitute alcoholism by any of its medical definitions, even if he did need to lie down now and again. For those wondering what is considered to be alcoholism, then the section on Musorgsky will reveal it in its full, destructive awfulness.

As to excessive drinkers (group b),[8] this diagnosis cannot be disputed in the case of Sibelius (Chapter 2). That he voluntarily and apparently easily refrained from alcohol and cigar consumption for seven years is as important for forming an overall judgement as his sporadic huge drinking sprees. Liszt for many years drank heavily. As the account of him in

Chapter 8 will show, he became increasingly infirm and lonely late in life, drowning his sorrows in cognac, a weakness he shared with his son-in-law, Wagner, and Tchaikovsky.

Of the possible alcoholics (group d), Warlock's substance abuse was not just with alcohol (Chapter 6).[9] Field will be dealt with shortly, as will Glazunov. Hugh Macdonald describes rarefaction in style and technique in Scriabin's later works,[10] which is hardly evidence for deconstructive influences on musical composition. Possible alcoholism is a just diagnosis for the others in this group, including two sons of J. S. Bach and also Otto Nicolai, from whom bright things were expected as he became chief conductor of the Berlin Philharmonic before dying young.

We turn now to those composers who, in their own way, are all exemplars of aspects of this complex and emotive subject.

Malcolm Arnold (1921–2006)

Arnold is not one of the greatest composers within these pages, but medically he is most illustrative and he did compose nine symphonies. Neither should we be snooty about film music; Prokofiev, Shostakovich and Vaughan Williams were not. At the age of twenty-one Arnold was diagnosed as schizophrenic.[11] His first marriage initially appears to have been calming, but in 1950 he attacked his wife, Sheila.[12] The question, over which he agonised, was whether this was because he had been drunk, or had he become psychotic? He was placed in an asylum for three and a half months where both insulin and electrical shock therapy (ECT) were given, and even restraint in a straitjacket.[13] This all indicates that his psychosis was more likely to have been schizophrenia than manic-depressive bipolar illness. Nevertheless, when he first went into Greenway Nursing Home it was to be dried out rather unsuccessfully of his alcohol dependence.[14] This was in the early 1960s, when Sheila divorced him at a time when he was also promiscuous.[15] In 1963 he married his second wife Isobel Grey, and the marriage was initially happy.[16] Although there were children, Arnold turned on her too, and he then made a serious suicide attempt. The years 1962–66 were lean years for composition.[17]

A second serious suicide attempt in 1975 could easily have been fatal had it not been for the fortuitous arrival of a friend at his home and the prompt skills of the Dublin ambulance service.[18] After another serious suicide attempt in 1977, he awoke in hospital with DTs (delirium tremens).[19] Shortly thereafter in 1978 he started composition of the *Symphony for Brass* and his Eighth Symphony, as well as the *Irish Dances*, the lattermost not finally completed until 1986. Then he went into Greenway again and new drugs were given. By June 1978 Isobel asked for a divorce. Having given up composition, Arnold considered starting again in 1979.[20] Then he was admitted to hospital in Northampton, where the primary diagnosis was alcoholism associated with schizophrenia and not bipolar disorder,[21] although the two may overlap. There was no serious composition between 1978 and 1982, whereupon the Trumpet Concerto came, and then silence again until an Indian summer of creativity from 1986 to 1990. His Ninth Symphony (1986) and the Cello Concerto in 1988 are especially noteworthy, along with a mixture of works with an emphasis on wind instruments: he had been principal trumpet in the London Philharmonic Orchestra. Arnold said the Ninth Symphony was a reflection on all his life, and he had contentedly worked for up to fourteen hours per day on its composition,[22] which in itself is not suggestive of alcoholism.

In the mid-1980s he vowed an abstinence from alcohol and faced up to the possibility of his long-term need for institutional care.[23] In his last fifteen to twenty years, Arnold became more settled after relinquishing further pretensions to compose and becoming fairly estranged from his two former wives and his children. Anthony Day was his companion for his last twenty years, conferring a stability and dignity upon his life, although by 2003–04 he had relinquished any attempt to compose, although significant composition had ceased by 1990.[24]

Arnold's prolific and highly successful career as a composer for the cinema, often with half a dozen scores annually, revealed his only partly fulfilled musical potential, although financially it secured his chaotic family life and the need for expensive long-term medical care. The periods 1962–66, 1978–82 and then 1982–86 illustrate the incompatibility of alcoholism and composition. Whether he was schizophrenic or had bipolar depression matters less than the fact that by the 1980s drugs were available which, along with Anthony Day, kept him on an even keel, even to the extent that he was knighted. He died of pneumonia in 2006, aged eighty-five, as a national treasure. Perhaps the key to this remarkable Indian summer is his strength of will to refrain from alcohol.

Constant Lambert (1905–1951)

An English composer not so lucky was Constant Lambert, a child prodigy who died aged forty-five and was best known for his expansive composition of 1927, *The Rio Grande*. He could be an acidic critic and an excellent writer, as his account of Satie shows.[25] His more exotic friends included Peter Warlock, by whose mysterious death in 1930 he was saddened (Chapter 6).[26] He also spectacularly fell out with Diaghilev, a case of biting the hand that sometimes fed him. Towards the end his health declined; he became irritable and drank to excess.[27] Perhaps this was a reason for his refusing to marry Margot Fonteyn.

Lambert's life slowly disintegrated. He composed much less in his last fifteen years, openly describing himself as a 'failed composer'. This has generally been attributed to alcoholism, but when he was admitted to hospital in 1951, apparently intoxicated, it was at last discovered that he was diabetic.[28] In the years leading up to this final and fatal illness he had been in a poor way, not least as his ballet *Tiresias* came to fruition with a discouraging reception at Covent Garden. Shead believes that exhaustion caused by criticisms of *Tiresias* hastened his end.[29] Erratic behaviour,

excitability and then slumber may have been due to previously undiagnosed diabetes as much as to alcohol,[30] as was also the case with Dylan
Thomas. That is the problem with diagnostic labels such as 'alcoholic',
and we have seen the dangers of being too judgemental. Lambert had
studiously avoided doctors, making himself the victim of his own fears.
It is sad that the combined blood levels of sugar and alcohol proved fatal
in so young a man. In 1946 he was described by Edward Dent as 'the
best all round musician in Britain'.[31] That he had an alcohol dependence
seems indisputable, and to it his sadly early death is usually ascribed. The
probable major contribution of diabetes is known, but mentioned much
less than alcohol; one wonders why.

John Field (1782–1837)

Another possibly alcoholic composer was John Field, to whom Chopin
expressed his debt. This Irishman went to London and there studied with
Clementi, by whom he was meanly treated.[32] He travelled widely and was
beguiled by St Petersburg, where for a time he settled. Piggott describes
Clementi placing his brilliant protégé in Russia to extend his own business
there and even taking Field's fees.[33] Field was said to have developed rectal
carcinoma in the 1820s, and he visited London to undergo surgery by Sir
Astley Cooper in 1831, apparently with some success.[34] He had been treated
with caustic potash earlier for piles by a London barber.[35] There was little
significant composition between 1823 and 1832. By the early 1830s he was a
sick man and sometimes a little confused. In Russia he became known as
'Drunken John'.[36] Clearly he had been drowning his sorrows and probably
numbing his pain with alcohol. The choice of analgesics in those days was
very limited.

In 1834–35 Field was hospitalised for nine months in Naples, where he
underwent several operations. By now he was very weak and walking with
a stick. His poor situation was discovered by some kindly visiting Russian
aristocrats called Rakhmanov, with whom he then returned to Russia;[37]
he even managed to then give three final concerts in January 1837.[38] His
Sixteenth Nocturne in F was probably composed and first performed in
1836, despite poverty, alcohol and advancing malignancy.[39] It is difficult to
judge now whether he was a true alcoholic or whether alcohol was the only
means to ameliorate his awful symptoms from cancer of the rectum. Like
Debussy, he could sit only on a rubber cushion.[40] The truth probably lies
in the middle, which in medicine is often the sensible bet. What is more

difficult to judge is the diagnosis of rectal carcinoma. Methods to treat that appropriately emerged only a hundred years ago, an early example of the treatment being Claude Debussy (Chapter 10). With Rossini (Chapter 10) we will see the awful results of attempting a piecemeal removal of the tumour. From the history available it seems that the diagnosis was made as many as ten or twelve years before Field's death.[41] His actual cause of death on 23 January 1837 seems to have been pneumonia.[42] If we accept that early in the nineteenth century any surgical attempt to extirpate the tumour was doomed to failure from the outset, then, on a balance of probabilities, the initial diagnosis of cancer is questionable. That Field survived more than a decade after the initial diagnosis leads to a strong suspicion that the true early condition was either a benign rectal polyp, or even haemorrhoids (piles). The former is the more likely, and it could have undergone malignant transformation as some do, something not recognised in the early 1800s. Surgical attempts to remove the polyp, especially if repeated, would damage the terminal bowel, causing strictures or incontinence or both, in which case poor John had ample reason to become 'drunken', although the Moscow musical world was greatly saddened by his passing.[43]

*

The worst has been left until the end, for there are two composers whose health was overwhelmed by alcoholism and whose musical output is reflected in this disorder, and a third with whom we may still hedge our bets.

Erik Satie (1866–1925)

Satie's Franco-Scottish parents went to live in Paris when he was four.[44] He was thenceforth very much a Parisian and a bohemian one, in keeping with that city in the late nineteenth century. From the Paris Conservatoire, which he had described as a 'sort of penitentiary', he was sent down, branded as lazy, untalented and worthless.[45] When he was readmitted in 1885 Satie did no better, so he tried the army. After a few months of that disagreeable experience he was able to simulate bronchial asthma, thereby effecting his medical discharge.[46] Then in 1905 he made a serious attempt to improve his technique by enrolling at the Schola Cantorum.[47] During the Great War he served in the home guard and questioned Debussy's reasons for not contributing more to the war effort.[48]

His unmistakable style, technique and personality flowered when he left his father's flat and moved to Montmartre. There he was a regular at the legendary café 'Le Chat Noir', meeting many of the *fin de siècle* figures from the arts and writing his *Gymnopédies*, by which today he is best known. By then he was a heavy drinker, with a preference for mixing his drinks, such as beer or eau-de-vie with calvados, or alternatively wine with cognac.[49] Nevertheless, Cocteau said that alcohol had no effect on Satie's work.[50] His quick mind and sense of humour combined to produce compositions such as *The Dreamy Fish* or writings like 'Mémoires d'un amnésique'. Intermittently he became interested in religion and politics.

When he came into a small legacy in 1895 he bought twelve (or seven) expensive purple (or grey) velvet suits, and the Velvet Gentleman was born.[51] Two years earlier he had been rejected by the painter Suzanne Valadon, probably the only known love or intimate of his life. Thereafter he spoke of sadness and icy-cold loneliness,[52] a rare, serious statement from this funny man. Orledge suggests that his lack of emotional fulfilment perhaps underlies his paranoid tendencies.[53] Like many such apparent dilettantes, he is easy not to take seriously, which may have been his wish. His long friendship with Debussy, as well as his work with Diaghilev and Picasso realised in the 1916 ballet *Parade*, indicate that people did then take him seriously, not least in his association with 'Les Six', whose numbers included Milhaud, Poulenc and Honegger but not Satie himself. Beneath all his amusing eccentricities, he became an increasingly tragic figure. His drinking became heavier and more dependent. Despite Cocteau's earlier opinion, his compositions diminished in number, length and recognition. In 1925 he died in hospital of cirrhosis of the liver.

Kessel and Walton identified several personality types predisposed to alcoholism.[54] The loss of Satie's mother when he was six and his immaturity with a self-indulgent narcissistic personality, as well as the possibility of his libido remaining unfulfilled, are all factors predisposing to alcohol dependence, leading as they do to a failure in learning skills for sorting out life's tribulations. Satie's early over-indulgence in alcohol was probably accompanied by fun and conviviality. That, in turn, reinforced the addiction. As the fun ebbed away, sometimes being replaced by that 'icy loneliness', the classic scenario for serious alcoholism probably became established. The intriguing question is whether, freed from alcohol and perhaps in the arms of a good woman, his undoubted talent might have given us more entertaining, if not truly great, music. It seems likely that the very frivolity and dilettante attitudes he always exhibited made greater and more substantial success improbable. He was his own *Jack in the Box*, wittily quipping that 'A composer should take no more time from his public than strictly necessary.' For all that, Lambert believed that he was a genuinely serious composer,[55] accepting that he clearly was not a serious person.

To encounter one whose music had a profound and lasting impact at the same time as he wrestled with a devouring alcohol addiction is almost unique, but it is fully and tragically met with our next subject.

✢ MODEST MUSORGSKY ✢
(1839–1881)

A man indeed is not genteel when he gets drunk
James Boswell, *The Life of Samuel Johnson,* 1791

And indeed the young, slender Musorgsky was genteel.* His mildly aristocratic family had an army tradition, and so Modest entered a crack regiment as a cadet. When he was seventeen years old he met Borodin,[56] who described a man then far removed from Repin's fearsome but sad portrait of Musorgsky in his last days. Borodin's picture was of a small, elegant, cultured man who spoke French with a slight lisp. Brown implies that the entire ambience of peacetime army life was decadent, sometimes violent, and that the role models encouraged impressionable adolescents to drink heavily, even competitively, be it with champagne or vodka.[57] Emerson believes that Musorgsky showed little enthusiasm for these antics at that time, but that the trigger into alcoholism was his mother's death.[58] Although Musorgsky left the army and became a civil service clerk, he may, nevertheless, have unwittingly acquired the alcohol habit from an early stage. He was a scant diarist, but wrote extensive letters to his musical mentor, Mily Balakirev. In one such letter written during 1859 he told Balakirev that he was 'tormented by a cruel disease: mysticism coupled with cynical thoughts of God'. He went on to say that he took measures to expurgate it altogether, but admitted to 'suffering terribly' and to 'associating with unworthy people'. He asked Balakirev to help curb his activities.[59] One inevitably wonders whether it was ladies of easy virtue who were unworthy, or were these just early features of dipsomania? It is known that he was a prude.

There is a Tolstoyan account of his trying to rescue a prostitute by offering marriage, but she drowned herself, adding to his mental anguish.[60] His first real love was a cousin who died young, but he probably fell for Maria Verderovskya, a wealthy patron of the arts nearly ten years his senior.[61] It was, he admitted, excessive drinking which dragged him down, and he told Balakirev that he had little faith in his own musical abilities. Balakirev, who was kindly disposed towards the endearing Musorgsky, nevertheless said he was a drivelling idiot.[62] Emerson believes that this refers to his

---

* There are several spellings of his name in use. That used by both Caryl Emerson and David Brown is employed here.

chaotic and naive behaviour, imputing neither his intellect nor that he was a holy fool. So by the time he was in his early twenties we find a mentally disturbed man with low self-esteem, little by way of achievement and a craving for alcohol as well as for human love and approbation. The miracle is that, despite these handicaps, great things were to follow. But what was his 'terrible illness'? Onanism has been inferred as a source of guilt.[63] Alternatively, his secret 'terrible illness' could have been epilepsy, as Seroff has implied.[64] The balance of probabilities does not incline one to a diagnosis of full-blown grand-mal epilepsy, of which there are no good accounts. That he did later suffer fits is certain,[65] but those on record all appear to have been associated with episodes of heavy drinking or subsequent alcohol withdrawal, a typical feature of late-stage alcoholism. There is nothing to suggest temporal lobe epilepsy in this conspicuously generous, mild-mannered and unaggressive man. He could have had petit-mal epilepsy, but clinical instinct leads us elsewhere. His periods of illness seem to have paralleled his alcoholic behaviour and were especially associated with his being alone, which he feared and hated.

It is relevant to his psyche and well-being that both company and physical occupation were good for him and for his health. Such happiness as he occasionally experienced was associated mainly with his three years in the late 1850s living in a commune, or a period in 1871–72 when he shared a flat with Rimsky-Korsakov.[66] The latter ended when Rimsky married Nadezhda Purgold, with Musorgsky as his best man.[67] We also return to a Tolstoyan view, this time of contentment when, after the emancipation of the serfs in 1861, he went happily to labour on the family farm, his sympathies clearly being with the peasants,[68] although economic necessity may also have led him to labouring. This is also musically relevant because by then he had adopted a Russian view of music, later drawing opposition from Tchaikovsky, who looked west, whereas the 'Mighty Handful' looked east.* Despite this musical preference for Russianness, in the spring of 1865 he continued with his early opera *Salammbô*, started two years earlier and based on Flaubert.[69] When, in 1865, his mother died, severing his final links with childhood and heritage, he went on a huge drinking binge and came out of it via DTs (delirium tremens).[70] From 1865 to 1868 Modest now stayed with his married and wealthy brother Filaret, which may have calmed down his increasingly erratic life. Early in January 1866 he was well enough to resume work, producing *St John's Night on the Bare*

---

* The group of five centred on Balakirev with Borodin, César Cui and Rimsky-Korsakov, as well as Musorgsky.

Mountain, which he unusually regarded as a fine work. The basis for this work reflects his febrile thoughts then: depravity was certainly a theme on that bare mountainside.

When Nadezhda Purgold described him in 1868 as a well-built man with an ugly red nose, but 'aristocratic manners' and 'beautiful hands – a splendid pianist',[71] she showed the dichotomy of this man's driving forces: one creative and refined, and the other intermittently and increasingly destructive. The obvious musical talent which later drove him to compose *Boris Godunov* was vying with a sometimes uncontrollable craving for drink. Perhaps it is no coincidence that the usually benevolent Borodin wrote to his wife that Musorgsky's earlier opera *The Marriage* was extraordinary, a 'paradoxical achievement teeming with novelties and humorous points, but as a whole a failure – impossible in practice'.[72] Musorgsky said that *The Marriage* was a cage in which he had become trapped.[73]

The escape from that cage was *Boris Godunov*, started in the autumn of 1868 and completed by Christmas 1869, while he laid the incomplete *Marriage* aside. Professor Nikolsky, a Pushkin expert, gave him the idea for *Boris*, assisting with historical aspects.[74] Almost inevitably it was rejected, and in 1871 the composer answered some of his critics. His revision became more tuneful and less gloomy and now introduced women. Three excerpts were premiered to acclaim at the Mariinsky Theatre in February 1873.[75] The premiere proper did not occur until February 1874. But then he started to exhibit dementia, also saying that he was not drinking much at the time. This is consistent with the established alcoholic, which by then he had become, since agitation, hallucinations (traditionally pink elephants) and delusions may be withdrawal phenomena.

In July 1873 Musorgsky's friend the artist Victor Hartmann had died, and Musorgsky hit the bottle again in his grief and sense of guilt. He had walked home with Hartmann just before his death, and his friend stopped, complaining of 'palpitatio cordis' (palpitations), which Musorgsky likened to his own experience.[76] There then occurred what was to become a regular feature, for he disappeared for a few days into the back streets of degenerate dissolution, to the consternation of his friends.[77] Then came another masterpiece, inspired by ten of Hartmann's pictures (four of which are now lost), the highly original *Pictures at an Exhibition* for piano, taking Musorgsky twenty days from conception to realisation.[78] Strangely, this wonderful music slumbered until it was orchestrated by Ravel in 1922.

Another distressing death was that in June 1875 of Nadezhda Opochinina, a mother figure whom he loved and commemorated in 'Epitaph'.[79] Throughout his life Musorgsky agonised over deaths even of mere acquaintances. A fateful year for what remained of his fragile health was 1875. Always dependent upon and often supplicant to friends, he fell in with a charming, wealthy, but fast-spending and rather dissolute naval officer, Pavel Naumov.[80] Naumov was not a malevolent man and neither was he an alcoholic, but when it came to drink he was free with his hospitality, which was the last thing Musorgsky needed, although Brown describes it as a congenial relationship.[81] Friends such as Glinka's widowed sister Shestakova tried to steer him away from Naumov,[82] as she feared that his living with the Naumovs was worsening his already frail condition. Now Modest's nocturnal habit of turning up very drunk at friends' houses worsened. At Shestakova's house he once vomited blood.[83] Such haematemesis is common in late alcoholic liver cirrhosis. The bleeding, which may be catastrophic, comes from varicose veins bursting in the gullet. In 1878 another old friend, the singer Petrov, died, and Musorgsky again was suffused by grief and inevitably a craving for alcohol.[84] Yet this was a time when people were still astonished by his musical memory.[85] Seroff believes that Petrov's death killed Musorgsky's enthusiasm for *The Fair at Sorochinski*, which he had started in 1874, whilst *Khovanshchina* remained incomplete. He fought back, attempting to improve his perilous finances by going on a concert tour in 1879 with an ageing diva, Daria Leonova, for whom he was mainly an accompanist.[86] Musorgsky had prepared assiduously, and for much of the tour he was musically, but not financially, a success. He often revealed continuing optimism in spite of everything, right up to the end. But again he became overwhelmed by a craving for drink and feelings of guilt in that once more he had relapsed. That innate drive to compose intermittently overcame this most disabling of diseases, although it was Rimsky-Korsakov who completed *Khovanshchina* after Musorgsky's death. After completing *Boris* in 1877, he composed little of consequence, apart from the still popular 'Song of the Flea', written whilst on tour with Leonova.

He was always generous. Even when broke, he refused payment for playing the piano at any fund-raising function.[87] When he appeared he was, or seemed to be, drunk. One Italian tenor, initially alarmed by Musorgsky's appearance, marvelled at his beautiful accompaniment, exclaiming 'Che artista'.[88]

Early in 1881 Musorgsky participated in a commemoration for Dostoyevsky. Then, on 23 February, he told Leonova that there was nothing left for him but to beg in the street. By then he was already in beggar's rags and short of food. That evening he was said to have suffered a stroke, although he quickly recovered.[89] A more probable diagnosis is that he had experienced an alcoholic seizure. He remained in a chair at Leonova's house, getting up cheerfully the next morning and eating his breakfast, only to suddenly collapse again. With the assistance of Cui, Dr Lev Bertenson, later to be intimately associated with Tchaikovsky's death, was called.[90] He promptly had Musorgsky registered as his 'employee', which entitled him to a private room in a military hospital on 24 February.[91] There Musorgsky was initially semi-comatose, then delirious, but within a few days he started to plan for the future. Over three weeks he ate well, regaining some of his former strength as well as reading Berlioz's *Treatise on Orchestration*.[92] Friends visited, one of whom, Repin, painted the famous, but incomplete, final portrait. Musorgsky was a popular patient; people had always liked him. As his birthday approached, a member of staff smuggled in a bottle of cognac, having possibly been bribed to do so.[93] Musorgsky's sometimes neglectful brother Filaret had for once visited, unwisely leaving money, whence probably the brandy came.[94] Sadly the contents of the bottle were quickly consumed, although the precise details have become the stuff of myth and legend. Musorgsky slept, and then awoke and is said to have cried out, 'Everything is finished. Ah, how miserable I am.'[95] Soon after that he died, on 16 March 1881. When Repin came in for the final sitting it was too late.[96]

In one sense Musorgsky is an exception. Whilst wrestling with over-whelming alcohol addiction he still produced great music. Rimsky wrote that his mental logic was growing dim, slowly and gradually.[97] These were triumphs over adversity because it is obvious that when he died, a week after his forty-second birthday, he had been a serious alcoholic for at least fifteen years. It is the optimism amongst the stupor and torture which one most greatly admires, conceding the admittedly short output. Yet all along there was an almost primal urge to get his music out: surely an ingredient of genius. Borodin should have the last word, not least because Musorgsky's case is almost unique in that he was chronicled by this friend, also a composer, physician and scientist. Borodin once wrote to his wife, 'This is horribly sad. Such a talented man and sinking so low morally. Now he periodically disappears then reappears, morose, un-talkative, which is contrary to his usual habit. After a while he comes to himself again – sweet, gay, amiable and as witty as ever. Devil knows what a pity.'[98]

✣ ALEXANDER GLAZUNOV ✣
(1865–1936)

There is Glazunov hence there is Russian music
> Boris Asafiev (critic and musicologist), 1920

In 1881, shortly after Musorgsky's death, St Petersburg welcomed the premiere of the First Symphony by a sixteen-year-old, Alexander Glazunov.[99] It is an amazingly assured as well as melodious work, seldom performed today. Glazunov donated his consequent prize money to the fund for erecting a memorial to Musorgsky.[100] Generosity was a theme marking the remainder of his long career, as he would often touch Russian musical history. After Borodin died in 1887, Glazunov and his friend Rimsky-Korsakov abandoned their own composition projects to complete or revise those which Borodin had left incomplete, such as the Third Symphony and *Prince Igor*, whose overture was set down by Glazunov entirely from memory years later.[101] Another and less rewarding personal characteristic was said to be revealed at the disastrous premiere of Rachmaninov's First Symphony on 15 March 1897, under Glazunov's chaotic baton.[102] Years later, Rachmaninov's wife suggested that Glazunov had been drunk at the time, she was the only one to do so.[103] Or did she say that others had said he was drunk? Rachmaninov himself never directly implicated him in the fiasco, despite criticising Glazunov's abilities as a conductor.[104] Glazunov never really mastered the art of conducting.[105]

Glazunov's star shone early after the First Symphony, seven and a half more symphonies following quite quickly. Apart from securing Borodin for posterity, he was an efficient and diligent director of the St Petersburg Conservatory, spending most of his time on academia and teaching. Amongst his grateful students were Prokofiev and especially Dmitri Shostakovich, for whose mother Glazunov raised funds to support the young Dmitri as he recovered from TB, saying the death of Shostakovich would be an irreparable loss for the world of art.[106] But his relationship with Shostakovich had become difficult. Wine and vodka, which Glazunov drank increasingly, had become hard to buy on the official market, and he obtained a regular supply of alcohol from Shostakovich's family.[107] As Glazunov had so helped to project Dmitri, so in turn young Shostakovich had wanted to advance on his own merits, and not because of black market booze from his father to his teacher,[108] not least because father Shostakovich was risking his own life with such a transaction.[109]

From 1917 onwards Glazunov had struck an accord with the communists, and he was anxious later not to disturb it. However accommodating the comrades may then have been, H. G. Wells found Glazunov cold, half-starved, sallow and wasted when he visited him in 1920,[110] a view substantiated in 1922 by Shostakovich.[111] How much this was due to drink or to the privations of communism we cannot know.

By the time Russia had stabilised after the civil wars which followed the Great War and Bolshevik Revolution, Glazunov composed little. There had been an earlier creative block in 1890–91, marked by depression and an assumed turning to the bottle. Compositions started to decline, if only in quantity, after 1910 when he left the Ninth Symphony unfinished, although the First Piano Concerto came in 1911 and the Second in 1917. By the 1920s his known weakness for alcohol may have become more serious. He spent most of his time teaching. It was noticed that he spoke increasingly briefly and quietly towards the end of lessons. The suggestion that there was an apparatus he installed, with a supply of liquor hidden in his desk and connected to tubing through which he could imbibe during the class, is regarded by Frolova-Walker as a 'joke'.[112] His health noticeably declined at this time.

He went to Vienna in 1928 to represent the USSR at the Schubert centenary and thereafter he stayed in the West. In 1929 he settled in Paris, where he married Olga Gavrilova, a woman ten years his junior.[113] It is probable that, in more congenial surroundings and with a new wife and stepdaughter, his drinking was moderated. He wrote the *Concerto ballata* for cello and orchestra for Pablo Casals in 1931. The last string quartet (Opus 107) was subtitled 'Homage to the Past', and its premiere by the Glazunov Quartet in the Glazunov Hall clearly was a deserved homage. He died in 1936. His contribution to Russian music is sometimes regarded as being that of a teacher, but his own compositions strangely are neglected today.

We cannot quarrel with the obvious picture of serous drinking, after the Great War, emanating probably from Shostakovich's testimony as reported by Volkov.[114] This comes with several caveats. Firstly, Fay has cast doubt as to how much of Volkov's book is an accurate account of Shostakovich's views or statements.[115] Secondly, it is clear from a number of accounts that Glazunov had suffered greatly during the Great War and Revolutionary period.[116] It is equally clear that during this period he had put the conservatory and its students first. He is crucial to the transition from traditional Russian Romanticism and nationalism to Prokofiev and Shostakovich, the latter declaring his teacher to be generous and dedicated.

Two things are strange. Firstly, Glazunov appears to have achieved a surprisingly relaxed relationship with the Soviets, which was to the benefit of others and the development of Russian music in the twentieth century. Secondly, few, if any, composers of his stature turned their efforts so selflessly and tirelessly to teaching and academic administration, again to the benefit of others. In the classroom Glazunov may have been supported by vodka. Was the vodka a sop to his dedication to a job which, viewed in terms of his legacy, may have been a comedown, or did an accommodation with teaching come from his drying up as a composer, with increasing lubrication from drink after 1908 as a cause? Teaching was possibly where, as a musician of integrity, he believed he should go after the prodigious early flow of composition, especially the symphonies.

His contribution and its relationship to his health and alcohol intake are crucial in understanding Glazunov. He seems to have gone through three phases. Firstly, there was the prodigy set upon a brilliant career at a time when both Rimsky and Tchaikovsky were pre-eminent. There followed the heavy-drinking academic and then his third late period, freed from academia and Petrograd winters, when he became a mature, restored composer. In retrospect, I suspect that Glazunov was an excessive drinker, rather than a true alcoholic. Although his last eight years after a late marriage were stable, his health weakened from the effects of early malnutrition because of his life in Petrograd from 1916 to 1923 and an excessive consumption of vodka over many years. He died in Paris in 1936 from kidney failure (uraemia).[117]

Conclusion

Diseases from syphilis to heart disease were savage in their depredations with many heroic composers. Of all the diseases, true alcoholism may have had the most negative effect on the historical development of musical composition, as witnessed by its infrequency in these musical pages. Having seen the effects of syphilis and alcohol on the creative mind, we must consider now the influence of neurological and then psychological illness in the next two chapters.

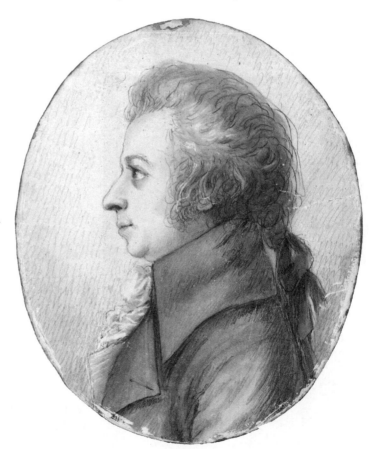

1 Mozart's ear compared with an ordinary ear.

2
Dorothea Stock's
Mozart portrait
– and not a lot of
ear showing.

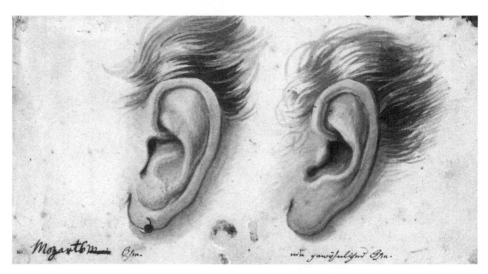

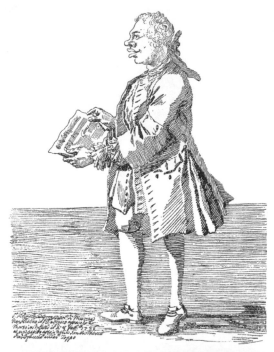

3 Pergolesi – A cruel caricature.

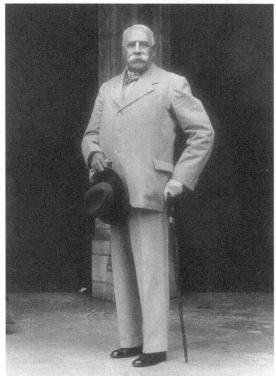

4 Elgar outside Hereford Cathedral – with a back like a ramrod.

5 Sibelius – That terrifying uncle to avoid at Christmas.

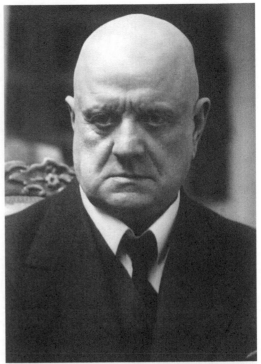

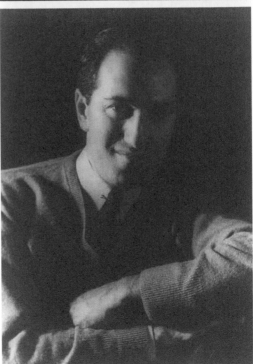

6 Gershwin – Before he was cut down in his prime.

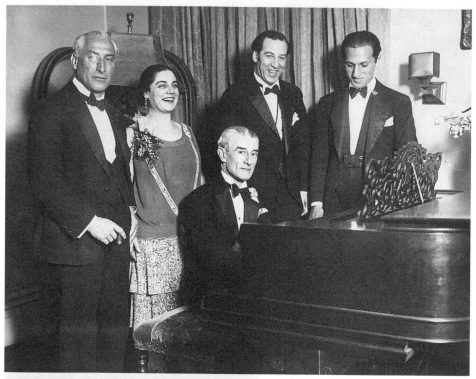

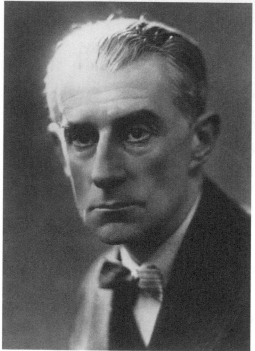

7 Ravel
(a) Playing the piano at his birthday
party, with (from *l.* to *r.*)
Oscar Fried, Eva Gauthier,
Manoah Leide-Tedesco and George
Gershwin, 8 March 1928, New York
City.
(b) Seven years later: an empty shell

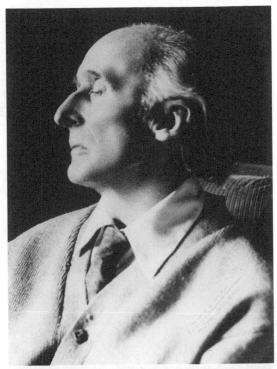

8 Delius – Blind, paralysed, but unbowed.

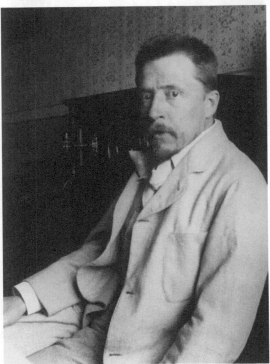

9 Wolf – In the asylum with the ravages of GPI.

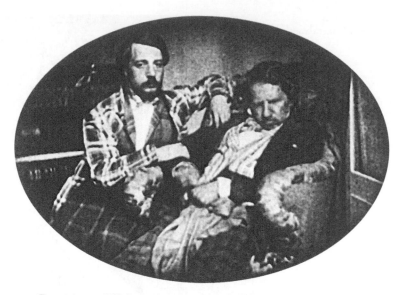

10 Donizetti – With nephew Andrea: a dribbling, babbling vestige.

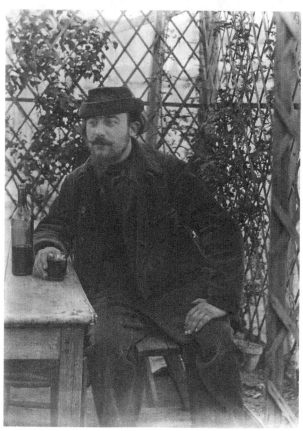

11 Satie – A most velvet gentleman.

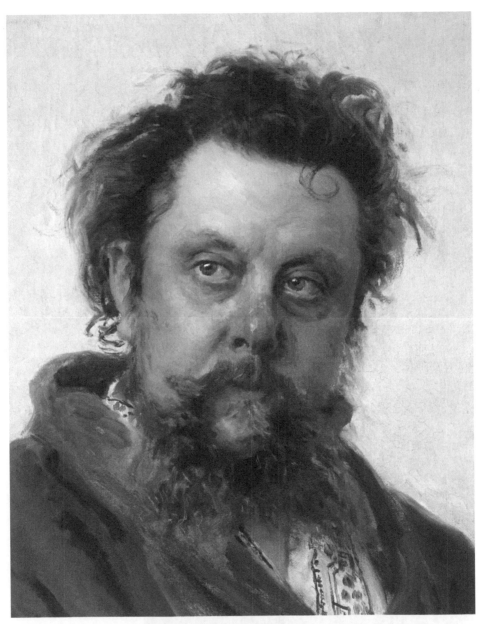

12 Musorgsky – The ravages of alcohol immortalised by Repin.

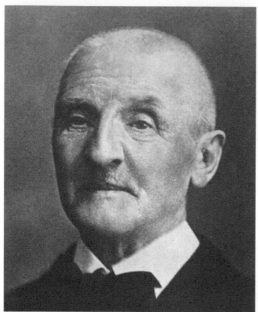

13 Bruckner – An orderly man …
obsessively so.

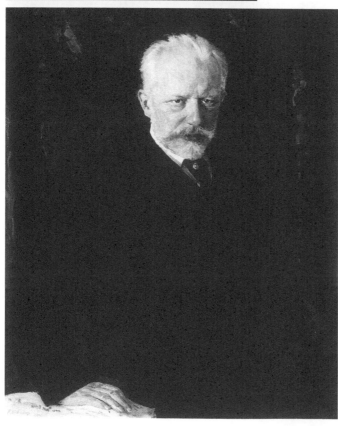

14 Tchaikovsky
– Kuznetsov's
realisation of a
prematurely old
man.

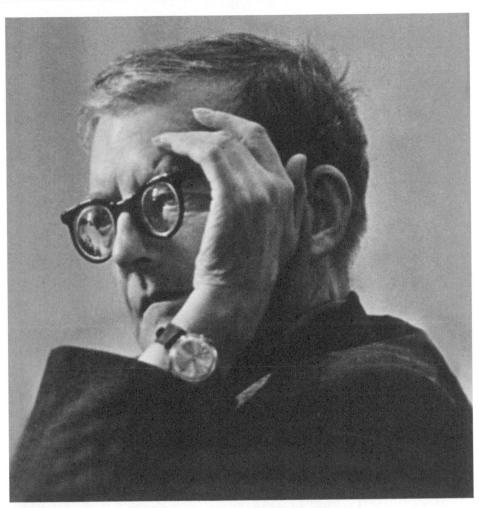

15 Shostakovich – Never not afraid.

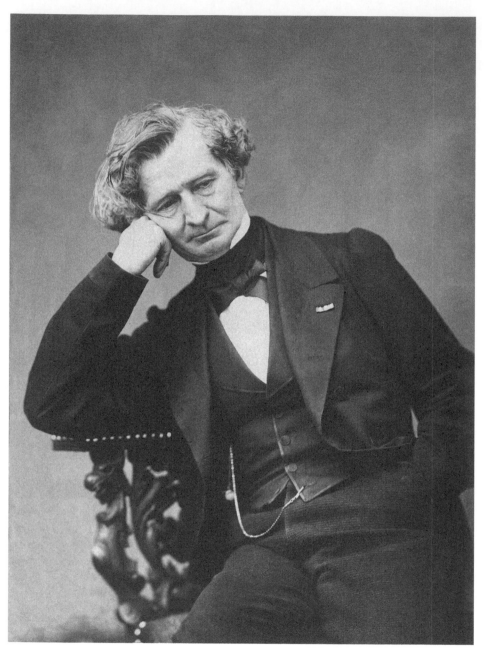

16 Berlioz – A life *fantastique*.

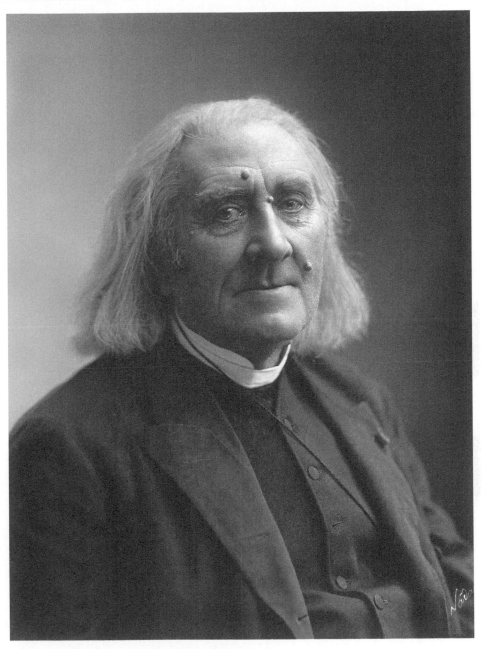

17 Liszt – Once film star good looks reduced to sad old age.

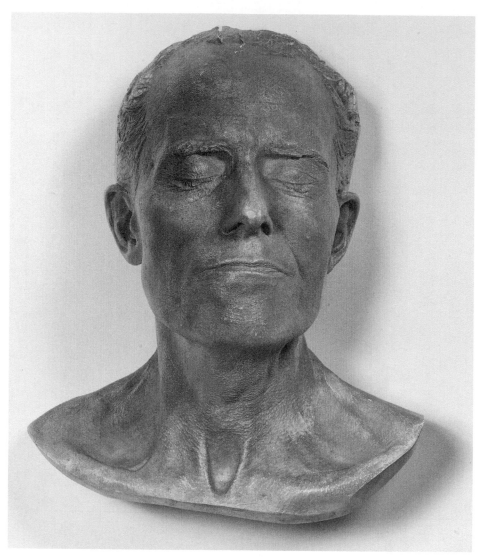

18 Mahler's death mask – Undaunted by death.

19 Britten – Aesthete and athlete

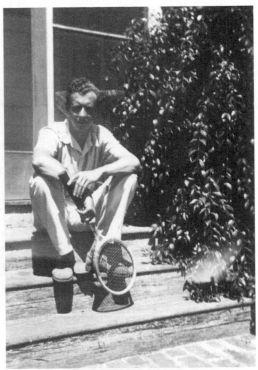

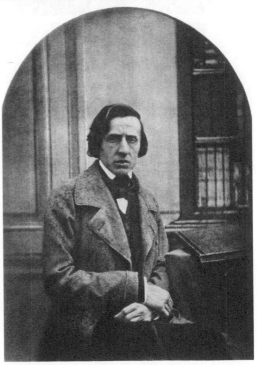

20 Chopin – The last picture.

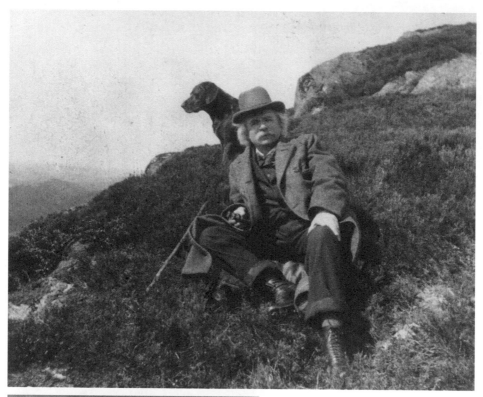

21 Grieg – A mountaineer with one lung.

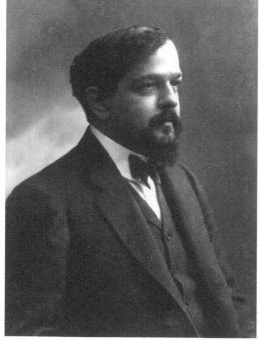

22 Debussy – The afternoon of an enigma.

23 Brahms – A scruffy intellectual.

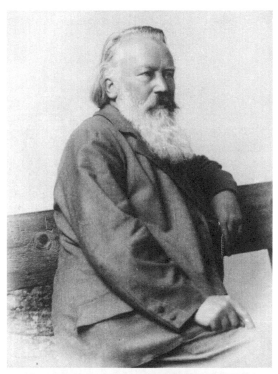

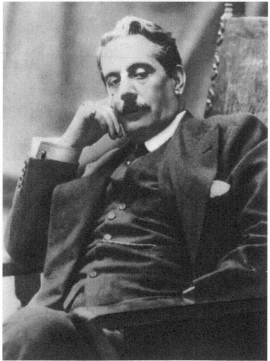

24 Puccini – Forever haunted.

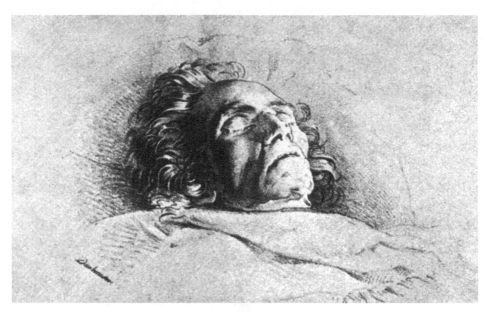

25 Beethoven – Josef Danhauser's death-bed sketch.

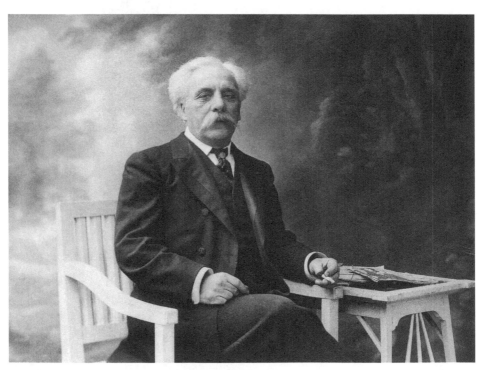

26 Fauré – Always a gentle man.

✝ **Chapter 6** ✝

Troubled Minds:
Mental Illness and Suicide

We poets in our youth begin in gladness:
But thereof come in the end despondency and madness
                William Wordsworth, 'Resolution and Independence', 1807

Some Psychiatric Disorders

A. Non-organic disease
  1 Neuroses
    • Anxiety
    • Depression
    • Obsessive-compulsive disorder
    • Paranoia
  2 Psychosis
    • Schizophrenia
    • Bipolar affective disorder (previously known as manic-depressive psychosis)
  3 Personality disorder
    • Alcoholism
    • Other addictions
    • Psychopathy

B. Organic brain disease
    • Dementias
      - Alzheimer's disease
      - Niemann Pick disease (aka Pick's)
      - Senile dementia (arterio-sclerotic)
    • Wernicke's encephalopathy (alcoholism)
    • General paralysis of the insane, or GPI (third-stage syphilis)

Diseases in group B, unlike those in A, are diseases whose consequences would be identifiable at an autopsy.

Introduction: Mental Illness

Having already regarded alcoholism as a mental disturbance, we now consider other psychiatric disorders. It is a complicated group of disorders and more difficult to categorise than physical diseases, but the list above attempts a simple, if somewhat dated, classification. At some stage in their lives at least 25% of the Western population will report psychological illness. The question is where variations within a socially accepted range of normality merge into an illness. There have been repeated attempts to assess the role of madness in creativity.[1] Is mental illness a positive driving force or an inhibition when considering the end product, be that a painting, novel or symphony? In a review of mental illness the names of great composers featured less than those of painters, poets or writers.[2]

If we consider composers discussed in other chapters, it is clear that many fit into the list. Ravel (Chapter 3) had pre-senile dementia, and Rachmaninov (Chapter 10) and Elgar (Chapter 2) were melancholic, if not frankly depressive. Sibelius (Chapter 2) sometimes drank too much. Musorgsky (Chapter 5) did suffer from alcoholic dementia. Donizetti, Smetana and Wolf (Chapter 4) developed general paralysis of the insane (GPI). This chapter is confined to composers with major non-organic psychiatric problems (group A) which were sufficient to affect their compositional abilities or become life-threatening and/or to require periods of institutional care.

It is interesting to reflect on past psychiatric care. Straitjackets and padded cells are all but gone, and with them immersion in hot and cold baths. The era of institutionalised long-term care is largely over. The modern trend is to rapidly ease people back into the community, sometimes for compassionate reasons, but possibly for economic ones too. The psychiatric wing of an acute teaching hospital from this author's professional lifetime is now the administrative block, and jocund remarks are made regarding the suitability of such transformation. Those now charged with care of the psychologically ill have excellent drugs at their disposal with much less tendency than in the past to make their poor recipients merely docile or stuporous.

Probably the most celebrated long musical history of psychiatric disorder is the sad case of Robert Schumann.

✢ ROBERT SCHUMANN ✢
(1810–1856)

A man haunted by genius
Hector Berlioz

On 27 February 1854, two fishermen rescued a bedraggled figure from the Rhine, whereupon he tried to jump in a second time.[3] It was Robert Schumann whom they had saved. That poor man, for many years intermittently visited by demons, had so lost the balance of his mind that he had jumped suicidally off a river bridge in Düsseldorf, having run away from the loving care of his family.[4] Another bridge in Schumann's tragic life was that between gentle innocence and deep dark torment. The image of this kindly man, often happiest with his loyal wife Clara and their children, was disturbed when papers left by Schumann's attending psychiatrist, Dr Richarz, were made public in 1991. These were abstracted by Rietschel et al. from Franken's paper in German.[5] That Schumann was suffering from the final stages of cerebral neurosyphilis evidently may have been Richarz's long-concealed opinion. Peter Ostwald, an American German-speaking psychiatrist, has thoroughly researched papers and correspondence that relate to Schumann and are now kept in Zwickau.[6] He believes that Schumann did not have third-stage neurosyphilis, although that suspicion persists and, in part, comes from Schumann himself.[7]

The certainty is that Schumann was often mentally sick. To dispassionately analyse Schumann's complex psychological and medical history we turn to his early life. Remaining dispassionate is difficult with the vision of a family fireside and children at their father's knee. Composers can be terribly vulnerable people; perhaps Schumann was even more so, especially as one remembers Clara trying to give him a posy of flowers as the men in white coats took him away for ever.

Early Years

In the year of Robert's birth, his father, a successful book-seller and publisher,[8] had been struck 'by a nervous disorder', something of which there was a family history. Initially the boy, whilst showing musical and literary talent, was not outstanding. His was a sensitive and cyclothymic disposition. In 1826 his sister, Emilie, who suffered from a skin disease, possibly

took her own life.[9] Schumann's father had died just before Emilie, and
Robert, then aged sixteen, became depressed by all of this. When he was
twenty he confessed to being haunted by fears of insanity, and when he
was eighteen he wrote that he thought he had actually gone mad.[10] He
then came under the tutelage of a piano teacher, Friedrich Wieck, whilst
supposedly studying law. He lodged with the Wiecks, promising to reduce
his champagne and cigar consumption, a pledge which was unfulfilled,
perhaps sowing the seeds of Wieck's disapproval of him. Eric Sams suggested that by 1832 Wieck may have suspected that Schumann had syphilis.[11] This was to re-surface as Wieck's daughter Clara grew into a lovely
young woman and one of Europe's most brilliant virtuoso pianists, to
whom Robert famously lost his heart, despite his earlier, possibly errant,
ways.[12] Wieck had spotted Schumann's potential, but doubted his resolution, although Robert was very ambitious.[13]

Injuries of Hand and of Penis

It may be that his ambition as a concert pianist led to the hand injury first
mentioned by Schumann in 1831 and causing weakness of several digits.[14]
Various consultations followed, at one of which he was advised to stick his
right hand into the entrails of a warm, freshly slaughtered animal, where
the 'good' from bodily juices might be beneficial to his hand.[15] Mercifully,
his well-known hypochondria took over, and he feared that the essence
might poison his system. He wrote to his mother on 6 November 1832,
'My hand is incurable.'[16] Henson and Urich gave a thoroughly researched
account of this in 1978.[17] The injury may have been caused by his using a
hand-strengthening device, a view firmly asserted by Jensen.[18] In his book
on piano technique, Wieck wrote in 1859 of a self-invented 'finger tor-
mentor' used by an unnamed 'famous pupil'.[19] A balance of probabilities
points to Schumann. The problem, as Sams indicated, is that Schumann,
a sometimes obsessive but constant diarist, did not mention an invention,
torment or serious injury to the hand.[20] In 1839 he said, 'Some fingers,
no doubt because of too much writing and playing in earlier years, have
become quite weak so that I can hardly use them.' Finger strengthen-
ers were quite common in the mid-nineteenth century; Sams quoted
Bötticher, who had recorded Robert Schumann ordering one, but not
until 1837, six years after the onset of this disability. Clara believed that the
strengthener did not cause his injury.[21] She attributed the problem to his
practising on a stiff dummy keyboard.[22]

The 'penile wound' is another totem in Schumann's history. Amongst neat and sometimes intimate diary entries made whilst in Leipzig during 1831, he confided that he had developed an exquisitely painful 'wound'.[23] Sams, in a personal communication with Ostwald, believed it was a syphilitic sore (chancre),[24] overlooking the fact that such sores are characteristically painless. Whether the wound was of his penis has nevertheless also been debated. The researches of Ostwald and Worthen leave me with little doubt that it was.[25] The records of hand weakness, which was non-progressive, are not redolent of neurosyphilis. Slater and Meyer charted composition and performance with Schumann's diary whilst commenting on the effects of his reported mood changes, delusions and worse.[26] They believed that the recorded progress of the hand condition reflected vicissitudes of his mood. But which was cause and which was effect? Moreover, the condition improved, and some piano playing therewith.[27]

A medical report written by Schumann's friend Dr M. E. Reuter in January 1841, when the composer was called to military service, is worth quoting.[28]

> In his youth he first noticed that the second and third fingers were less strong and agile than the others.* Prolonged use of a machine with which fingers were forcibly dorsiflexed [bent back] led to a paralytic state of these fingers, in which there was only weak sensation and their movement was not subject to military control. He was compelled to give up a virtuoso career, but the fingers have remained in the same paralytic condition despite repeated attempts at treatment so that, in playing the piano, he cannot use the middle finger at all and the index finger only partially. He is incapable of holding objects in his hand.

Dr Güntz for the militia was of a similar opinion six months later, concluding that 'He cannot carry out arms drill reliably.'[29] In 1842 Dr Brachman was instructed by the military authorities to prepare a further report.[30] He opined, 'The paralysis of the index and middle fingers of the right hand is only partial and does not prevent him from playing the piano as is generally known. By the same token it should prevent him even less from handling a gun.' Subsequently, Schumann was rejected by the military for other medical reasons, such as short-sightedness or hypertension, which Dr Brachman had suspected.[31]

Talk of guns recalls another unusual diagnosis. Carerj has claimed that

---

* He almost certainly meant second and third digits, not fingers. The second and third digits are the index and long fingers; the thumb is not a finger.

Dr Richarz's autopsy of Schumann had revealed a trigger finger which caused Schumann's hand problem.[32] Trigger finger is a common condition in which a tendon for bending a finger becomes stuck, leaving the finger locked in a flexed position. It is easily relieved by a small operation. In a nineteenth-century autopsy, conducted by a psychiatrist, the balance of probabilities has to be enormously against evidence for it being found. The diagnosis is about the easiest in all of clinical medicine, provided the patient is still alive. Henson and Urich conclude: 'There seems little doubt that the condition was neurologically determined.'[33] They diagnosed that a branch of the radial nerve (posterior interosseous nerve) had become compressed in a muscle tunnel within the forearm.

Compression of peripheral nerves is quite frequent: that of the ulnar nerve, behind the 'funny bone' at the elbow, and of the median nerve at the wrist (carpal tunnel syndrome), is common. That of the posterior interosseous nerve is uncommon and nebulous in its random presentation,[34] although it has been described amongst musicians.[35] If only extension (straightening) of the index and middle (long) fingers was affected, then posterior interosseous nerve compression is a good suggestion. Henson and Urich explain why the cause of the problem did not lie further up the 'electronic circuit' of nerves which 'wire up' the locomotor system.[36] On that basis, disease in the spinal cord or brain can be discarded and, with it, so can syphilis.

Mention of strengthening machines evokes a suspicion that Schumann could have developed an overuse syndrome, perhaps by using a dummy keyboard,[37] as he and Clara did. A characteristic of overuse syndromes, not unusual amongst musicians, is that the onset is often insidious. Much the same can be said of that recent and litigious group of disorders known as repetitive strain injuries (RSI) with which secondary gain is often associated,[38] as are psychological factors. There has been surprisingly little attention to either a psychological component or RSI as it may have affected Schumann's hand, despite his psychiatric history. For all his problems with the piano, Schumann continued to write copious letters in a good hand.

When the hand problem first obtruded, Schumann was a sensitive, highly-strung individual with serious mood swings. He was passionately in love with Clara. She was a greater pianist than he ever would be. For an ambitious man in a male-dominated profession, perhaps a sick note for a hand injury let him bow out from the concert platform without losing face and do what ultimately he did better than Clara, and that was composing. In March 1834 Schumann had written of his hand that he could 'compose without it', reflecting that life as a travelling virtuoso concert pianist could not be any happier than it was now.[39] Was it all 'creative malady'?[40]

More Depression

In about 1830 Schumann had talked of jumping into the Rhine,[41] whereafter he always tried to occupy ground-floor rooms. He became seriously depressed again in 1833 after another double death: those of his sister-in-law, and then his brother Julius, from tuberculosis.[42] Also in 1833 Robert contracted malaria, from which he made a good recovery.[43] In 1836 Wieck severed all relations between his family and Robert. There were periods of frenzied activity, and passionate despair generally followed such bursts. In 1837 he, or 'Florestan' (representing heroism) and 'Eusebius' (suffering) – alter egos who appear in *Carnaval* – composed the F sharp major Sonata Opus 11 for Clara. During that year, Clara contacted Robert, whereupon Wieck took her away on a seven-month concert tour. Robert despaired again. The story of how Robert and Clara fought their way through the courts before marrying in 1840 has been told many times.[44] With it went recurrent depression and intermittent elation, and probably some heavy drinking, which had been part of the basis for Wieck's opposition to Schumann.

That the marriage at times became difficult was inevitable, but it was also filled with the love and domestic security which Schumann probably craved. In his elation shortly after marriage, Robert quickly sketched the First Symphony, followed by what was to become the Fourth Symphony as well as the A minor Piano Concerto. In this state during 1842, he started to compose the Piano Quintet. That is a piece of such radiant vigour that it is hard to imagine its composition other than by a person who was self-confident, if only at the time, and yet, as he completed it, he admitted to feeling melancholy again.[45] Just before that, an elated Schumann had rapidly composed three string quartets.[46] Schumann himself said that, whereas outwardly he seemed lacking in confidence, inwardly he felt much more confident. Yet when the couple toured in Russia, he was depressed again. Ostwald believes this may have been a reaction to press notices of concerts, at which he was 'Clara Schumann's husband'.[47] During October 1844 Clara found him 'swimming in tears' whilst they were in Dresden.[48] There he consulted two homeopaths, namely the Drs Müller, and then the court physician, Dr Carl Gustavus Carus, because of the gross fluctuations in his mood and thoughts of suicide.[49] He was given cathartic salts, with hot and cold baths and various medications.[50] In February 1846, whilst working on his Second (C major) Symphony, he complained of tinnitus (ringing in the ears);[51] and nearer his end this complaint was repeated, although deafness was never recorded. Tinnitus is a very common complaint, usually with no demonstrable cause.

Schumann had written that his 'semi-invalid state' might be divined in the Second Symphony, which reminded him of dark times, probably resulting from the depressive end of his bipolar disorder in 1844. Composition had ceased in 1845. The Second Symphony seems (to this ear) more an acclamation from a recovery in his spirits. He recorded the commencement, 'when I had hardly got over my illness'.[52] The first movement is redolent of struggle, but the complex scherzo second movement may owe much to Schubert's 'Great' Ninth Symphony, also in C major. There is a relentless affirmative bustling energy with both Schubert's Ninth and Schumann's Second. The symphony comes to a seemingly contented resolution in its final movement, which he marked 'Allegro molto vivace'. He had reported musical excitement in the last movement.[53] Could the Second Symphony's programme be one of 'I was down and ill; I then started to energetically recover'?

1848 was the year of revolution, not least in Dresden. The Schumanns' response to this disturbance is revealing. Robert, who had little interest in politics, left very rapidly with Clara and their eldest child by train, leaving the other children with servants in Dresden. Once Robert was settled in Mügelen, Clara, although seven months pregnant, two days later returned to Dresden at 3.00a.m. with two women to retrieve the rest of her brood, leaving Robert to record these events in his diary.[54] Subsequently they returned to Dresden, where Robert did not obtain the leading posts he desired and felt snubbed. So in 1850 they finally left for him to become music director in Düsseldorf, where early success was mixed with his apparent lack of vigour, which was especially noted after 1850.[55] He was not a good conductor, and there were difficulties between the Schumanns and both the chorus and the music committee.[56] However his symphonic masterpiece, the Third ('Rhenish') Symphony, composed in only five weeks, had its successful premiere there, greatly raising Schumann's spirits.[57]

In 1852 Clara noted a 'rheumatic attack', with further insomnia, dizziness and depression. The onset of some hesitancy of speech and of apathy was more ominous, as were 'serious giddiness and remarkable aural symptoms' in the autumn of that year.[58] In July 1853 Schumann even suspected that he had suffered a stroke.[59] Yet he then went on to compose for Joachim the *Fantasie* for violin and Violin Concerto. It was Joachim who, in September 1853, brought young Johannes Brahms to the Schumanns.[60] Thereafter Brahms was seldom far from their affairs or place in musical posterity. Curiously, Schumann referred to Brahms and Joachim as his 'demons'.[61]

Disintegration

In 1853 Clara had been indulgent towards Robert's 'table moving', feeling that the cheering effect it had upon him outweighed the oddity of his moving tables by 'personal magnetism'.[62] That year Robert became quite vituperative about Clara's success, and one turns for an explanation to his own professional decline. There are accounts of him reacting strangely and of his failing in rehearsal to pick up glaring errors.[63] It is now hard to judge whether Schumann was a bad conductor because of his fragile, worsening health, or whether conducting was just not his forte; possibly both were true. Yet in late 1853 the Schumanns toured Holland successfully: he with the baton, she playing the piano, both for music by Robert. Ostwald has commented that, away from home, Schumann was better able to keep his psychosis under control.[64] Early in 1854, he started to catalogue his own music and, it was noticed, in a neat hand, revealing no evidence of organic brain disease, tremor or a chronically disabled hand.[65]

On 10 February 1854 Schumann recorded 'very strong and painful aural symptoms', then wonderfully beautiful music constantly sounding in his head. Sadly, the wondrous company of angels was soon to be joined by demons.[66] Two weeks later he asked to be sent to the asylum.[67] Instead, Clara sent him to bed; he said he was unworthy of her love. Two days later the boatmen rescued him from the Rhine and, for a short time, he was nursed at home, where Clara was not allowed to see him. On 4 March 1854 he was admitted as a voluntary patient to Dr Richarz's Endenich asylum near Bonn.[68] There he had his own room and access to a piano, exercised daily and was visited by Joachim and Brahms, but again Clara was forbidden access to him.[69] There seems to be a division of opinion here over whether she was prevented from seeing him on medical advice or was just too busy with the children and her own career. It seems that the cause lay with Dr Richarz, who would not permit Clara to see him,[70] and not with Clara, who surely wanted to play Leonora to Robert's Florestan in that romantic age. Richarz could have been concerned that Schumann might harm Clara, about which Robert had dreamed. This was a good wife who had already shown herself lovingly lacking in objectivity about her Robert.[71] One wonders whether it occurred to Clara that Robert really was not a good conductor, teacher or communicator. Richarz was gauche in his dealings, informing Clara that Robert did not recognise her exist- ence,[72] which in reality could have implied several things without meaning he did not love her.

Clara made repeated agitated complaints, particularly about getting no information from the staff regarding her husband's condition, although Richarz and his assistant, Peters, did write to her from time to time. By the spring of 1854 Robert had improved, and it was then that their last child, Felix, was born.[73] After six months Robert was still incarcerated, possibly for his own protection, enjoying his view of Bonn and affably communicative, but he was forgetful and easily agitated. In September 1854, he wrote his first letter to Clara for months, or at least the first that has been available to historians. It was lucid, well written and full of both questions and affection. He exclaimed, 'Oh! If only I could see and speak to you again.'[74] Not only was her visiting forbidden, but Ostwald reports evidence that the doctors actually withheld letters between them;[75] however, he is equivocal as to whether Richarz prevented her visiting or whether she, in fact, distanced herself from a problem that was now out of her hands. Staff scrutinised, even restricted, all correspondence,[76] which may be an explanation for her passing close to Endenich on her own travels and not visiting. To know that the poor fellow was there must have been agonising enough, without having the door politely closed in her face had she tried to see him.

At Christmas 1854, those two stalwarts Joachim and Brahms became dissatisfied with Schumann's care.[77] Robert himself confided that he wanted to leave Endenich, where he said the staff completely misunderstood him. Thereafter clearly he deteriorated, although in the spring of 1855 Bettina von Arnim, a poet and friend, demanded to see him.[78] She reported that he spoke as he often spoke, in almost hushed tones, although this may have been to avoid being overheard by the staff. He commenced by saying that it had become difficult to speak, whereafter he conversed loquaciously with her upon many topics. Sams suggested that Schumann's voice was affected by syphilis.[79] Von Arnim described Schumann as being 'the only rational human being' at Endenich and tried to have him discharged or transferred elsewhere,[80] as Robert had requested.

Clara received her last known letter from Robert on 5 May 1855.[81] He had shown some improvement over several months and he was even working on the Paganini Caprices, although when he ran out of paper he was not always given more until Brahms visited. The Caprices were originally a composition from 1853, and there was little evidence of fresh musical input to them at Endenich. It was just encouraging to see him attempting to work again. The reason why Dr Richarz did not discharge his patient then remains elusive. Perhaps Richarz was protecting Clara and not Robert.[82] Instead, he advised Clara that there would never be a full recovery.[83] Then Robert became more incoherent and somnolent, possibly because of sedative medication.[84] Lederman, like Ostwald, believes that this sedated pattern at Endenich was due to the administration of drugs such as chloral hydrate, morphine and even chloroform.[85] By the time Brahms visited him in April 1856, Schumann spoke continuously, but almost incomprehensibly. He had been busy listing names of towns and countries in a good hand. He had become alarmingly thinner, probably because he had gone on hunger strike, which Richarz had recorded in his diary.[86] Jensen comments on Richarz's lack of compassion.[87] By this time Schumann was restless, occasionally aggressive, and for this he was 'punished', as for example by confiscation of his books and other possessions.[88] Ostwald found evidence from Richarz's papers of 1871 that several inmates at Endenich had died by going on hunger strike, something which Richarz had reported in a professional journal.[89] At last, on 14 July 1856 Clara went to visit Robert, but did not see him. Dr Richarz evidently 'could not' and thus did not 'allow' her to see him, but told her he could not promise that her husband would be there in another year's time.[90] Clara returned with Brahms on 23 July, having been warned that Robert was close to death but, once more, Richarz could not allow her to see her husband.[91]

The End

She was called back, and on 27 July those two nineteenth-century romantics Robert and Clara Schumann met for the first time in two and a half years. It was to be almost their last meeting. Clara recorded the moment: 'He smiled at me and then embraced me with great effort, because he could no longer control his limbs. Never will I forget it, for all the world's treasures I would not exchange this embrace. My Robert, that's how we have to meet again.'[92] That he had lost control of his limbs was probably due to his advanced state of emaciation and weakness. Clara tried to feed him herself and, on 28 July, persuaded him to take some soup and wine. The next day she and Brahms went to the railway station to meet Joachim. When they returned, Robert Schumann, aged forty-six, musical scion of German Romanticism, was dead, relieved of the mental torture by which his whole being had been increasingly consumed.[93]

Richarz conducted an autopsy, something for which psychiatrists and neurologists seldom have natural gifts. At best, their interests were with the central nervous system. Dr Ostwald examined Richarz's report in detail.[94] He regarded comments about the skull, the meninges and the brain itself as inconclusive and inevitably so, not least because microscopy at that time was very primitive. Richarz did report the brain as being slightly lighter than expected.[95] From the recorded observations, there was no obvious evidence of pathology in the brain, and nothing to support a diagnosis of cerebral atrophy, neurosyphilis or chronic alcoholism (Wernicke's encephalopathy). Dr Richarz recorded that the body was emaciated and that the heart was both enlarged and thin-walled, indicating heart failure. It has been suggested that Schumann was hypertensive,[96] but without measurements we cannot take that further, although it is a possible cause of heart enlargement, a more likely cause for which was malnutrition. Such changes, which become irreversible, are often the cause of death in people with severe anorexia nervosa or after hunger strike, as well as with prisoners of war. The report does not mention the liver, kidneys, the gastrointestinal tract or the genito-urinary system (i.e. guts and waterworks).

Syphilis or Not?

A probable origin of the syphilitic diagnosis was the teenage wound assumed by Sams to have been a syphilitic chancre,[97] but painful tears of the foreskin, especially in those who remain uncircumcised, are common amongst sexually energetic men, and chancres are painless. Moreover, in his extensive study of all the Schumann papers, Ostwald said he could find no evidence that the painful wound was of his penis anyway. In Jensen's view that evidence is inconclusive.[98]

Ostwald conducted an analysis of Schumann's hair, locks of which Clara had preserved. Only small traces of mercury were found.[99] These were of an order which one might encounter from the wearer of a hat whose band had been treated with mercury, or alternatively in the case of someone who took any of the tonics and general medicines that were then commonplace. This is quite strong circumstantial evidence against syphilis. The clinical point at which the prescription of mercury was reduced in the treatment of syphilis was when excess salivation or the shakes occurred or teeth fell out. Of that there is no recorded mention in the diaries or correspondence between Schumann and his immediate circle. This is not an assured exclusion of syphilis, but makes it highly improbable. If Schumann was syphilitic, why did Dr Richarz not treat him with mercury, as would have been standard practice in the 1850s? Of mercury prescription there is no apparent evidence either, within the limitations of incomplete medical records available to Ostwald.

O'Shea reports that after analysing Schumann's remaining letters,

Ostwald found his intellectual faculties to be well preserved until 'shortly before his death'.[100] Worthen opines similarly regarding his physical symptoms.[101] 'Shortly' may be inconsistent with Robert's last known letter to Clara having been written more than a year before he died. But then how extensive was Richarz's censorship of correspondence between Robert and Clara? On the basis of statements by Richarz, Ostwald argued that Schumann's late mental features were not typical of third-stage syphilitic dementia (GPI).[102] There is a famous sign in the eyes with syphilis, the Argyll Robertson (AR) pupil. The pupil or pupils become small and often irregular, reacting to light but not to variations in near and distant vision (accommodation). Worthen quotes a German paper which described Schumann's pupils at Endenich being of unequal size, irrespective of ambient light.[103] This was a decade before Argyll Robertson described his sign, which is now always associated with syphilis. Furthermore, Worthen's description could be one of several other conditions (e.g. Adie's syndrome). Moreover, syphilis is not the only cause of AR pupil; it may be seen in diabetes. On the evidence, were there to be an otherwise stronger scenario of tertiary syphilis, one would be very suspicious. What deflects us from that course can also be found in Worthen's book, for he points to Schumann's physical and intellectual symptoms until shortly before Endenich as being vague.[104] Those of late syphilis would have been preceded by features whose description is sparse or absent from available accounts. Most importantly the features recorded are insufficient to sustain a diagnosis of AR.

Jensen quotes Schumann as having said to Richarz on 12 September 1855, 'I was syphilitic and was cured by arsenic in 1831.'[105] That surely amounts to *mea culpa* – or does it? It would be another fifty-two years before a reliable blood test for syphilis was introduced. Moreover, it was not until 1830 that syphilis became diagnostically disentangled from other venereal diseases. Treatment with arsenic became common only in 1908. Did Schumann say this because he deduced it from past misdemeanours, or because a doctor had told him? Someone with a cyclothymic personality, such as Schumann, may have expressed guilt from a conscience which had long since weighed heavily upon him. Jensen describes him in Endenich as a man burdened by guilt. How sound his state of mind was at this time would be a court's first question. Even upon a balance of probabilities, this judgement at best remains uncertain.

In the absence of a Wassermann test and an up-to-date medical examination, we shall never know whether, like Schubert, Schumann died *with* syphilis, let alone *of* it. Writing over fifty years ago from the Maudsley

Neurological Institute In London, Slater and Meyer reviewed the information available then, concluding that Schumann had a personality disorder and was not schizophrenic but that he was bipolar. Syphilis was unlikely to have killed him but could not be excluded, although the symptoms before he was admitted to Endenich were atypical.[106] They concluded that the most likely cause of death was emaciation induced as a result of his supposed psychiatric treatment. It seems very improbable that he died of, or even with, syphilis. His treatment latterly may have been force-feeding by a nasogastric tube, even purgation by enemas.[107] Blood-letting was almost inevitably used, and hot and cold baths were fairly routine then. But at that time perhaps it was accepted use and custom, although not everywhere. It should not prevent us considering what effects this might have had on his heart, and above all else the balance of his metabolism, let alone that of his mind. To this care we may attribute the accounts by Brahms or Joachim of his exhibiting malcoordination or 'seizure'.[108] It was the latter which provoked the final call for Clara to visit her beloved husband.

It is instructive to briefly digress and ask how unwelcome diagnoses become attached to great people. An ardent claim that Schumann may have been syphilitic came from Sams,[109] whose ardour in pursuing the diagnosis is surprising after his more scholarly work with Schubert's case (see Chapter 4). He did not primarily base his diagnosis on the clinical features, although some were suggestive, but upon his conviction that the hand condition was due to nerve damage (neuropathy) caused by mercury.[110] As to neuropathy, two eminent neurologists, Henson and Urich, aver that 'Mercurial neuropathy is so rare as to raise doubts as to causation.'[111] They continue: 'We have been unable to trace a recorded example of isolated mono-neuropathy because of mercury poisoning.' Sams's claim that, as lead causes neuropathies, then mercury, which is similar to lead, must do so too is stretching attribution too far.[112] Furthermore, neuropathy due to poisoning is progressive, which Schumann's hand condition was not. Sams continued that Schumann went to Leipzig – 'a notorious source of syphilis' – and then asserted that Schumann was very short-sighted (uncertain anyway), egregiously concluding that 'Severe myopia at 30 is consistent with syphilis.'[113] His rejection of mechanical causes for Schumann's hand injury, in that 'nothing less than a thumbscrew' might have caused it,[114] has no basis in current knowledge of hand conditions. Sams also suggested that Schumann's mention in 1831 of his hand 'trembling' was an example of 'hatters' shakes',[115] a classic feature of mercury poisoning, immortalised by Lewis Carroll's Mad Hatter. This too should be discarded. Such shakes are neurologically progressive, whereas Schumann's 'accurate and precise' cataloguing of all his compositions was completed in January 1854, just weeks before the admission to Endenich.[116] Eric Sams's judgements regarding Schumann's illness and death may be disregarded.

Conclusion

By today's standards the treatment of Robert Schumann is open to serious criticism. But let us remember what a 'reasonable body of doctors would have done at that time'. The easiest way usually to exonerate (or sometimes condemn) a doctor's care of a patient is to examine case notes. In the story of Robert Schumann that is impossible. Attempts have been made. Unlike records regarding other inmates at Endenich, many of his are missing.[117] Ostwald implies they may have been destroyed, perhaps by Richarz himself, suggesting either that there may have been anxiety regarding a charge of malpractice, or alternatively that Richarz was protecting a great man's reputation.

The question as to what Schumann might have achieved had he not become psychotic is straightforward to answer. He would have been a totally different person and composed accordingly. What is clear is that Schumann intermittently drank heavily, as alleged by Wieck,[118] causing composition to be suppressed; but which was cause and which effect is unclear. Slater and Meyer's diagrammatic correlation between mood and composition vividly leaves little doubt that depressive episodes were passages of musical silence.[119] The lingering and tantalising issue is: what did Schumann's periods of elated mania do? It is an important question because Schumann's case is most unusual in this study, in that his was not an organic brain disease, as the autopsy confirmed.

The most revealing and happy period was 1841–42, after his marriage, when music quickly flowed. However, there seems no reason to judge these works any differently from similar works from other composers. Little substantial music came after 1853, and the quality of the last pieces may be questioned. Significantly, Clara is reputed to have suppressed, even destroyed, some late compositions as unworthy.[120] Schumann's was a classic case of bipolar affective disorder, as first described in 1906 by Grühle, who rejected Möbius's diagnosis of schizophrenia.[121] For all the lingering doubts, it must be said that to totally separate a sometimes deeply depressed but loving man from his family was, at the best, inhumane. His institutionalised treatment must have had a devastating effect upon a partly broken mind and have gravely assaulted his physical well-being to the point of chronic anaemia and emaciation. As Dr Richarz himself observed, Schumann died in 'a state of extreme emaciation'.[122] At Richarz's asylum he was a captured bird, at times wildly irritable and at others inconsolable, in a captivity for which he himself had asked. This paradox, like the question as to whether syphilis was the last scorer against his name, remains buried with him.

✢ ANTON BRUCKNER ✢
(1824–1896)

Half god – half imbecile
Gustav Mahler[123]

Bruckner's biographer Karl Grebe said, 'His life does not tell us anything about his work and his work does not tell us anything about his life.'[124] An essentially inoffensive man, Bruckner evoked vituperative controversy in his own lifetime. Brahms described 'symphonic boa constrictors'. Admittedly, Bruckner preferred the waltzes of the younger Johann Strauss to the symphonies of Brahms.[125]

Bruckner became intimate with death as six of his eleven siblings died in infancy, and his father succumbed to tuberculosis when Bruckner was only twelve. Thereafter he sought, as fatherless boys often do, alternative father figures. Later they even included his friend the conductor Hermann Levi, who was fifteen years his junior. Bruckner became an assistant schoolmaster in Windhaag, earning a pittance,[126] which perhaps explains his lifelong preoccupation with financial security. When he was nineteen he moved to a more congenial post in Kronstorf.[127] There his formidable abilities at the organ became clear. But it was during these experiences that his tendency to be pedantic, subservient and especially deferential to authority figures developed. The borderline between orderly pedantry and pathologically obsessive behaviour became indistinct.

In 1845 he returned, as organist and teacher, to the great Abbey of St Florian, where he had been a chorister.[128] It remained a spiritual home for the rest of his life. During 1855 he finally decided to become a composer and became cathedral organist in Linz.[129] He continued his counterpoint studies with Simon Sechter; Sechter was generally a hard taskmaster, but he noticed that Bruckner worked obsessively hard and uncharacteristically warned him not to overwork. He had never before had so dedicated a pupil.[130]

The 1860s had already revealed a cyclothymic tendency, accentuated by his wish to marry. In 1867, the year in which Sechter died, one of Bruckner's many offers of marriage was again rejected. His diary recounted a succession of failures with 'dear young ladies'.[131] A period of severe depression and nervous collapse followed. He spoke of impending madness and even threatened suicide.[132] During 1866 he had already experienced delusions that he was to bail out all the water from the Danube.[133] Gross features of numeromania followed, when he counted the stars, leaves on trees, even grains of sand.[134] One day he met a grand lady wearing a complex pearl necklace, and asked her to leave for fear that he would obsessively count the many pearls with which her bosom was emblazoned.[135] His compositions and scores bear musical inscriptions revealing his compulsion for numerical ordinance. Horton, clearly depending on Foucault, states that 'Compulsion is not manifest in thematic, tonal or harmonic elements of the music.'[136] He separates counting pebbles from musical repetition, which he reasonably describes as a basic trait of Western music, his example being Beethoven's Fifth Symphony. He reasonably infers that the frequent and intense revisions of Bruckner's work arose from insecurity. Redlich implies that Bruckner had a sexual inferiority complex.[137] To play devil's advocate, if he had, would he have blithely dressed up to go dancing and to pay court with obvious pleasure?

As a result of the turmoils which by May 1867 had overwhelmed him, he had himself admitted to a hydropathic sanatorium; he stayed there until August,[138] by which time his health had greatly improved. When he was discharged his benefactor, Bishop Rudigier of Linz, detailed a priest to stay with Bruckner as a minder,[139] whereafter he composed the F minor Mass. Another friend, the conductor Herbeck, was keen that Bruckner should succeed Sechter as professor of harmony and counterpoint in Vienna. When things were set up for him to do so, Bruckner dithered and then quibbled over money.[140] Here we see that Bruckner's problem could have been one of indecision rather than low self-esteem. Ultimately, he accepted the post and set up house in Vienna with his sister 'Nani'.[141] At first the over-powerful critic Hanslick was quite supportive. Then the naive Bruckner, who worshipped Wagner, joined the Wagner Society. Inevitably, the anti-Wagner pro-Brahms faction, led by Hanslick, identified him as an enemy, whereafter he was for many years caught in the web of Viennese musical politics.[142] Nani died in 1870, and so he engaged a housekeeper, Frau 'Kathi', who remained his faithful servant for the rest of his life.[143] Away from Vienna he met with more ready success in Paris and London during 1870–71, but that was as an organist rather than a composer.[144]

The later middle period of his life revealed other psychological peculiarities beyond numeromania. Although not a man of broad interests despite some university education in law and physics, Bruckner became preoccupied with death. He pulled strings to view the body of the Emperor Maximilian after it was returned to Vienna following his assassination in Mexico, having written to a friend that a wish to see the corpse was 'the only thing dear to my heart'.[145] Later, after a serious fire in Vienna, he gained access to view the charred corpses of the many victims.[146] Of particular interest to him was the re-interment of the mortal remains of Beethoven and Schubert. Indeed, so closely did he peer at these gruesome relics that his pince-nez fell amongst the dust and bones. This remained an intermittent dark corner in Bruckner's life, but does not seem to have been true necrophilia.

The premiere in 1877 of his Third Symphony, dedicated to Wagner, was planned under the baton of Herbeck, who then died before it took place. Bruckner himself conducted the first performance, which was a fiasco. Most of the audience left in protest before the end, but not a seventeen-year-old admirer called Gustav Mahler.[147] After this failure we encounter a recurrent theme in that Bruckner carried on regardless, starting promptly on the next symphony, sometimes even before completing its predecessor; this was the case with the Fourth ('Romantic') Symphony, which became a success. Well regarded as a university teacher, he proved popular with students and was always happy to retreat to the pub with them at the day's end. Although he enjoyed beer, there is no evidence that he drank excessively.

In 1881 Bruckner recorded that he was suffering from 'leg troubles',[148] particularly with swelling (oedema), the first harbinger of heart disease. By this time he was again mentally disturbed. His regard for Wagner by any criterion was obsequious. By his death Bruckner was again cast into despair, to which the Adagio of his Seventh Symphony bears testimony. It also reveals that, unusually for Wagner, the admiration was mutual: as Wagner said, 'I know only one who comes close to Beethoven and that is Bruckner.'[149] Bruckner had begged that, despite a successful premiere at the end of 1884 in Leipzig, his Seventh Symphony should not be performed in Vienna before the critical eye of Brahms and the vituperative pen of Hanslick,[150] who predictably poured venom after the first Vienna performance in 1886: 'unnatural, bombastic, sickly and decadent'. Worse was to come, for Bruckner immediately passed to the Eighth Symphony, which he gave to his friend Hermann Levi, who was to conduct the premiere, although Levi was confused by both its length and its complexity. He tried unsuccessfully to shield Bruckner from these concerns, but Bruckner despaired and thoughts of suicide recurred.[151] Again, a familiar pattern re-emerged as a determined but obsessional and compulsive Bruckner responded by revising not only the Eighth, but also the Third – again – with the First Symphony and F minor Mass both similarly treated.

Multiple revisions incorporating friends' suggestions and attempting to respond to criticism have baffled subsequent custodians of Bruckner's legacy, forming part of the 'Bruckner problem'.[152] As a generalisation, it seems that his low self-esteem was partial. Close attention to his approach to composition could perhaps show a lack of confidence in Anton Bruckner the man, but not in his music. However, correlating periods of mental breakdown with circumstances affecting Bruckner at the same time does not readily evoke a picture of cause and effect. Perhaps these compulsive repetitions were a response to more arcane inner compulsions. Watson inferred that Bruckner's periods of psychopathology, worst in 1867, 1887–91 and 1895–96, were not necessarily related to bad times professionally.[153] He was ill again during 1892 with shortness of breath and 'dropsy' as his legs became swollen,[154] as they first had done in 1881. This was the year of his final pilgrimage to Bayreuth. On 18 December, the premiere of his Eighth Symphony with the Vienna Philharmonic under Richter was an unqualified success. However, Bruckner, despite declining health and energy, was already writing his final and Ninth Symphony, which remained incomplete at his death. Professor Leopold Schrötter was treating him for fluid accumulation in his legs, liver and lungs, clearly a case of gross heart failure. Rest, less exertion and reduced fluid intake (especially beer) were sensible recommendations, possibly with digitalis.[155] That there were intermittent periods of recovery during the last five years makes digitalis treatment likely.

In the spring of 1893 he was much better and was able to go, as was his habit, to Steyr for an August holiday, only to be ill again. There are clear reports of breathlessness on exertion, and also of liver and stomach complaints for which a diet was prescribed.[156] The replacement of beer by milk was not to his liking. Aware that his end was approaching, he made a will with clear instructions.[157] He wished to be embalmed and placed in a casket with a glass top so that his face could be seen. Where is the low self-esteem there? These instructions also revealed an anxiety, said to be common in the nineteenth century and shared with Chopin and Mahler, that he might be buried before life was extinguished. The casket was to be placed beneath the organ at St Florian surrounded by a generous heap of skulls of the late lamented brothers. Death was a lifelong preoccupation.

In 1891 he had met a chambermaid, Ida Buhz, in Berlin to whom he became engaged in 1894; initially he was accepted but in 1895, with a typical Brucknerian mix of indecision and stubbornness, he broke off his engagement because she refused to convert from Lutheranism to his own Roman Catholicism.[158] His devout belief in God and Catholicism was probably the greatest constant throughout his life.

As was his tradition, he played the organ at Christmas in 1894, although his famous supremacy at the keyboard seemed to be in decline.[159] This was when a needle was passed into the membranes surrounding his lungs (pleura) to drain off accumulated fluid.[160] He was too ill in 1895 to attend the first performance of his Fifth Symphony under Schalk. Neumayr's review of Bruckner's diaries reveals clear evidence of increasingly fervent religious observation and accurate accounts of the number of Hail Marys, Our Fathers and Ave Marias offered.[161] Freud once said that neurosis was a private religion and religion a public neurosis, which resonates with Bruckner's obsessive-compulsive disorder and its consequences. He was known to pray whilst working not only at composition, but even on hearing church bells whilst he was lecturing.

Despite his declining cardiac condition he continued to work on the Ninth Symphony, but it had become a painstaking labour and one which was often shelved as he returned to revisions of earlier works. He went out and about less, retreating into his own little world. In 1895 Emperor Franz Josef heard of Bruckner's indisposition with typical symptoms of breathlessness and difficulty on stairs. Accordingly Bruckner, with Frau Kathi and frequent visits from his brother Ignaz and Dr Zorgo, was re-accommodated in the lodge of the Schloss Belvedere in Vienna, thanks to the emperor. In January 1896 Bruckner attended the Musikverein for the last time, hearing a performance of his *Te Deum*, to which he was carried in a sedan chair.[162] In July he nearly died and received the last rites, but again he rallied. By the end of the month he was up and about and eating well.[163] His prayer was excessive. In August he was taking little walks but, when Hugo Wolf called in early October, Bruckner was gaunt, somewhat wasted and confined to bed.[164] Bruckner realised he might not live to complete the Ninth, in which case the *Te Deum* was to substitute as the final movement, but only as a makeshift solution.[165] On the morning of 11 October 1896 he worked on the Ninth Symphony. The doctor advised against a walk that cold and windy day. At 3.00p.m. he complained of feeling very cold. Frau Kathi made him some tea, with which he was put to bed. He took a few sips, rolled over and painlessly expired.[166]

Throughout his career there were repeated episodes of composition abating as mental illness overwhelmed him. Then he returned to work, but with periods when he was driven by inner anxieties to revise earlier work, suppressing progress in developing new ideas. Cooke reflects that Bruckner's innate insecurity, worsened by harsh criticism, caused the 'Bruckner problem' with its multiple revisions and versions.[167] The genius is that, from such mental disturbance, there emerged nine cathedrals of sound, always measured and often on an epic scale. In the Ninth Symphony there is much which is tranquil, showing little sign of the inner turmoil which drove him to those revisions. Peace is supreme at the symphony's incomplete ending, and perhaps in his home, made cosy for him by Frau Kathi, so it was for the dying man too.

✣ PYOTR ILYICH TCHAIKOVSKY ✣
(1840–1893)

I would go mad were it not for music
    Letter from Pyotr Ilyich Tchaikovsky to Nadezhda von Meck, 1878[168]

During late autumn in the St Petersburg of 1893, in a downtown apartment, three figures appeared: the opera singer Nikolai Figner, Diaghilev and Rimsky-Korsakov, lifting a dead body from a bed to the table.[169] The corpse was that of Pyotr Ilyich Tchaikovsky. His life's end has been subject to delving scholarship, some coloured by bitterness and sometimes unsubstantiated claims. We will consider Tchaikovsky's life and health before turning to the great questions which remain regarding the last two weeks of his life.

A Lifeline

Born in 1840, he was sent ten years later to boarding school in St Petersburg, where he was distraught to be separated from his mother.[170] In 1850 he wrote to his former nanny that he found solace at the piano when he was sad. Later he survived scarlet fever, whilst the child of the friends with whom he lodged died of it, an event about which Tchaikovsky later experienced a strange sense of responsibility.[171] Guilt would haunt the rest of his life. His distress was even greater in 1854 when his mother died of cholera, which his father survived.[172]

He went to the St Petersburg School of Jurisprudence in 1850. From there, aged nineteen, he entered the civil service, showing little interest in his work.[173] By then he was probably actively gay, although he fell in love with a Belgian opera singer, Désirée Artôt, in 1868; she was probably the only woman he loved, apart from close relatives. Garden discards this as 'puppy love'.[174] They even became engaged, although she threw him over for a Spanish baritone.

Behaviour patterns emerged in the 1860s, including his solitary tendency, despite an elegant, courteous charm. He was easily tipped into depression, not least by adverse criticism, which there was with 'Winter Daydreams', his First Symphony, in 1868.[175] But perceptions of his own sexuality became an increasing source of introspection, to be dealt with separately. Tchaikovsky had lodged with Anton Rubinstein in Moscow as well as spending time with his own sister, Sasha, and her family in the Ukraine. In 1871 he moved into his own apartment,[176] and great compositions followed, including the successful Second ('Little Russian') Symphony at the end of 1872 and the First Piano Concerto two years later, as well as the first two string quartets. He was clearly restless and sometimes depressed, and, for most of his adult life, he suffered from 'catarrh of the stomach', which he self-dosed, usually successfully, with castor oil.[177] Here is another consistent but contrasting theme, because he avoided doctors and feared death. Despite Holden's claim of 'a lifetime of heavy drinking',[178] there is little to support a diagnosis of true alcoholism. Tchaikovsky had been depressed by the initial lack of success with *Swan Lake*. It was his marriage to Antonina Milyukova in July 1877 and the flowering of his intimate friendship with Nadezhda von Meck which both coloured and adumbrated the following years and their music.

Antonina Tchaikovskova (née Milyukova), homosexuality and Nadezhda von Meck

Tchaikovsky often wrote of his 'tendencies'. In a letter to his brother Anatoly of January 1875 he confided, 'My damned pederasty does form an unbridgeable abyss between me and most people.'[179] On 10 September 1876 he wrote to his brother Modest that after a lot of thought he had concluded that 'Our inclinations are for both of us the greatest and the most insurmountable obstacle to happiness and we must fight our nature with all our strength.'[180] Poznansky, reviewing much correspondence, claims that the issue of homosexuality became an issue of self-torment largely in 1876–77.[181] Poznansky also assesses the place of homosexuality in late nineteenth-century Russian society, revealing that there was no prosecution for homosexuality of a high-ranking official or a member of the cultural elite during that half-century.[182] He describes its cultural acceptance especially in high society. The unpopular Prince Vladimir Meshchersky, although known as the 'Prince of Sodom and citizen of Gomorrah', was variously exposed as having had sex with an itinerant cast of soldiers, actors and others.[183] This did not affect his rise through the political ranks to enjoy high office with two Tsars, who appear to have been unconcerned about homosexuality.

There are two crucial issues here. Firstly, until Tchaikovsky married he assumed, or perhaps just hoped, that his 'tendencies' could be controlled, even altered. Before his disastrous marriage he had neatly compartmentalised his 'pederastic activity'. Intercourse occurred generally with members of the lower social orders,[184] whereas he was careful whilst indulging his impulses amongst the aristocratic and cultural company with whom he associated. Poznansky infers that, as Tchaikovsky grew older, 'his homosexual anxiety' diminished. In the works of authors such as Brown or Holden, that remains uncertain, not least in relation to an attraction to his nephew 'Bob' Davidov, with its lack of reciprocal affection.[185] It was his marriage which erased any lingering association with heterosexuality.

Antonina Milyukova was an attractive music student whom Tchaikovsky had known slightly for several months when he received several letters of adulation and unrequited love from her.[186] At that time, whilst working on the Fourth Symphony and *Eugene Onegin*, he had been considering his ability to control and modulate his 'natural tendencies', which led to his contemplating marriage, to assuage rumours and please his elderly father.[187] Initially he regarded Antonina's entreaty as absurd and impossible to nurture. Then eight days later he proposed to her – perhaps an example of his innate, even impulsive, fatalism. Naturally he was accepted, despite his profession of nothing more than the platonic love of a man approaching middle age. Antonina would not have been the first woman to believe that her female charms might 'cure' a man's homosexuality.[188] The key question is whether Tchaikovsky conjectured similarly. He wrote to his brother a few days after the wedding, confiding that some 'bedtime intimacy' had occurred, although 'defloration had not'.[189] Sleep had come as 'a blessed relief', and within days he was writing from their honeymoon in St Petersburg that he had seen his wife in the bath and found her repellent.[190] Consequently he went directly to church to pray and later fled to his sister for nearly a fortnight, working again on the Fourth Symphony. She looked after him but was unsympathetic, speaking of his 'debauchery' when he promptly had a fling with his brother-in-law's manservant.[191]

After returning to Antonina he had waded into the Moscow River, wondering if the cold might induce fatal pneumonia. That he immersed himself only up to the waist calls his suicidal resolution into question.[192] Was this an attempted suicide, a *cri de coeur* or an invitation for fate to direct his own future? Curiously, he had written on the score of his Fourth Symphony, 'In the event of my death. Deliver this to Madame von Meck.'[193] After returning from the river he told Antonina that he had been fishing, and he then is said to have had a nervous breakdown.[194] Garden describes a 'coma' for forty-eight hours,[195] which is very improbable, although he may have been sedated and accordingly become stuporous. Tchaikovsky's brother Anatoly took over at this point, having also been left to look after Antonina within hours of the marriage. He saw to it that she was financially looked after and took Pyotr Ilyich to see a psychiatrist. The specialist advised total rest and that he was never to see Antonina again,[196] advice which Tchaikovsky found congenial. Despite Anatoly's firm and considerate stage-management of the brief but disastrous marriage, Antonina was not a problem which went away easily. She demanded money and moved into a flat next door to Tchaikovsky with her illegitimate child by another man. Further lovers and children followed. In 1896 she was admitted to a mental asylum in St Petersburg, where she died twenty years later.[197] Through his publisher Pyotr Jurgenson, and despite his inadequacy as a husband, Tchaikovsky did try to treat her well financially. Garden describes their marriage as a 'maliciously capricious trick of fate'.[198] Tchaikovsky was fearful of a scandal and exposé from Antonina,[199] and the borderline between maintenance and hush money may become blurred. Through this haze we see the period from the late 1870s to the early 1880s when he socially and professionally withdrew, firstly to Switzerland.

To return to the music, it is hard to conceive how the Fourth Symphony (composed May 1877 to January 1878), *Eugene Onegin* (May 1877 to January 1878) and the Violin Concerto (March to April 1878) were composed at all. A probable clue is the symphonic transition from the first three symphonies, in their often warm and reflective manner, to portents of tragedy foreshadowed in the Fourth Symphony and plangently manifest in the last two, which were composed between the summer of 1888 and early 1893. Between them came the enigmatic, unnumbered *Manfred Symphony*. Tchaikovsky appears to have entered into a period of superficial pragmatism after the delayed December 1881 premiere of his Violin Concerto. Hanslick gratuitously said of it he could 'hear the stink',[200] wounding further an always sensitive man. In the early 1880s came pieces such as *Capriccio italien*, *Mazeppa* and the '1812' Overture. Of the last, its composer said it was 'loud and noisy', having been written 'with no warm feeling of love' and with 'no artistic merit'.[201] These pieces are interesting in that there was little of the inner Tchaikovsky in them, highlighting the intense intimacy of the later and greater works. He claimed to have composed the Second Piano Concerto to stave off boredom.[202] Had boredom come of true endogenous depression, there would not have been a prompt surge of composition; the two are incompatible.

To introduce the equally important Nadezhda von Meck, we turn the clock back again to the end of 1876. Tchaikovsky had received a letter from this rich and cultured widow of a railway tycoon, who was nine years his senior. She had written to solicit some pieces for violin and piano from the composer and was to become his wealthy patroness until 1890.[203] Von Meck and Tchaikovsky deliberately never met, although their huge correspondence spared no detail or expression of intimacy. She wrote that the more fascinating he became, the more she feared his acquaintance.[204] To this day their relationship remains the subject of translation and interpretation. Above all, the Fourth Symphony, dedicated to von Meck, mirrors these turbulent times. For Tchaikovsky this was the confessional by proxy, or was von Meck a mother figure, or just Tchaikovsky's 'beloved friend', who said she loved him?[205] That he became emotionally hugely dependent upon the correspondence is beyond doubt. Nadezhda von Meck had eleven surviving children of the eighteen she had borne, and was in her forties. They clearly both wanted and needed a relationship upon a spiritual, intimate and cultured plane. The sustenance of their deep and trusting friendship probably reflected their very special needs and was a tribute to their respective skills with the written word. Review of their correspondence reveals an epistolary romance.[206] In 1882 Tchaikovsky told Modest of a mad desire to be caressed by a woman.[207] Was it the caress that he craved, or did he crave the idea of wanting to be caressed by a woman? They are two very separate issues. There is evidence that, despite his active homosexuality, he envied boy–girl love.[208]

After his first and successful visit to London in 1888 he at last took possession of a house that he could call his own, at Frolovskoye near Klin. It was there that he settled into comfortable, even contented, routines,[209] especially of composition, the triumph of which was his second ballet, *The Sleeping Beauty*, premiered at St Petersburg in January 1890 and regarded by Brown as a high spot in Tchaikovsky's composition.[210] Then came a severe shock. After upholding their intimacy for nearly fourteen years, von Meck's sudden withdrawal in October 1890 was a blow from which Tchaikovsky never fully recovered. There has always been speculation as to why the abrupt and brutal severance occurred. One view is that von Meck said her money had run out,[211] although there has been little other evidence for this, and Tchaikovsky was comfortably off by then anyway. Her children may have been concerned regarding future legacies, which presumably would have been split eleven ways, even without Tchaikovsky. Had they threatened to reveal the peculiarities and peccadillos of mother's strange friend? They may, but there is no surviving evidence to support such a theory. A few months later *The Queen of Spades* was a triumph, although it had been composed before von Meck's rejection. In 1891, whilst preparing *The Nutcracker*, he became depressed once more, retreating to Paris. By now he considered opting out of his only trip to the USA. However, Tchaikovsky had already benefited from a hefty advance of funds so there was no turning back, even when he was downcast again by the news of his sister Sasha's death.[212] America became a good distraction with dynamic schedules and great hospitality, although he promptly wept after checking into his hotel in New York.[213]

In 1893 he finally returned to Klin after another successful tour of Russian and European opera houses. Later he had abandoned his plans for an E flat minor symphony for one in B minor, which he started sketching on his return from Hamburg. He wrote to Bob on 11 February that this was to be his 'Programme Symphony'.[214] By 24 March he had finished the composition, proceeding to orchestration in July and August. Another potential title was 'A Life Symphony', before he settled on 'Pathétique'. For all its magnificence this Sixth Symphony seems to be self-engrossed music, in contrast to the late courageous works of Beethoven.

During May 1893 Tchaikovsky was in London and then in Cambridge to receive an honorary doctorate. His correspondence then affords insight into the man's cyclothymic peculiarities. He complained about the weather, although people were kind to him and he charmed his hosts. But he wrote to Bob that there were no pissoirs.[215] During that summer he was ill with abdominal pain, diarrhoea and weakness, symptoms then diagnosed as cholerine.[216] One is aware of the generally perceived persona of Tchaikovsky as a solitary, overwrought neurotic. Equally, there are accounts of his overcoming shyness and becoming sociable, witty and, with those he liked, gregarious.[217] As he became a distinctly elderly fifty-three, he may have become a calmer and less anguished person. Not long before he died he said in a letter to the poet Daniil Rathaus and to his friend Kashkin that he was a happy person.[218] In contrast, whilst in England in 1893, Tchaikovsky had expressed a readiness to quit life then,[219] although he wrote that he was glad that he had been liked, and he developed a passion for English novels, especially those of George Eliot. Tchaikovsky even considered turning a story from Eliot's *Scenes of Clerical Life* into an opera.[220] In contrast to many biographies, Tchaikovsky's friend Herman Laroche described him at this time as 'a Renaissance man contemplating life and people with love but without agitation',[221] clearly not the typical perspective of one contemplating suicide. A letter from Tchaikovsky at that time claimed he had never been happier or healthier, and in another he wrote that he believed he would live a long time.[222]

1893: Cholera, 'Pathétique' and Death

Before analysing the tragic events of October and November 1893 we must consider cholera, which is an infectious disease of the gastrointestinal system caused by the bacterium *Vibrio cholerae*. It is typically associated with poverty and poor sanitation. The usual cause is a failure to physically separate sewage from drinking water. In late nineteenth-century Russia this was well known, and for the rich and middle classes, boiling tap water before drinking and customary hand washing with toilet hygiene were regarded as conferring immunity. Herman Laroche maintained that Pyotr Ilyich was always scrupulous with his own personal hygiene.[223] That custody of water supplies was woefully inadequate became clear shortly after Tchaikovsky's death when *Vibrio cholerae* was found in the water supply to the Tsar's Winter Palace.[224]

Holden took information procured from Russian medical literature in 1903.[225] The epidemic in which Tchaikovsky died lasted from 14 May 1892 to 11 February 1896, affecting half a million people, of whom 45% died, mostly amongst the poor,[226] although cholera was not the sole province of social class five. In the week of Tchaikovsky's passing, eight people died in St Petersburg, and he was the eighth.[227] There is a typical medical picture of cholera and, to avoid repetition, the following description of Tchaikovsky's last few days illustrates it almost perfectly. The incubation period may vary from a few hours to five days, something not fully appreciated by David Brown.[228] Clinical medicine is usually based upon trends and seldom upon absolutes.

What of the Sixth Symphony? In a letter of 20 September to Jurgenson, Tchaikovsky had now come away from earlier titles; he had named it *Pateticheskaia sinfonia*.[229] Poznansky says the true translation implies 'impassioned' rather than 'pathetic'.[230] That he dedicated the 'Pathétique' to his beloved nephew Bob Davidov is clear from Tchaikovsky's own inscription upon the score, which had been used at the world premiere in St Petersburg on 28 October 1893. Correspondence between Tchaikovsky and Jurgenson reveals that 'Pathétique' had been suggested a month earlier, discrediting Modest,[231] who claimed that the title had been his brainwave the morning after the premiere. Of more importance medically is a belief that the 'Pathétique' was meant as a personal requiem, but for whom? Perhaps it was for his friend the poet Apukhtin, who had recently died.[232] Another close friend, the music critic Herman Laroche, affirmed after the composer's death that, in the time leading up to it, Tchaikovsky recounted his numerous future musical plans,[233] a view conflicting with notions of suicide.

Poznansky has researched Tchaikovsky's movements in the days leading to the final illness day by day, hour by hour. Only on 31 October does Tchaikovsky seem to have briefly disappeared from view. On the following day he met a friend, the lawyer August Gerke,[234] and then had lunch with Bob's aunt Vera.[235] That evening Tchaikovsky went to the theatre, after which he went with a group of friends to Leiner's restaurant.[236] He arose the next morning, 2 November, at Modest's flat, refusing any breakfast and complaining that he had an upset stomach.[237] He attended lunch with Modest and friends at the flat, again eating nothing. Later that day he experienced diarrhoea and vomiting, but refused to see a doctor. In the evening Pyotr Ilyich had so deteriorated that Modest sent for Dr Vasily Bertenson, the brother of Dr Lev Bertenson, who was a court physician.[238] When Lev Bertenson arrived later, he declared Tchaikovsky to be in the 'algid phase' of cholera, a condition which the brothers had never actually seen, as was often the case with society doctors at that time.[239] Characteristically, Tchaikovsky's extremities were cold and blue with lividity and black spots upon his face. He was belatedly given the traditional hot bath treatment. Despite a profound thirst, any water ingested was quickly spewed back and the diarrhoea was copious. Even so, the patient felt and looked better on 3 November. By the 4th, his doctors were worried by Tchaikovsky failing to produce urine. Today that is recognised as an inevitable consequence of gross fluid depletion and also of circulating toxins, which may cause acute kidney failure. During 4 November, Tchaikovsky deteriorated with frightening speed, becoming delirious and then comatose, and he finally died in the early hours of 5 November.[240]

Within hours of death a procession of visitors came to pay their obsequies. Rimsky-Korsakov, who had been in close attendance, expressed horror when a drunken cellist, Verzhbilovich, kissed the just-dead Tchaikovsky.[241] Rimsky questioned the application of health regulations, especially in relation to the corpse of a person who had just succumbed to cholera. Poznansky has researched those regulations, showing that they had recently been altered.[242] Thus the use of antiseptic vaporisers and the wrapping of the body in a sheet soaked in mercuric chloride, plus avoiding contact with mucus membranes (those of Verzhbilovich apart), had all complied with these rules. On the second night after death, Tchaikovsky was interred in a hermetically sealed lead-lined coffin as statutes then required.[243]

Shortly after the death rumours were abroad in St Petersburg as to the cause of death. The press assumed it was cholera and vituperatively criticised the Bertensons' clinical competence.[244] It was fair to comment that the brothers had no experience with cholera and to suggest that an experienced doctor from a public hospital should have been consulted. The faith many people have in doctors is touching. Even in the late twentieth century Poznansky implied the possibly malign effects upon Tchaikovsky of the Bertensons' delay in attending to subsequently apply the hot bath treatment.[245] However, it is also fair to say that the treatments available in 1893 were, at the best, blandishments and, at the worst, actually counterproductive, such as the notorious hot bath treatment to which Tchaikovsky's own mother had fatally succumbed.[246] Until the advent of intravenous fluids and then antibiotics with other supportive medication, the outcome from cholera was death in nearly half of all cases. It mattered little as to which doctor attended.

The Likely Cause of Death

Fig. 2 summarises the various permutations which available evidence may suggest. From the clinical descriptions it is really a contest between cholera and arsenic poisoning. The primary evidence obviously comes from Russia and the former USSR, in which both suicide and homosexuality were forbidden and unmentionable. So it is all questionable.

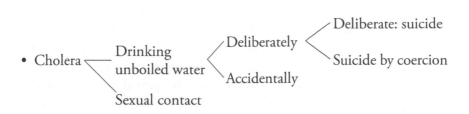

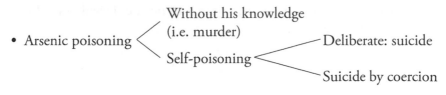

Fig. 2 Tchaikovsky's death: differential diagnosis

As a cause of death cholera is immediately obvious, with an epidemic in St Petersburg during 1893. Furthermore, Tchaikovsky's clinical course, as described by the Bertensons and their assistants, substantiates that diagnosis perfectly. The only other plausible diagnosis is that of arsenic poisoning, apart from other gastroenteric infections, which are very improbable. The question is whether the death was caused by another person or by suicide. The subsidiary question is: if it was suicide, did that come of his own free will, or was it by coercion?

It may be helpful to briefly mention the chief protagonists:

1   **Anthony Holden** discredits much of Modest Tchaikovsky's testimony, clearly believing that Pyotr Ilyich committed suicide, possibly in response to the fable of the so-called 'court of honour' (see below). He is inclined to arsenic rather than to the deliberate ingestion of unboiled, cholera-contaminated water.

2   **David Brown** appears to have been swayed by the 'court of honour' fable, speaking of a 'conspiracy of silence' in the USSR. He claimed that the inescapable conclusion universally held and unspoken in the USSR was that Tchaikovsky had committed suicide.[247] As he said, 'The story that he died of cholera from drinking unboiled water is a fabrication.' He concluded that his suicide 'could not be doubted', attributing it 'almost certainly' to arsenic.[248] Ten years later, Brown clearly remained uncertain as to whether poison or contaminated water was the culpable agent, but inclined towards poisoning. However, he promised us a revelation: 'Soon it will be disclosed in print in the USSR that the circumstances of Tchaikovsky's death are unclear.'[249] Well, bravo! Finally, in 2006 he decided that none of this mattered much, but the music did.[250] This is an understandable view, but leaves one unclear as to the standing of historical biography. Clearly, people do want to know what happened and why, as the ongoing controversies over the deaths of Richard III, JFK and Hitler demonstrate.

3   **Alexander Poznansky**'s two books after communism's fall, disappointingly, have not assuaged Russia's paranoia and addiction to secrecy. He presents vigorous research to defend Tchaikovsky from the charge of suicide.

Scenarios

To account for Tchaikovsky's last days and death, the scenarios in which these terminal events may have occurred must be considered.

1. The Court of Honour

Of this possible fable there are two accounts, with variations.

a. The Jacobi–Voitov–Orlova Version

In 1917 or possibly 1913, an old woman, Ekaterina Jacobi, told a young man, Alexander Voitov, that she had a story to publicly disclose before she died.[251] Her lawyer husband, like Tchaikovsky, had been an alumnus of the School of Jurisprudence. He had called some fellow alumni and Tchaikovsky to attend a 'court of honour' at his house in Tsarskoe Selo, sixteen miles south of St Petersburg. This kangaroo court was to protect the reputation of the School of Jurisprudence, in that it was claimed that Tchaikovsky had experienced a homosexual liaison with the nephew of Count Alexey Stenbock-Fermor. The Count was a courtier to the Tsar and, in this version of the story, these circumstances had been brought to the Tsar's attention. After five hours of interrogation, a clearly distressed Tchaikovsky left in a hurry, having been told to take his own life so as to avoid public disgrace and a possible Siberian exile, and to protect the school's honour and reputation. Jacobi said the Count had asked him to take a document regarding the affair to the Tsar's court.

Ekaterina Jacobi had been sitting with her needlework for five hours outside the door, and just happened to overhear these proceedings. In 1966 a now very elderly Voitov, who, by coincidence, had been the unofficial historian of the School of Jurisprudence, confided this story to Alexandra Orlova, the very much younger widow of Gyorgy Orlov, who had been an archivist at the Tchaikovsky museum in Klin during the 1930s.[252] In 1969 Orlova had tried unsuccessfully to publish the court of honour history, which had been censored by the Soviet authorities. In 1979 she fled to the USA, where in 1980 she published her story initially in Russian. It is now available in English.[253] Wiley quotes Voitov's widow, who denied knowledge of a court of honour.[254]

b. The Mooser–Drigo Version

Holden believes that the first account of Tchaikovsky's death came from R. A. Mooser, a Swiss musicologist who, whilst studying with

Rimsky-Korsakov and Balakirev, was friendly with Riccardo Drigo, the resident conductor of the Russian Imperial Ballet.[255] Drigo told Mooser that Tchaikovsky had seduced the son of Modest's caretaker,[256] news of which reached the Tsar, who subsequently directed there to be a court of honour, with Tchaikovsky being told to take his own life or risk shame and Siberian exile. Curiously, Mooser's memoirs have remained unpublished, although allegedly he was so astonished that he told Glazunov, who he claimed wept as he heard the story.[257] When in 1930 Nina Berberova was writing Tchaikovsky's biography, she interviewed Glazunov at length, and he made no mention of these revelations ascribed to him.[258] However, in 1990 Woodside had seen Mooser's unpublished memoirs,[259] from which Glazunov is alleged to have confirmed Drigo's account, wherein the Tsar is said to have declared that the man 'must disappear immediately'. But by then the Stalin Terrors were approaching. A variant on this theme was that Tchaikovsky had an affair with the Tsar's nephew and that the Tsar had prescribed poison or a revolver.[260]

2. A Fateful Glass of Water

What cannot be doubted is that Tchaikovsky's last few days read like a textbook account of a man dying from cholera. Tchaikovsky's well-described clinical features fit cholera so well that their being disregarded can only be on sound evidence. The question is where and how it might have been contracted, for which there are several accounts, as follows.

a. Leiner's Restaurant
On 1 November 1893 after the theatre, Tchaikovsky and some friends had retired to Leiner's restaurant on Nevsky Prospect.[261] As was his habit, Tchaikovsky drank white wine and mineral water with pasta and fish. When he asked for a further glass of water the waiter apologised, saying that the restaurant had neither mineral nor boiled water left. So impatiently Tchaikovsky ordered unboiled water, the waiter initially refusing. Finally the glass was brought, so the account goes, at which point Modest joined the party just in time to unsuccessfully prevent his brother drinking contaminated water. Perhaps significantly, Modest never mentioned this aspect of the episode.[262]

b. Modest's Flat
The following day Pyotr Ilyich arose at Modest's flat complaining of a stomach upset, but initially not conspicuously ill, although he declined

lunch.[263] According to Modest, he drank unboiled water from a carafe on the table. Tchaikovsky became severely ill the same evening and within three days he was dead.

c. Other Cholera Stories

Other cholera stories include a British theory as to how Tchaikovsky might have caught cholera through homosexual practices.[264] As a recent documentary demotically put it, 'perhaps he snogged the wrong bloke'.[265] We cannot deny this but, on a balance of probabilities, it seems unlikely. So let us instead look at the conflicting evidence and try to forensically analyse it within the limitations of not just the USSR, but modern Russia. The four key components to doing so are the court of honour, arsenic, suicide and cholera.

Scenarios Analysed

I. The Court of Honour

Both the Jacobi–Voitov–Orlova and the Mooser–Drigo versions can be despatched together. Here my dependence upon Poznansky is gratefully acknowledged. With the relaxed attitudes towards homosexuality in late nineteenth-century Russia, one questions whether the Tsar, at the time overwhelmed by vast problems, would have been too bothered about what 'the greatest of our composers' got up to with Count's nephews or a care-taker's boy. After all, at this time the Tsar's brother Grand-Duke Sergei had left his wife to keep house with his adjutant. Tchaikovsky was also a close friend of Grand Duke Konstantin: perhaps intimately so. Tchaikovsky had little to fear, being very well connected in high places. And why would Count Stenbock-Fermor, who was a high courtier, have asked a more lowly official (Jacobi) to deliver a letter to the very person with whom he himself regularly worked?

As to the court itself at Tsarskoe Selo, Poznansky has charted Tchaikovsky's known and recorded movements on the day in question. Given that the alleged overheard deliberations took five hours, and then adding a minimum of two hours' travelling time, Poznansky concludes that quite simply Tchaikovsky did not have time to get there and back on the date claimed by the court's proponents.[266] There was not a sufficient window of time. Moreover, why would the School of Jurisprudence have been so keen to distance itself from the alleged scandal of homosexual-ity when, in doing so, attention might be drawn rather than diverted?

Amongst its convivial collection of collegiate songs were ones celebrating the pleasures of sodomy.[267]

2. Arsenic

The attraction to the arsenic story is that it is tasteless and odourless, and drinking contaminated water could perhaps be a smokescreen for arsenic poisoning. More important is that, taken in the right dose, arsenic can quite closely and clinically mimic cholera.[268] So far, so good, but what is that right dose, remembering too that individuals' reactions to ingested chemicals vary enormously and unpredictably? Traces of arsenic can be found in drinking water today. None of 149 people who accidentally consumed an ant-killer containing arsenic became seriously ill.[269] Of course, a large dose can cause almost instantaneous death. So how did Tchaikovsky's assailants deduce an appropriate dose to mimic death from cholera? If he had died too suddenly or blithely survived, then the plot to kill him by simulating cholera would have been a fiasco. Had Tchaikovsky himself wanted to die, he would assuredly have taken a hefty dose incompatible with survival.

But who was to administer the fatal dose? Poznansky has deconstructed the poisoning theory,[270] which had Modest or the Bertensons as murderers by proxy. What would Modest's motive have been? The answer is hard to find, and jealousy is too weak an explanation. Then why would four doctors at the pinnacle of their profession associate with potential scandal, sexual or otherwise? Why would they collude in conspiracy to murder and flagrantly ignore all the tenets of their honourable profession?[271] Unless the Tsar told them to do this, promising immunity from prosecution, then the whole business seems quite absurd. For reasons previously outlined, it seems highly improbable that the Tsar was involved in any such devious plot. There is an allegation that the poisoner was Tchaikovsky's lawyer, Gerke, in spite of future lucrative contracts from which he could benefit, having just been successfully concluded by them both.[272] The motive remains elusive, and by the time of Gerke's visit to Modest's flat, Tchaikovsky was already ill. So we can now disregard this theory too.

At first sight it might appear that the issue of arsenic poisoning could be resolved by toxicological analysis of Tchaikovsky's remains, such as hair, usually one of the best-preserved human parts. Here again we need to be cautious. Analysis of hair is an excellent test for chronic arsenic poisoning, but in the case of the type of acute poisoning to bring about the composer's death over a few days, little arsenic would have reached the hair.[273] Bone analysis would be fraught with similar difficulties.

Proponents of the poisoning theory have relied on the testimony of Orlova. As long ago as 1966 she allegedly said that she had 'incontrovertible evidence' that Tchaikovsky had died by poisoning.[274] David Brown stated that death by suicide is undoubted, proposing arsenic as the likely agent.[275] 'Undoubted' is undoubtedly a risky description to use when discussing suspicious deaths a hundred years later. A court would not accept it as being beyond all reasonable doubt, and even a balance of probabilities would be hard to achieve. Anyway, Brown subsequently backed off this probable fiction.[276]

A curious piece of evidence advocated by the poison school of thought is the troupe of mourners who filed through Modest's flat to pay their final respects to Tchaikovsky. To argue that they would have taken this potential health risk only if they had *all* known he had *not* died of cholera is ludicrous. Had they all known that, then they would have surely speculated wildly as to what he *had* died of. Supposing that they knew it was not cholera, then how could such a diverse group have known so soon, unless the Drs Bertenson had trumpeted their complicity, which clearly they did not? It is too ridiculous to consider further. We can be certain that if there had been the merest rumour, then the newspapers, who were immediately active in reporting Tchaikovsky's death, would have pursued the matter remorselessly. Instead it was the medical competence of the Bertensons to treat cholera which they criticised.

3. Suicide

The body of evidence favouring suicide is more substantial, although it was not considered at the time.[277] Tchaikovsky had for so long been a melancholic man, frequently despondent and often self-pitying. That he was beset with feelings of guilt over 'my damned pederasty' over many years is abundantly clear.[278] Writing of his love for Bob shortly before his death, Tchaikovsky commented, 'What a monster of a person I am.'[279] Whilst in Cambridge his host, Sir Alexander Mackenzie, had been aghast at Tchaikovsky's haggard appearance, describing him as 'a spent man'.[280] This was when Tchaikovsky told the singer George Henschl that he was ready to meet his end.[281] But that was only shortly after he had told Rathaus that he was a happy man. Importance has been attached to his last journey from Moscow to St Petersburg, when he had looked out of the train window and indicated to a companion where he would like to be buried.[282] Did this reveal suicidal intentions? People often cheerfully direct where their final resting place is to be, without contemplating suicide.

There are other pointers against the case for suicide. On that fateful morning at Modest's flat, his giving directions with Gerke for future professional success was hardly a suicidal prelude. A suicide note is a frequent accompaniment of an actual suicide, and there was none. Above all, it seems totally inconsistent with intended suicide that, on the third day of his grave illness, he had appeared to improve and so thanked his doctors for 'snatching' him 'from the jaws of death'.[283] Although uncertainty will continue, there is no clear balance of probabilities in favour of suicide, let alone its being beyond all reasonable doubt. That with which we are left is cholera.

4. Cholera – a Fateful Glass of Water

We might first ask why, if Tchaikovsky intended suicide, did he choose contaminated water, an agent with only a 45% chance of fatality, rather than arsenic or a revolver? Of crucial importance are the two scenarios where this ingestion is claimed to have occurred:

a. Leiner's Restaurant
Leiner's restaurant is easily disposed of. If when Modest entered the room Tchaikovsky was drinking water, which he tried to prevent, then how did Modest, who had only just arrived, know that it was unboiled water? Poznasky has traced the origins of this story,[284] firstly indicating that Modest made no mention of it in his memoirs. The story originated from Bob Davidov's younger brother Yuri and his friend Yury Yuryev in the 1940s. In 1992 Poznansky met Yuri Davidov's daughter, who explained that her father had been perturbed during the Soviet era by rumours of suicide and homosexuality, both of which had been unmentionable and forbidden in the USSR. Thus, he had fabricated the story with Yury as a second witness to support the account of a fatal accidental drinking of infected water, thereby protecting his uncle's reputation.

b. Modest's Flat
Even if Modest did originally claim that Pyotr Ilyich had poured himself a glass of unboiled water, then is that not quite absurd? Firstly, did he really keep flasks of water whose ingestion could so easily cause death conveniently in the dining room?[285] We are back to motive and jealousy, a fragile argument. But maybe Tchaikovsky had gone to help himself from the kitchen tap. If so, then would Modest not have tried to prevent him and then have described the event in his diary, which he did not? Perhaps

Tchaikovsky had helped himself, unbeknown to Modest. If so then how did the glass ever enter the public domain at all? Years later Galina von Meck (Nadezhda's grand-daughter and Tchaikovsky's niece by marriage) suggested that in fact Tchaikovsky had drunk tap water.[286] Having logically pursued this case almost to the end, Poznansky concluded that cholera *was* the cause of death, as opposed to poison. In finally resolving the issue, he strangely stated that 'In the final analysis the entire question of how or when Tchaikovsky became infected is irrelevant.' He called it the 'Fortuitous Tragedy'.[287] Quite simply, without the how, where or when, then a confident diagnosis of a deadly infection becomes impossible or, as a law court would say, unsafe, and, without an assured diagnosis of infection, opinion will inevitably revert to suicide and poison.

Brown rejected cholera as the cause of death partly because of quibbles about incubation periods.[288] Whether one follows a figure of one to three days or a few hours to five days is uncritical; either is an acceptable estimate. Anyway, his statement, that the period between the alleged ingestion at luncheon and the onset of illness was four hours, is inaccurate. Tchaikovsky declined breakfast that day because of an upset stomach. Brown rightly pointed to a 'conspiracy of silence', and from the beginning there were probably vested interests anyway. Modest seems to have claimed to be the owner of the fateful glass of water, and importance has been attached to the discrepancies in the chronology of events as written by both the Bertensons and Modest.[289] Speaking as a doctor, I believe that is not unusual. When one has read case histories recorded by various conscientious doctors, especially of different specialties, and then those left by nurses for the same patient, one has often found a discrepancy. That is neither deceit nor nefarious; it is human nature reflecting different focuses and perhaps human fallibility. Furthermore, there were pressures on both parties. Modest would look to the reputation of his revered brother. The Bertensons were treated savagely by the St Petersburg newspapers and had their professional reputations to defend.[290]

Conclusion

The literature on this subject is labrynthine with, in many places, variations on a theme. Poznansky ultimately avoided the issue of how Tchaikovsky died; after all, it was the music that mattered. But surely the historian's duty is to the truth in all aspects of a great person's life, including his or her death. The foregoing has been an attempt to distil the most salient features and to conclude by analysis. There are several points about which we can be almost certain. Tchaikovsky was riven by guilt over both his sexuality and its promiscuity. Zajaczkowski has suggested that Tchaikovsky's tragedy was his inability to form an integrated relationship with another man.[291] That is not grounds for suspecting suicide. Secondly, the contemporaneous records of the clinical features are a perfect fit with cholera, during an epidemic which affected nearly half a million people, and common things are common. Unlike the sound basis for cholera, that for arsenic is flawed. Murder can be eliminated in the absence of motive, opportunity or just likelihood. The court of honour story is persuasive, but of questionable foundation. So we return to cholera. The suggestion that Tchaikovsky may have put himself at risk with a sexual liaison, proposed by Stuttaford,[292] is as difficult to disprove as it is to prove. In St Petersburg during 1893 any departure from customary hygienic practices ran the grave risk of death.

It may all have been an example of Russian roulette. Tchaikovsky tended to vacillate and dice with fate, as when he capriciously decided to marry, or later waded inconclusively into the river. He once said, 'I think in one direction and act in another,'[293] describing the Fifth Symphony as a 'surrender to destiny'. So perhaps he lowered his normally scrupulous levels of self-care, allowing fate to decide his own destiny – and it did. As a St Petersburg newspaper said, 'The cruel epidemics have not spared even our famous composer, P. I. Tchaikovsky.'[294] Prosaically, this melancholic fatalist may just have surrendered his tortured soul to the risks of catching cholera as it raged through St Petersburg. Even more prosaic is the possibility that he had accidentally and unwittingly fallen short of his own standards of hygiene; it only takes one careless mistake to contract this often fatal illness. How sad it all was. As Tsar Alexander III himself declared, 'We have many Counts and Barons, but only one Tchaikovsky.'[295]

Carlo Gesualdo (1560–1613)

The story of Carlo Gesualdo, Prince of Venosa, might have been co-authored by Bram Stoker and Sigmund Freud. There is no darker nor more morbid a figure in music. He was born into the aristocracy. Aged twenty-six he made a political marriage to Donna Maria, who, at twenty-one, was already the survivor of two earlier marriages.[296] In 1590 Gesualdo discovered that Donna Maria was having an affair with Don Fabrizio Carafa, third Duke of Andria. One day Gesualdo told her he was going hunting. Instead, he returned with three hired assassins to find his wife in compromising circumstances.[297] Gesualdo was said to have been a proficient swordsman, with which skills he not only murdered the lovers and their child but, with particular ferocity, dismembered those parts by which he had felt cuckolded.[298] Gray and Heseltine comment that he took seriously to music only after he gave up murder.[299] He re-married with a duke's sister, with whom there were three children, all of whom he outlived, despite his being asthmatic.

Gesualdo was a leading composer of madrigals and an exponent of dramatic counterpoint.[300] His madrigals are said to leap from joy to death, always with the language of pain.[301] He endowed a monastery and commissioned great paintings within which he had himself favourably portrayed. These are seen as acts of expiation in atonement for earlier acts of painful violation.[302] But then in his last decade he inclined to sadomasochism. Indeed, a severe beating, which he enjoyed daily, was the surest way to make him smile. Glenn Watkins's biography was apposite: 'The Prince of Venosa, one of the best musicians of his age, was unable to go to stool without having been flogged by a valet kept expressly for the purpose.'[303]

Ober believes that he had latent trends under reasonable control, thereby preserving some heterosexual competence, until Donna Maria's infidelity.[304] That then released sadomasochistic tendencies which would increasingly dominate his life, and which scholars assert are the theme of his mature, albeit perverted, musical compositions.[305]

His own death is controversial. That he may have been murdered is a predictable view.[306] Watkins reviewed the likely suspects and found little evidence for murder.[307] It is tempting to suggest that his colourful, gothic life, like that of his great contemporary Caravaggio, was coloured by his time and background. Then one encounters the lavatory attendant, whip in hand, and realises that Gesualdo was mad.

Suicide

Is suicide an act of courage?
The Times, 1786

In the 1960s the suicide rate in England and Wales was one in every 10,000 of the population.[308] For those who have dealt with suicide there can be few more tragic causes of death, if any. Freud believed suicide occurred because instincts of self-preservation break down. The post-Freudian Austro-American analyst Otto Fenichel suggested that innate in every person there is an instinct to kill, be killed or kill oneself. That suicide may result from bipolar depression is clear in that, before effective medication became available, the mortality rate due to suicide was 20%. Less obvious are the factors which suddenly tip a seemingly happy and successful individual towards this awful end. That the inner torment was there, hidden and suppressed, can often be supposed, but mysteriously it was not always conspicuous.

The English Suicides

Lastly, we briefly consider two English composers, separated by two centuries but with aspects in common, of which the most solemn is suicide. **Jeremiah Clarke** (1674–1707) and **Peter Warlock** (aka **Philip Heseltine**) (1894–1930) followed in the footsteps of two famous English composers, Purcell and Delius, respectively. Warlock was Delius's first biographer.[309] Clarke and Warlock both drew inspiration from England, with its rich heritage of religion, legend and folk music. Clarke, unlike Warlock, went in accordance with his times. *Praise the Lord, O my Soul* celebrated the coronation of Queen Anne in 1702. *The Lord is my Strength* in 1706 was a tribute to Marlborough's great victory at Ramillies in the War of the Spanish Succession.[310] Now similarities cease.

Warlock was a hard-drinking extrovert. It is suspected that during his time in Kent, sharing a house with the composer E. J. Moeran, alcohol may not have been the only substance which they abused.[311] Gray affirms that Warlock's experimentation with hallucinogenic drugs such as cannabis was short-lived,[312] whilst also affirming that his being alcoholic was very dubious.[313] Heseltine dabbled with the occult and allegedly with sadomasochism, echoing the account of Gesualdo which he co-authored with Cecil Gray. Warlock married an artist's model known as 'The Puma' in 1917, but it was an unsteady union.[314] He had little basic musical training, and it was perhaps this and his waywardness which halted his ambitions to regenerate English music. Before Christmas 1930, when he was re-working 'Bethlehem Down', he returned to his London flat with friends. On the following morning, 17 December, he was found dead in a room with a gas fire turned on but unlit.[315] The tap was subsequently found to have been very loose by one account,[316] but that was denied by a plumber at the inquest.[317] Some assumed that he had committed suicide, not least because the cat had been turned out, although the coroner returned an open verdict.[318] His alleged inebriation makes the diagnosis of suicide more suspect, although the autopsy revealed little evidence of either recent excessive alcohol ingestion or chronic alcoholism.[319] Maybe he had tried to light the gas fire, fumbled, stumbled and fatefully slumbered. Gas fires can blow out just as cats can stay out. But he had talked earlier of death by coal gas poisoning and had just re-written his will exclusively in favour of Winifred Baker, a nurse with whom he had been close.[320] Warlock's life in 1930 was a mess personally and professionally, and he had been depressed, twice returning to live with his mother. From 1929 there had been little composition. The balance of probabilities is that he committed suicide.

Warlock still evokes controversy and hostility. His illegitimate son, the late respected art critic Brian Sewell, wrote in a tabloid newspaper in 2011 'Why I will Never Love my Father'.[321] The day before, a newspaper had carried an article proclaiming that Sewell's father was a sadist.[322] Sewell's basic point seems to have been that his Roman Catholic mother refused to have an abortion, Warlock not desiring a child. This led to Sewell being born, about which his parents had a blazing row, possibly provoking Warlock's suicide.

The verdict of suicide is clearer with Jeremiah Clarke. 'A Sad and Dismal Account of the Sudden and Untimely Death of Mr Jeremiah Clarke' appeared in a broadsheet in 1707, stating that he had a violent and hopeless passion for a very beautiful lady of superior rank.[323] This caused him to shoot himself, having first considered hanging or drowning, the decision allegedly being made upon the toss of a coin. Suicide was a crime in England until 1961 and subject to criminal prosecution, in spite of which he was buried in the crypt of St Paul's Cathedral. Wikipedia has published a list of famous 'suicides by firearms' in the UK in which Jeremiah Clarke is the only composer to have so died.[324] There is nothing today to suggest that Clarke, unlike Warlock, was an unstable character. Perhaps this too is evident in their respective outputs: where Clarke's bears a mark of celebration and establishment, Warlock was a rebel, once pursued by the police whilst speeding naked on a motorcycle.[325] More importantly, his music seems to reveal a retreat into the past, overshadowed by something a little mystical.

Postscript

It would be silly to imply that within this chapter repose all composers with mental problems. Below is a list of others in whom depression, if only at times, was a problem. Perhaps, above all else, this list illustrates Jamison's proposition that creative people experience greater highs and lows than more mundane mortals.[326] Beware the man who says he wishes he was dead before having a good dinner and then going on to the theatre, or the wife such as Alice Elgar, who recorded that Edward was 'very depressed'; he had been doing his tax return![327] Nevertheless, the great psychiatrist Anthony Storr believed that artists used their work to save their souls and their minds.

Composers with Significant Episodes of Depression

Monteverdi
Joseph Haydn
Beethoven
Rossini
Berlioz
Mendelssohn
Chopin
Liszt
Wagner
Saint-Saëns
Bizet
Tchaikovsky
Rimsky-Korsakov
Elgar
Puccini
Debussy
Sibelius
Rachmaninov
Schoenberg
Holst
Bartók
Lambert
Shostakovich
Arnold*

---

* Possibly bipolar, although schizophrenia seems more probable. The two may co-exist or overlap.

Chapter 7

Nerves Beyond the Edge:
Other Afflictions
of the Nervous System

It is in the brain, and the brain only, that the great sins of the world take place

Oscar Wilde, *The Picture of Dorian Gray*, 1891

Introduction: The Nervous System

I N OUR EPOCH of rapidly evolving medical science we can look forward to a time quite soon when cancer and heart disease might often be little more than interruptions to our lifestyles and not threats to life itself. So much more of the human system has become accessible, reparable and controllable. A major exception is the nervous system, with its difficulties of surgical access but, above all else, an inability to repair itself or to be repaired, which makes diseases such as motor neurone disease, multiple sclerosis and the aftermath of head injury or stroke still so devastating. There are now some encouraging signs of progress born of genetic engineering and microchip technology.

The nervous system is enormously complex. There are many millions of nerve cells (neurones), some highly specialised, in our brains, and they are all interconnected. Of prime importance is the central nervous system, which consists of the brain, the repository of our higher functions (e.g. sight, hearing, speech, emotion, memory, intellect and voluntary movement), and the spinal cord. The latter is the main electrical pathway to and from the brain. The knowledge that our foot is too hot is carried in the sensory nerves to the brain via the spinal cord, and the impulse to quickly move it away from the heat source returns down the spinal cord, passing messages to motor nerves via the peripheral nervous system. When these systems are disturbed, diseased or destroyed, then human life can become truly awful.

We have already encountered neurological disease in earlier chapters. George Gershwin died rapidly from a malignant brain tumour (Chapter 3). Maurice Ravel's brain prematurely atrophied as he developed pre-senile dementia (Chapter 3). A whole chapter is devoted to the dreadful effects of syphilis (Chapter 4), with some of which it was the brain itself which functionally disintegrated, as was the case with Donizetti, or with Smetana, whose auditory nerves were also affected, hence his deafness. It was Delius's optic nerves which were affected, along with the spinal cord. His brain and thus higher intellectual functions remained unimpaired until his death.

In this chapter we will look at a variety of neurological conditions and their impact on several composers. After Shostakovich, much of the rest of the chapter will concern strokes. We have already encountered Verdi and Sibelius (both Chapter 2), whose ultimate and rapid cause of death was a stroke, in different contexts.

Stroke (or cerebro-vascular accident, CVA) is one of the commonest causes of death in the UK today. Strokes fall broadly into two groups. Between 85 and 90 per cent are caused by a blood clot (thrombus) occluding part of the circulation to the brain, whereas the remainder are due to haemorrhage within the brain substance or into the membranes (the meninges) which surround the brain (subarachnoid haemorrhage).

✢ DMITRI SHOSTAKOVICH ✢
(1906–1975)

I don't know how not to be afraid
Dmitri Shostakovich to Igor Stravinsky, 1960

Of all the most tortured of composers' souls few, if any, surpassed the inner torments of Shostakovich. For an explanation of Shostakovich's inner turmoils one should read Figes's masterpiece *The Whisperers*.[1] Here is a fly-on-the-wall account of relationships between ordinary people in Stalin's savage and unpredictable police state. His career seems to have been a balancing act in which he often had to curb his natural creative instincts and pay obeisance to his Soviet masters. That he paid a devilish price in subverting his own loyalties cannot be questioned.

He was born in the dying years of the Romanov dynasty to a middle-class musical family. The First World War started when he was eight. For his last fifty-eight years Shostakovich's health and fortunes were intimately and fatefully entwined with those of the USSR. There can be few, if any, composers who have resonated more constantly with the political times in which they lived and worked than Shostakovich. Having attended the Leningrad Conservatory as Glazunov's pupil,[2] he became short of money after his father died and accordingly worked as a cinema pianist. Early in 1923 he had complained of neck pain. Swellings, due to enlarged lymph nodes, were discovered, and the diagnosis of TB was sustained by microscopic examination after the nodes were surgically removed.[3] He had insisted upon first taking his public piano examination before the operation in late June. The ever-generous Glazunov raised the money for his convalescence by the Black Sea, where he had his first passionate love affair. When he appeared at the Warsaw piano competition his health again let him down, eventually leading to the removal of his appendix in late April 1927,[4] although he still received a commendation.

In 1926 his First Symphony was a success, establishing him as a composer showing precocious maturity. The pro-Soviet Second Symphony ('To October') followed. In 1930 he wrote a satirical opera, *The Nose*, based on a story by Gogol, which was not well received. His most famous opera, *Lady Macbeth of Mtsensk*, was premiered in 1934. Then, in 1936, Shostakovich was at a performance also attended by Stalin.[5] This was the year in which the Great Terror started, and it was clear that the dictator was not enjoying *Lady Macbeth of Mtsensk*. Shostakovich was seen to become visibly ashen, and to sweat and twitch as he beheld the dictator's displeasure and then early departure.[6] Two days later *Pravda* published an article describing it as coarse, primitive and vulgar.[7] The memorable headline was 'Muddle Instead of Music', and it is suspected that Stalin himself may have written these criticisms. In 1936 Shostakovich's daughter Galina was born, and he voluntarily withdrew his Fourth Symphony, which was not premiered for almost another quarter of a century.[8] Such pragmatism may have saved his life, but the toll upon his inner harmony was clear to those close to him.

The motif for Wendy Lesser's account in *Music for Silenced Voices* is that symphonies were inevitably very public and thus had to be politically tailored.[9] In 1937 the popular Fifth Symphony was described to the composer's pleasure as 'an artist's creative response to just criticism',[10] and, in turn, Kabalevsky congratulated him for 'overcoming mistakes and following new paths'.[11] Lesser's theme continues with the string quartet as a more intimate and significantly less scrutinised art form, and so she charts the relationship between the true Shostakovich and his music through this medium. Lesser acknowledges that it is a difficult course to follow, for her subject was a man of stark contrasts; a funny melancholic or a courageous coward. His poker-playing friend, the writer Mikhail Zoshchenko, said that in Shostakovich one quality obliterates the other.[12] So, with his apparent rehabilitation after the Fifth Symphony, we enter the spring of 1938, when his son Maxim was born and he composed the First String Quartet with its simple themes of springtime, even childhood.[13] Clearly, he wanted to be merry and lyrical although, as with much Russian music, we are seldom far from melancholia in the second movement.[14]

When the Great Patriotic War started in 1941 Shostakovich volunteered for the Red Army. He was rejected, mainly because of his poor eyesight, and so he became a firefighter. There is an iconic propaganda picture of him in spectacles and a tin hat. Ironically, his eyesight had not prevented him from officiating as a football referee, but then referees' eyesight is often called into question. He was very keen on soccer and even played on Sunday mornings himself. By now Shostakovich was an important cog in the Soviet wheel and, accordingly, was evacuated with his family to Kuibyshev on the Volga once Leningrad was encircled.[15] Before this, he had started composition of the Seventh ('Leningrad') Symphony. Delving into Shostakovich's memoirs is not cheerful work, describing as they do his often drab, grey life. In 1943 his tide turned, as did the Wehrmacht's as they retreated after Stalingrad and Kursk. So came the Eighth Symphony, sometimes subtitled the 'Stalingrad', dedicated to Mravinksy. The authorities may have had a point when they asked how he could have been so upbeat in Leningrad during 1941 and so gloomy after the Red Army's victory at Stalingrad. The Eighth was effectively banned until 1956.[16] In 1944, after the death of a friend, he fell into another depression. Shostakovich was a man of strange contrasts. Maybe that is why the cheery Haydnesque Ninth Symphony is said to be a paradox going to the heart of the Soviet-Marxist aesthetic.[17]

In 1948 Shostakovich was again denounced by the Supreme Soviet (under the Andrei Zhdanov decree); he lived in dread of a knock on the door in the night,[18] and spoke of the loss of his spiritual youth. Often in mortal fear, he adopted three phases of composition. The first was for films and for the money. Second came official pieces to keep the commissars happy. Thirdly, he kept serious compositions in his desk until better times. In 1949 Stalin ordered him to New York for the World Peace Conference. The journalist Nicolas Nabokov wrote that 'he was not a free man but an obedient tool of his government'.[19] Shostakovich even became cornered into giving a public denunciation of Stravinsky, one of many occasions when his accommodations with the Soviets caused him great distress. Nabokov claimed there were times when Shostakovich considered suicide, particularly in 1948 after he had been denounced by Zhdanov.[20] On his return from the USA he was assigned to an instructor in Marxism-Leninism.

When Stalin died in 1953 Shostakovich's life became easier, although his wife, Nina, died in 1954 and he missed her greatly. He had spent the spring of 1953 at a sanatorium in the Caucasus for rest and recuperation.[21] Two years later, Shostakovich married Margarita Kainova, a party activist, the unhappy marriage ending in divorce in 1959.[22] Then, inexplicably, during 1960 he at last joined the Communist Party. Reviewing the reasons for this step, Fay considers that some form of coercion seems likely.[23] His third wife, Irina, years later shared with Lesser her own suspicions of blackmail.[24] It is certain that he experienced an emotional breakdown over this issue. Then he finished the Eighth Quartet, dedicated 'To the memory of the victims of fascism and war'. He hinted that it was to be his last work as he contemplated suicide, although Maxim later denied such contemplation.[25] Fay, who spoke at length many years later with Irina, writes of the family confiscating his sleeping pills.

By the late 1950s Shostakovich's always fragile health and weakness had deteriorated further. In 1958 he commented on the 'high priests of medicine', his frustration directed at their inability to come up with a diagnosis over 11 years.[26] Elizabeth Wilson charts the weakness of his right hand, which had affected his playing in Paris whilst on a concert tour.[27]

She describes symptoms which betray weakness of the right shoulder, for example difficulties in raising the arm in the customary position whilst cleaning his teeth. In his paper on Shostakovich's weakness, Pascuzzi produced correspondence which suggests that the weakness may have started as early as 1954 and in the legs.[28] He had spent a month in hospital for 'treatment' of weakness in the right hand during 1958 and again in February 1960.[29] Later that year his legs collapsed at Maxim's wedding and he fell, breaking his left leg.[30] The fracture was probably to his hip bone (neck of femur), for by now his weakness and consequent inactivity would have predisposed him to brittle thinning of the bone known as osteoporosis, which is typically associated with hip fractures. Nevertheless, he continued to play the piano privately in chamber works and he still composed quickly. More importantly, he now wrote his Twelfth Symphony with its dedication to Lenin. In June 1962 he went into hospital again for treatment to his right hand, whence came his Thirteenth Symphony, 'Babi-Yar'.[31] In autumn 1962 he married Irina Supinskaya, an intelligent and caring lady; she was twenty-seven and he fifty-six.[32] Their marriage was a happy one. In 1966 he decided with trepidation to accompany the singer Galina Vishnevskaya (Mrs Rostropovich). In rehearsal he was very nervous and made mistakes. On the humid night in late May all was well, but the next day he suffered a heart attack (myocardial infarct).[33] He had already been in a cardiology clinic for three weeks in January 1965. After his discharge he was pronounced a 'Hero of Socialist Labour'.[34]

Further periods of hospitalisation followed, all of inexplicably great length, for investigation and treatment of his weakness. The doctors professed themselves 'pleased with him'. He scoffed that, after eight years, this was a little hard when all he wanted to do was to get upstairs unaided and play the piano. He was ordered to relinquish smoking and alcohol.[35] The impracticality of such advice was revealed when, cheered up by brandy, he set verses by Alexander Blok to music, yet another work started in hospital.[36] Although no alcoholic, Shostakovich did tend to drown his sorrows. By September 1967 he had been taking country walks, but then wrote that his legs were once more worsening.[37] Again he fell, and this time he broke the other leg (or perhaps his ankle), after which there was an extraordinarily long post-operative hospitalisation. He was in plaster for two to three months.[38]

After another prolonged period of hospitalisation in 1969, he was said at a Moscow hospital to have a rare form of poliomyelitis.[39] This is interesting because variants of the disease do exist, as do secondary relapses with deterioration years later from the effects of an earlier attack of polio. Shostakovich's known clinical features could fit into a diagnosis of post-polio syndrome. The only problem is that there is no evidence of a previous attack of polio (which would typically have been fifteen to thirty years earlier). It is much more likely that Shostakovich was suffering from amyotrophic lateral sclerosis (ALS), known now as motor neurone disease.[40] The most famous case today is that of Professor Stephen Hawking, himself a triumph over almost overwhelming physical odds. In this condition the nerve nuclei in the tracts of the spinal cord and sometimes of the brain degenerate, leading to paralysis of all those muscles whose controlling nerve or nerves originate in those nerve nuclei.[41] Pascuzzi suggests that the condition is much commoner than is popularly supposed.[42] This, in turn, implies that there are milder variations of motor neurone disease which do not rapidly or inexorably lead to rapid total paralysis and death. In 1969 Shostakovich decided to treat death musically after hearing Musorgsky's *Songs and Dances of Death*. He had recently said that if he could turn the clock back, he would live his life differently.[43] Also that year came his Fourteenth Symphony, a fifty-minute epic of soprano, bass and chamber orchestra in eleven movements. Shostakovich regarded it as the pinnacle of his career. He was more impatient by then to hear his recent compositions performed. Doubtless he was becoming aware that his days might be numbered. The Thirteenth String Quartet is a disturbing, even harrowing, work, although Irina said that her husband was quite a settled person and not a melancholic man.[44] Such are the perceptions of loving spouses.

To an orthopaedic surgeon it is fascinating that Shostakovich in 1969 first consulted Professor G. A. Ilizarov at Kurgan in Siberia.[45] The composer had heard of near-miracles worked by this world-famous surgeon in treating broken bones which had healed in bad positions or not at all. Under Ilizarov's care, Shostakovich had a small operation to his right hand and then started on a fixed and healthy regimen of general rehabilitation, including country walks. Shostakovich said the treatment was working miracles. He started to play the piano louder, faster and more often. Interestingly, he could now shave with his right hand. Several long periods in hospital followed, and clearly Shostakovich had an almost child-like faith in Ilizarov's powers. What is mysterious is the nature of the wonder operation. The answer is unavailable, and, in speculating, the options are limited. It may be that the muscle-tendons activating the back of his hand were weakened more than those for the front of the hand, giving him a dropped wrist. Re-routing a spare stronger muscle-tendon unit to compensate for the weaker ones can be very effective. However, motor neurone disease is progressive and inevitably any surgical success would be transient, as the transferred muscle-tendon unit succumbs, as did its predecessor.

In 1970 Shostakovich was working with the film director Kozintsev (composing *Hamlet*, 1963, and *King Lear*, 1970), who noted that, as the car came for Shostakovich, he struggled to get in and out of it. When occupied for nine hours at the studios he then became alert with nervous energy.[46] Such occupation and the positive rehabilitation programmes worked wonders with his morale. Many excellent physiotherapists are also good amateur psychologists.

Shostakovich suffered his second heart attack in September 1971,[47] and it is difficult to know how much his overall weakness was due to his progressive motor neurone disease and how much was breathlessness on exertion, which characterises progressive heart disease, as we will see with Benjamin Britten (to whom the Fourteenth Symphony was dedicated). Earlier in September 1971 he finished his Fifteenth Symphony, which was premiered under the baton of his son Maxim on 8 January 1972. Shostakovich was a keen exponent of irony, and it cannot have been lost upon him that, by the time of the final four symphonies, he was all but the darling of Soviet music, whilst the West by now rather rejected his allegedly gloomy Soviet formalism. Both Britten and Shostakovich were by then in declining health, and their relationship had an intensity born from apprehending the transience of life. He was keen for the Fifteenth to be played in Leningrad, his spiritual home, under the baton of the great Evgeny Mravinsky, chief conductor of the Leningrad Philharmonic for forty-nine consecutive years. The two men, who had done so much together, had become estranged over disagreements about Mravinsky's interpretation of the Thirteenth Symphony.[48] On hearing the ailing Shostakovich's wishes, the conductor promptly visited Shostakovich at his dacha. The rift was healed. The first performance of the Fifteenth in Leningrad was a success. Most significantly Shostakovich, although far from well, had energetically started to compose the more cheerful and melodic Fourteenth Quartet the day after Mravinsky's visit.[49]

By now ill health was catching up with him, and it was in December 1972 that, to add to his troubles, lung cancer was diagnosed during investigations for kidney stones.[50] He had always been a heavy smoker. In February 1973 he had his first course of radiotherapy, after which another prolonged creative block developed. It was also in 1973 that he publicly deplored the anti-Soviet pronouncements of the nuclear physicist Andrei Sakharov.[51] In this episode we possibly see the labyrinthine circumstances within which this frail man wrestled. Was the signature on the document deploring Sakharov actually his? Then he also criticised Solzhenitsyn – 'a filthy slander'.[52] Alternatively, if the signature was his, then was it willingly given? He, of course, was condemned for his condemnation, whereupon he condemned himself saying, 'I won't forgive myself until the grave.'[53] Stradling regards Shostakovich as having been a lifelong communist.[54] As Churchill said of Russia, this was 'a riddle wrapped in mystery inside an enigma'. In June 1973 he had sneaked an American second opinion whilst receiving an honorary degree in the USA. 'Heart trouble' and a 'progressive neurological disorder' should not have been too taxing a diagnosis for the American doctors to make! They said he was 'incurable'.[55]

When Rostropovich with his wife, Galina Vishnevskaya, emigrated to the USA in the spring of 1974, Shostakovich knew he would not see them again. He and Galina said a tearful farewell at his dacha, and Shostakovich's parting words were 'Come back Galya, we'll be waiting.'[56] He was too unwell to go to the airport himself, although Irina bade them farewell. Despite increasing weakness in the right hand he completed his fifteenthth and last quartet, which Lesser describes as having an overall atmosphere of other worldliness, especially as it ends with the instruments in turn fading away into silence.[57] It was this and the lack of a dedication for the first time that led Eugene Drucker of the Emerson Quartet to suggest that this was a valediction, or 'an elegy to himself'.[58] Again impatient, Shostakovich could not wait for the Beethoven Quartet, one of whose members had just died, so the premiere was given on 15 November 1974 by the young Taneyev Quartet in Leningrad.[59] His very last composition was the Viola Sonata Opus 147. In contrast to the Fifteenth String Quartet, it is not a sombre work; perhaps it was a serene farewell. So his last few months were punctuated by intense episodes of composition, even hopes of a miracle. In August 1975, still seeking that miracle, he was re-admitted to hospital. On 9 August he awoke and enjoyed his breakfast, and Irina read Chekhov to him. Then he experienced respiratory seizures which allegedly caused another heart attack,[60] and in the afternoon he choked and died. In a delayed bulletin, the Soviet authorities gave heart failure as the cause of death. In 1991 Irina told his biographer Laurel Fay that cancer was his primary cause of death.[61] I just wonder. The muscles of breathing and the gag reflex which prevents choking can be affected in motor neurone disease. But then perhaps no-one choked to death in the Soviet utopia, and they did declare him to be 'a loyal son of the Communist Party'.

To assess Shostakovich's psyche is difficult. He showed some neurotic traits and at times he drank heavily. Were they coming to get him? Quite simply 'they' certainly contemplated doing just that. He had always been an anxious, nervous and diffident person. There were also obsessive-compulsive disorder (OCD) traits, just as there were depressive ones. He was fastidiously clean and a mighty hand-washer. He also sent postcards to himself to check whether the postal service was working. For most observers Shostakovich remains a complex, fragile person. His great achievement was that, for fifty years (1925–75) of Stalinist and post-Stalinist Russia, he was one of the three greatest Russian composers. And that too was his stifling, frightening and at times unsustainable burden. Lastly, we see that his often indifferent health was not always an impediment to composition. Whether it actually engendered the conceptual side of the composition seems improbable. He composed in spite of, not because of, his often awful life circumstances. In 1979 Solomon Volkov published *Testimony: The Memoirs of Dmitri Shostakovich*,[62] although whether the memoirs were totally Shostakovich's has been questioned (see Chapter 5). But Volkov's testament is one in which, beyond the grave, Shostakovich leaves us in no doubt as to his hatred, not for Russia or even communism, but for the hideous Soviet apparatus. Apart from his heart disease, today revolutionised by minimally invasive surgery, it is doubtful if twenty-first-century medicine would have radically altered his other diseases.

We will now attend to composers who died of strokes. As an approximate contemporary, Prokofiev is irrevocably linked with Shostakovich.

✣ SERGEI PROKOFIEV ✣
(1891–1953)

The air of foreign lands does not inspire me because I am Russian
Sergei Prokofiev, 1933

It was 5 March 1953 and much of Russia was in turmoil and draped in black. Two Russians who, in their different fields, had ridden in triumph over the first half of the twentieth century, had died within an hour of one another. Both had been unwell for some time and had, in the opinion of their respective physicians, suffered fatal brain haemorrhages. It was the death of Joseph Stalin, 'Father of Mother Russia' and also its greatest murdering tyrant, who had brought about the mass mourning which poured onto the streets of Moscow and beyond. If only those people had known what Stalin had done. He had, of course, unscrupulously interfered with the creative arts in theUSSR. Like writers, composers had been mendaciously persecuted. Along with Shostakovich and Khachaturian, Sergei Prokofiev was sometimes officially defiled. He had died just an hour before Stalin, and his passing, for all his fame and the prestige he brought to Soviet culture, was marked with little more than a bough of pine laid upon his coffin by his immediate family in a city apartment. All the flowers had decked the course of the mortal remains of Comrade Stalin.[63] Just as there often had been no bread, now at the end there were no flowers. So full were the newspapers of eulogies for the great tyrant that the death of the composer of *Romeo and Juliet*, *Cinderella* and *War and Peace* hardly had a mention, and then only several days later.

A major difference between Shostakovich and Prokofiev is that the former understood and dreaded the evil potential of the communist apparatus. It seems that little of this dawned upon Prokofiev until he became a prematurely elderly and sick man. When he returned to live permanently in Russia in 1936 he assumed that the comrades would be thrilled to have him back amongst them and that they would leave him alone to get on with composing.[64] They didn't, although, like Shostakovich, he seems to have enjoyed some of the perks of perhaps being more equal than others. He believed that his place was in Russia, as he was Russian. This was deeply felt, but without any vestige of self-promotion as a patriotic scion of the Bolshevik Revolution. Unlike Shostakovich he never joined the party.

There had been earlier health problems. Whilst preparing his First Piano Concerto, whose reception was very mixed despite its humour, he had succumbed to pleurisy.[65] Later, with the same work, he won the Rubinstein Piano Competition. It remains unclear how he avoided conscription during the Great War. Jaffé, whose biography used interviews with Prokofiev's son Oleg, implies that his concern during the 1917 Revolution in St Petersburg was for his own safety.[66] As Kerensky tried to forward democratic socialism and the Red Army collapsed on the Eastern Front, Prokofiev retired to the Caucasus with his mother, completing the 'Classical' Symphony there.[67] In September 1918 he left for New York, via Vladivostok.[68] He also met Carolina (Lina) Codina, a singer of Spanish, Polish and French origin. In 1919 he came close to death with a febrile illness reported as scarlet fever with a throat abscess, possibly diphtheria.[69] Prokofiev and Lina were to meet again in Paris and married after she became pregnant in 1923,[70] although Sergei was perhaps a reluctant husband. The following year they went to live in Oberammergau.

When Prokofiev returned to the USSR in 1927, having made a lot of money in America, it was to a generous reception, and herein probably lay his failure to grasp the Faustian dilemma he faced in supping with the comrades. In June 1927 there was the delayed premiere of his 'Bolshevik ballet' *Le pas d'acier*, although biographers imply that, even in the 1930s, he knew little of Soviet reality, let alone life for the poor under their alleged 'saviours'.[71] He had returned to the Soviets to teach them, and not the opposite.[72] Dressing like Bobby Jones and sipping champagne were unlikely to endear him to the workers.[73] In October 1929 he was involved in a car accident when a wheel came off his car. Lina said he was semi-conscious for several hours.[74] He injured both his hands, and for several months excluded engagements as a pianist, before making a full recovery.

The late 1920s and early 1930s were an itinerant time in Paris, the Americas and Germany, where he played his Fifth Piano Concerto with the Berlin Philharmonic under Furtwängler in 1932.[75] What seems clear is that he was becoming homesick, never more so than on his return visits to Russia, but it was Mother Russia, and not Marxism or the Five-Year Plan, which called him back. He finally returned to live in his native land in 1936.

From the late 1930s and certainly after 1941 it becomes increasingly difficult to explain Prokofiev's revisions, withdrawals and subsequent re-submissions of works. They may have been due to the eternal attendance of the 'cultural police', or to artistic compromise, or perhaps to his health. I am not immediately inclined to blame 'the system'. Very unusually it had allowed him out of the USSR to tour the USA once more. Yet when he returned to America in 1938 Nabokov reported a 'profound and terrible insecurity' in his manner. When the Americans tried to persuade him to emigrate he said, 'I have to return to Moscow, to my music and my children.'[76] Prokofiev wrote *Zdravitsa* (sometimes subtitled *Hail to Stalin*) to command and had been very uneasy about it. His response was to write three very personal piano sonatas to express his true feelings,[77] possibly illustrating Wendy Lesser's proposition with Shostakovich.

When Prokofiev went to Leningrad in 1940 to prepare *Romeo and Juliet*, a prima ballerina, Galina Ulanova, described the composer as a haughty and unapproachable man.[78] Or was this the advent of ill health? But he then turned his attention to R. B. Sheridan's *The Duenna*, which he set as a humorous and romantic opera,[79] suggesting that, despite ill health, his talent for romantic flourish and rasping wit remained undiminished.

In 1941 the Nazis were on the outskirts of Leningrad. Prokofiev was by then entangled with Mira Mendelssohn, whom he had first met in 1938. She was a card-carrying party member, and one of Soviet Russia's cultural elite. His marriage to Lina had been deteriorating for some time before that. Mira was more submissive than Lina and, unlike Lina, able to help Sergei's career, if only politically.[80] The Prokofievs were evacuated in 1941, and he wanted to take both Lina and Mira with his party to Nalchik in the Caucasus.[81] Marriage with Lina had by then passed a point of no return.[82] Lina, understandably, was unenthusiastic at being accompanied by Mira and went into limbo, ultimately being sent via the Lubyanka to Siberia for eight years.[83] Prokofiev ultimately married Mira on 13 January 1948, just six weeks before Lina's arrest and banishment.[84] To return to 1941, Prokofiev perhaps now had recognised the worldly circumstances surrounding him as he composed a symphonic suite, *The Year 1941*. His next major project was the great opera *War and Peace*, which was to occupy him intermittently for years. In that fateful year of 1941 his health deteriorated so much that he stopped giving concert performances.[85] This followed further evacuation to Tbilisi, where food was scarce and expensive. There he suffered a heart attack. However, he continued to play privately but, according to friends and colleagues, did so with less accomplishment than before.

In October 1943 Sergei and Mira returned to Moscow as the German army retreated to its Armageddon. *War and Peace,* still incomplete, was withdrawn from the Bolshoi that autumn, to be replaced by *Cinderella*. Ballerina Ulanova noted that Prokofiev's attendance at rehearsals became rarer.[86] Sometimes he was ill and hospitalised. The evidence suggests that his earlier heart attacks were associated with high blood pressure, as he increasingly complained of headaches, nosebleeds and dizzy spells. Hingtgen, who has researched this epoch, affirms that he continued with his practice of working on several pieces simultaneously. At that time no

focal neurological features such as weakness, speech impairment or disturbance of intellectual or cognitive function were recorded.[87] *War and Peace*
was given in the spring of 1944. He revised it intermittently until almost
the end of his life, with an increasing tendency towards the parallelism
between the Great Patriotic War of 1941–45 and the events immortalised
by Tolstoy. The first complete staged performance was in Leningrad, six
years after his death.[88] He spent the summer of 1944 at Ivanovo, a country
retreat outside Moscow run by the Composers' Union. Typically, reports
of Prokofiev's time there vary. Gutman recounts him being comradely, but
then snubbing Shostakovich.[89] His health seems to have improved at that
time, and Jaffé even describes him playing volleyball,[90] as well as working on the Fifth Symphony and Eighth Piano Sonata at Ivanovo. A year
later this fiercely competitive man was medically forbidden even to play
chess.[91] In January 1945 he conducted for the last time with the premiere
of his Fifth Symphony. Whilst with Mira after this performance, he was
overtaken by dizziness and fell down some stairs, banging his head.[92] Jaffé
believes that the fall occurred several days after the episode of dizziness.[93]
According to Gutman, he was knocked unconscious and sent to hospital,[94]
where he rambled incoherently for several days thereafter, presumably due
to concussion. His high blood pressure was probably treated, although
symptoms of it continued to afflict him.[95]

In the latter half of 1945 he worked with Eisenstein on the 'Boyar Plot',
that being the second episode of *Ivan the Terrible*, which Stalin hated.[96] He
also sketched the Ninth Piano Sonata and the Sixth Symphony, although
that was not finished until February 1947. During the winter of 1946–47
he was often too ill to attend preparations and rehearsals of *War and Peace*,
yet he continued to revise that work and also to sketch a cello sonata. Mira
recorded that, for all his ill health, the one driving constant was work, and
that, even away from a desk or piano, he would continue to compose,
whether in a railway carriage or a hospital bed. She said, 'The illness which
overshadowed the last years of his life did not lessen his capacity for work;
on the contrary, because of it all his mental and physical energies were
concentrated on his art.' So when the doctors (with those orders again)
allowed him to work only for twenty minutes twice a day, Prokofiev said
that he 'vegetated'.[97]

On 11 October 1947 he joined Evgeny Mravinsky on the podium in
Leningrad to share enthusiastic applause for the premiere of his Sixth
Symphony, often regarded as his greatest work and a requiem for his
health.[98] Despite his infirmity, he later composed what he described as a
'simple symphony for young listeners'. This, the Seventh Symphony, was

premiered in 1952. This late premiere came after his prudently fallow period following Zhdanov's cultural purges of 1948, and even then Prokofiev feared that he might be misunderstood. Whilst confined to bed he confided to his friend Kabalevsky that he was extremely anxious whether his intentions had been understood.[99] It is fascinating that, despite Zhdanov, his concern with Kabalevsky was about his intentions regarding artistic interpretation rather than the 'thought police', by whom much of Prokofiev's work in 1948 had been condemned, especially his opera *The Story of a Real Man*. Jaffé believes the authorities were determined to break him one way or another.[100] His last ballet, *The Stone Flower*, based on Ural folk legends, was started in 1948 but premiered only in his last year. It drew criticism, and he was cast low by this as his health and strength ebbed. In the winter of 1948–49 he was very ill and went into the Kremlin hospital. With one hand they gave, having with the other already taken away. When his Cello Concertino was premiered in February 1952 by Richter and Rostropovich, he was too ill to go on the platform. He had also pragmatically written an upbeat third movement to his Seventh Symphony, to replace a sadder one.[101] But he told Rostropovich to lose the Soviet ending after he had died.[102] Early in 1953 he insisted that Mira catalogue his last works (Opus 132 to 138) – probably the prescience of a dying man.[103]

On 5 March 1953 he was working on a duet. By now he and Mira were living in relative poverty. Having suffered a bout of 'flu, he staggered out of his study complaining of a crashing headache and saying that he felt nauseated and dizzy; he then lost consciousness and died within an hour.[104] The doctor attending diagnosed a stroke due to a massive cerebral haemorrhage,[105] which is likely to be correct on a balance of probabilities. There was no autopsy, and forty-eight hours later he was buried. Hingtgen records that the Prokofiev archive, not assembled until 1994, was 'unable' to provide her with any more information regarding his medical condition.[106] It is fascinating, given many similarities in their lives and backgrounds, to contrast Prokofiev's persistence with a melodic, sometimes romantic and un-Soviet genre with Shostakovich's increasingly heroic astringency. Although both were humorous and witty men, even in their music, Prokofiev was seldom bleak or ascetic. There is something Mahlerian in his description of the Fifth Symphony as 'a symphony of the greatness of the human spirit'.[107] Shostakovich understood and was overwhelmed by the Soviet system; perhaps Prokofiev's often lighter genre was because he never fully grasped its realities, despite being worn down by them.

✢ HECTOR BERLIOZ ✢
(1803–1869)

Remembrance of Things Past
Marcel Proust

Without good contemporaneous and preferably medically recorded observations, especially with an autopsy report, musical pathography can readily descend into a murky brew of speculation, hagiography or demonology; and to what purpose? The best of all endeavours is when we are able to present fresh research from a sound basis, so it is with some apprehension that one approaches Berlioz, that giant of nineteenth-century Romanticism. Berlioz's life from beginning to end was touched with pathos, irony and sadness, based in part upon his own impulsive fatalism as well as poor health. Much remains elusive, including his medical conditions. What cannot be doubted is his mental disturbance, which is almost emblematic of his creative career. His life and his medical history often became indivisible.

A Sad and Troubled Pathography

So what do we know? Firstly, he may have suffered several strokes near to the end of his life,[108] possibly dying from another. Secondly, in common with many inhabitants of these pages, his life was seldom free of money worries, unhappy and unsuitable romances and sometimes a failure of public recognition. Thirdly, there can be no doubt that from the late 1840s, if not earlier, until his death, he was increasingly tortured by abdominal pain often referred to at the time as 'intestinal neuralgia' or 'grippe', which was sufficient to force him to relinquish engagements. Today this diagnosis only infers serious abdominal pain. As a consequence, he was often dependent upon laudanum, although there is little firm evidence that he became fatally addicted to opiates, or to alcohol. Lastly, in response to all of these afflictions, although basically a passionate man, he became increasingly sardonic, desolate, despondent and lonely. His mood changes too could be extreme and sudden. An ability to bounce back as a young man receded as he aged. At the end of 1831, back in Rome, he took to wearing a hooded greatcoat. It was perhaps so garbed that he accompanied the corpse of a young woman to a communal grave.[109] Perhaps, like

Bruckner, he held a morbid fascination not just for death, but also for the dead. In 1864 he wrote of death, 'Take me when you will! What is he waiting for?'[110] Thereby we can attempt to imbricate his often tortured psyche with an unknown intestinal affliction and then the final presumed strokes. He distinguished two types of mental 'spleen'; the first frenetic and potentially creative, the other passive – just sleep.[111] This is evidence of a manic-depressive cyclothymic tendency. Creativity and the depressive component of bipolar disorder are mutually exclusive.

As early as 1828 we read of another round of illness, including bronchitis which troubled the rest of his life.[112] This pattern had three components. He was chesty, but the 'angina' described as early as in his twenties and thirties was not the angina of coronary heart disease that we know today. Had it been, he would probably have died much younger. The scant descriptions, reinforced by his build and colouring, suggest that he was possibly asthmatic. When reluctantly based in Rome, he claimed that the city 'threatened his lungs', and even got himself a sick note to excuse him from living there.[113] In common with Mozart, Bizet, Elgar and Mahler he suffered from recurrent septic throats, and he is reputed to have once lanced a tonsillar abscess himself.[114] Like Liszt and Lord Nelson he had such poor teeth that, by early middle age, very few were left.

His sometimes febrile attraction to women was first manifest when, as the twelve-year-old son of a doctor from near Grenoble, he fell for a girl six years older.[115] The sweet Estelle Duboeuf in pink boots was probably his first fulfilment of a developing ideal of womanhood whilst he approached puberty. As his story starts with Estelle, so it ended with her more than half a century later.

When he was seventeen Berlioz went to Paris to study medicine. He stuck it for two years and even passed the examinations,[116] but loathed it. He then thought of studying law. Instead, he enrolled at the École Royale de Musique, despite paternal disapproval. He went on to discover the Paris Conservatoire library in 1826,[117] and it was shortly after, pursuing his lifelong love affair with Shakespeare, that he went to see a travelling English theatre company under Charles Kemble. Its leading lady had been replaced by a bonny young Irish actress, Harriet Smithson, about whom Berlioz famously developed his *idée fixe*. He was enchanted by her Ophelia in *Hamlet* and it became 'the supreme drama of his life'.[118] In 1829 she was told he was epileptic and possibly mad.[119] I can find no evidence of his suffering from true epilepsy. It would be several more years before they actually met properly. The *idée fixe* emerged musically during 1830 in his first major success, the *Symphonie fantastique*. This was when Berlioz finally won the Prix de Rome, but with a piece little known today, *Sardanapale*.[120] By then he had become engaged to the very suitable Camille Moke. With Camille he now wanted to remain in Paris, but was not excused from his obligatory two-year domicile in Rome.

In 1831 he heard that Camille Moke (or her mother) had broken their engagement in favour of the heir to the Pleyel piano empire.[121] Armed with two pistols, poison and a female disguise to gain entry to his beloved's boudoir, he set off for France. He would do away with her and also an innocent man (possibly Pleyel), then finally himself.[122] Whilst in Nice on his way back he mislaid his disguise and guns, so went to the beach instead, where it is generally surmised that he went nocturnal swimming with a girl he had just met. He explained, 'As you see, I am cured.'[123] The story is related if only to illustrate his capricious tendency.

On 9 December 1832 he gave a concert consisting principally of the *Symphonie fantastique* and *Le retour à la vie*, also known as *Lelio*. His symphony was inspired not just by his *idée fixe*, but also by his reading of De Quincey's *Confessions of an Opium Eater*.[124] It was a great success, and he received many notes of congratulations from prominent audience members including Chopin, Liszt, Paganini – and Harriet Smithson.[125] A week later they met, she speaking very little French and he even less English. On 1 March 1833 she broke her leg,[126] from which she never totally recovered. Against the wishes of both families and the friendly fatherly advice of Liszt, they married on 3 October 1833.[127] She was thirty-four, he four years younger. Their only son, Louis, was born ten months later.[128] Even before they married, Berlioz took an overdose of opiates, only to quickly change his mind, taking ipecacuanha to successfully induce prolonged, life-saving vomiting.[129] Here we see again his impulsive approach to and quick withdrawal from the abyss, not to mention his skills in self-treatment. Holoman judges that from the beginning of their marriage there had been little evidence of mutual support. They even had separate bedrooms. Nevertheless, there followed in the mid- to late 1830s a lull, a period of stability, if not mutual happiness. It was a fecund period of composition. The first major piece to follow his marriage was *Harold in Italy*, after Byron's *Childe Harold*. By now, under Berlioz's influence, orchestral composition and playing were being revolutionised, in fact modernised, as was conducting.[130] With Berlioz we approach the era of von Bülow and Wagner, both of whom admired him. Then, in 1838, the completion and the rehearsal stages of *Benvenuto Cellini* were torrid and he fell violently ill, possibly because of overstress. Berlioz withdrew the work after six performances, only three of which were complete.[131] In late summer he went down with severe bronchitis, which lingered until that year's end.[132] On 18 December Berlioz was in bed with bronchitis when Paganini sent a gift of 20,000 francs, saying, 'Beethoven having left us, only Berlioz can make him come alive again.'[133]

By 1840 his career was established, whereas Harriet's had disintegrated. She had become impossible to live with and lost her looks, becoming stout, disorganised and often drunk. In 1844 they separated, although materially he cared for her until she died in 1854 after several disabling strokes.[134] He was saddened and emotionally disturbed by her death despite the separation. When she was a semi-paralysed and aphasic, drunken wreck, he never quite relinquished the *idée fixe* of his idealised memories. Even before their separation he had begun his affair, probably in 1841, with the singer Marie Récio, a woman of limited ability beyond the predatory, but of erotic bearing, described by the young Hanslick as 'Berlioz's fiery-eyed Spanish lady'.[135] Berlioz dedicated the fourth song of his cycle *Les nuits d'été* to her. In 1842 he had been ill again with tonsillitis accompanied by tinnitus and a transient deafness, and spasm of the right hand.[136] The following year, during a tour of fifteen concerts, his throat troubled him once more, but this time he noticed weight loss and complained of abdominal colic,[137] which was to become his life's burden for the next twenty-six years. It is difficult to separate the physical from the psychosomatic with Berlioz. When he was preparing a concert for 8,000 people during the 1844 International Festival of Industrial Products he became ill with 'nervous agitation', accompanied by chills and sweats. Typhoid was diagnosed, for which he was bled during the concert interval by his old anatomy teacher.[138] It is interesting that he sometimes continued working whilst allegedly ill, claiming that conducting improved his health. Conversely, whilst he was truly unwell, composition was often temporarily put aside. By 1849 the 'intestinal disorder' had become much more established. From now on it was worsened by stress and improved by holidays, which usually were no longer than a week. That year he was hard at work on the *Te Deum*, which he said lifted his spirits and improved his health; the two probably were interrelated.

Eight months after Harriet's death in 1854 he married Marie, and seven weeks later his cantata *L'enfance du Christ* was an immediate success. Once more his abdominal symptoms were severe, so much so that cholera was diagnosed.[139] Indecision at the time as to whether it was cholera or a milder version known then as cholerine implies that it was not cholera. As we saw with Tchaikovsky (Chapter 6) the clinical course of cholera is an easily recognised pattern. This diagnosis, however, implies that he had experienced copious diarrhoea. Holoman states, 'Everything we know of this problem suggests a diagnosis of ulcerative colitis – a condition aggravated by emotional stress.'[140] About this diagnosis we should also be sceptical. This section concludes with a brief analysis of the likely diagnosis. Nevertheless, this was the time when Liszt's mistress, Princess Carolyne Sayn-Wittgenstein, encouraged him to continue with the mighty task of setting the second and third books of Virgil's *Aeneid* for the musical stage. In the manner of Wagner, Berlioz also wrote the libretto. He finished the two-part magnum opus *Les Troyens* in April 1858, composition having been interrupted by days or weeks in bed. The first part, 'La prise de Troie' (Acts 1 and 2), was not performed in his lifetime. Acts 3, 4 and 5, 'Les Troyens à Carthage', were not premiered until 1863, when recurrence of his chronic bronchitis caused him to miss half of the twenty Paris performances.[141] From contemporary accounts we learn that he likened his abdominal pain to a band around his middle effected by sitting forward.[142] His protégé Camille Saint-Saëns noted that Berlioz was a gourmet, but that when he refrained from rich food he was better.[143]

In the 1860s Berlioz became increasingly dependent upon laudanum, although he said that sometimes it did little for the pain, but at least made him dopey and allowed him to sleep.[144] As early as 1859 the singer Pauline Viardot, who coveted a role in *Les Troyens*, had been horrified by Berlioz's appearance when visiting him and later wrote not only of his 'intestinal illness' but of his 'life hanging by a thread'.[145] She said he would not be at *Les Troyens*.[146] But it was Marie who died of a heart attack in 1862 and, although he had told his son, Louis, that marriage had been a millstone around his neck,[147] he was again grieved by this loss, and Marie's mother became his faithful carer for the rest of his life. He became lonely and in the evening would sometimes walk through the Montmartre cemetery, where both his wives were now buried. At the cemetery he mysteriously met a girl of twenty-six, and with this Amélie he briefly fell in love. She too was unwell and ended this affair, although that too may only have been a theatrical concept in Berlioz's mind. Later, by chance, he was devastated to discover that Amélie too had been lying in the Montmartre graveyard for six months. He told Princess Carolyne that she wrote like an angel.[148]

After *Les Troyens* he retired from both musical politics and composition, although he still travelled abroad to conduct when he was well enough and taught a little sometimes. His 'intestinal neuralgia' led him to say that he felt as if he had spent his whole life in bed.[149] Increasingly ill, edentulous and lonely, he reawakened his childhood infatuation with Estelle Fornier (née Duboeuf), now a respectable widow of sixty-seven.[150]

Re-acquaintance with Estelle seemed to enliven him. Once more the burden of remembered imagery, which he cast over this worthy widow, only caused her to mark out the boundaries of their relationship. They last met in September 1867, by which time he had long since stopped proposing marriage. Macdonald states that her attitude moved from incomprehension to sympathy.[151] He still wrote to her lovingly and regularly until his death, and he dedicated his *Mémoires* to her.

A little earlier, in the spring of 1865, feeling more invigorated, he went to see Louis, whose ship had docked at St Nazaire. On the way he became violently ill with the severest attack of 'intestinal neuralgia' he had hitherto endured. Worse was to follow for, as his strength ebbed in 1867, he received the tragic news that Louis, by now a sea captain of whom he had become proud at last, had died of yellow fever in Havana.[152] He was now alone. So he burned a lot of his memorabilia and correspondence, for there was no longer anyone for him to leave them to. His doctors became anxious about the obvious increase in his frailty and weakness. He hated the cold and longed for the warm days of summer and of the south. An engagement to conduct the *Damnation of Faust* in Vienna before Christmas 1866 had caused him fatigue but excitement, both of which weakened him further.[153]

Whilst Berlioz was in Russia for a handsome fee, a journalist said his body was as thin as his baton, so audiences were uncertain as to which he used to beat time.[154] In February 1868 he was back in Paris, only to re-pack his bags and go on to the warmth of Nice. Just before leaving, Dr Nélaton, who had attended to the dying Rossini, declared that 'No cure is possible.'[155] Shortly after arrival, he fell down some rocks by the beach on a vist to Monaco and gashed his face open. It is assumed that this was the first of several mini-strokes that he suffered.[156] That seems likely, in that when he returned to Nice he took a stroll on the promenade, where there was nothing upon which to stumble. But once more he blacked out (perhaps a drop attack or TIA) and fell. As Berlioz had so often done before, he retired to bed for a week, refusing to see local doctors. On returning to Paris he was kindly nursed by his mother-in-law and manservant and was visited by his own doctor.[157] It was noted that now he had difficulty in writing. Uncertainty remains whether this was simply due to weakness or was in fact dysgraphia, which is the written equivalent of dysphasia and a possible neurological consequence of a stroke. The point is of relevance in that, when he was to be a guest of honour at a choir festival with a banquet in August that year, he was unable to speak. Fortunately he had made notes and, using them, someone else addressed the guests on his behalf.[158]

He returned to Paris for the remainder of his life. Of this coda reports are mixed. Generally he went for little strolls, often thought of the past, fed the birds and felt lonely. But there are also accounts of his calling on friends and going out for bibulous dinners until 2.00a.m.[159] From December 1868 until his death three months later, Holoman describes him as withering away.[160] On 3 January 1869 he wrote his last letter, although by then his powers of speech were poor, as was his ability to hold a pen. Increasingly he stayed in bed and, on 8 March 1869, he babbled a little and is alleged to have said, 'All is emptiness.'[161] So it was that he just faded out like a guttered candle.

Conclusion

Berlioz's cause of death remains uncertain. It is convenient to speak of a stroke or strokes, for at least two seem well-described episodes which preceded his death by only a few months and thus raise this possibility. These were probably mini-strokes, although his final days and weeks sound more like an inexorable decline unmarked by a sudden event such as a stroke. Nevertheless, a couple of drop attacks, followed by difficulty in writing, speaking and possibly partial paralysis, make that diagnosis in 1868 likely. But by March 1869 the ultimate cause of his death may have been atherosclerosis of the cerebral circulation slowly clogging up the blood supply to his brain. additionally, he clearly had a lifelong predisposition to asthma or chronic bronchitis, perhaps both, not helped by his weakness for cigars.

The interesting question is: what was the cause of his 'intestinal neuralgia' or 'grippe'? We can only speculate but, upon a balance of probabilities, the descriptions which we have deflect us from the upper gastrointestinal tract, where we can safely bid farewell to peptic ulcers, even gallstones, and concentrate on his bowels. The history is far too long to encourage a diagnosis of cancer. So, to generalise, we are left with inflammatory bowel disease. Berlioz's highly strung personality fits well with the allegedly psychosomatic and modern diagnosis of irritable bowel syndrome, which, nevertheless, is improbable as the pain seems to have been too extreme. The severity of his symptoms and wasting might suggest ulcerative colitis, as proposed by Holoman,[162] or Crohn's disease. Typically, ulcerative colitis is not particularly painful; Crohn's disease may be. Also rectal bleeding, a prime feature of ulcerative colitis, is never mentioned. Severe pain makes either less likely than diverticulitis, which fits the known clinical facts

neatly. In that condition pouches (diverticula) of the bowel lining pro-
trude through the muscular bowel wall and become inflamed. Areas of
bowel become constricted leading to disturbed bowel habit and pain,
sometimes severe and colicky and often cramp-like. Episodes of fever
and general malaise as well as weight loss may occur. Any relationship
between exacerbations of this condition and emotional stress remains tenuous. Today medicines and even surgery to resect loops of affected large
bowel in diverticulitis may relieve symptoms, if not being curative. We
may speculate: if better therapy had been available then, would Berlioz
have continued composing for longer? On balance, that seems improbable because his melancholic and then impetuous temperaments were the
weather vanes to his late musical silence, and it seems likely that it was
Estelle, Harriet, Marie, Amélie and Estelle again who charted the course
of his music through all the other afflictions which frequently beset him.

Finally, there is another condition which satisfies well the doctors' principle of never making two diagnoses where one will suffice. The pancreas is
a large structure lying between the duodenum and the spleen (see Brahms
in Chapter 10). With acute inflammation of this organ, the sufferer will
either quickly die or recover. Chronic pancreatitis, however, can ensue
and today is due to excessive alcohol intake in 80% of cases. There is little
convincing evidence to label Berlioz as an alcoholic, although substance
misuse may enter his history. His symptoms included severe pain effected
by bending forward, intolerance to rich food and gross wasting, which all
resonate well with features of chronic pancreatitis. Even the drop attacks
could be attributed to disturbance of insulin secretion, which often occurs
in chronic pancreatitis. Today the diagnostician would wrestle with diverticulitis versus chronic pancreatitis, both of which remain very difficult to
treat.

Had there been no Berlioz, then the coming of the golden age of French
music would have been uncertain. One even questions whether the epic
scale of sometimes programmatic music by Bruckner, Mahler or Richard
Strauss would have been less likely and the era of the 'Great Conductors'
less probable. Hector Berlioz is as intrinsic to the development of musical
composition and performance during the last 175 years as the Stephensons
are to high-speed mass travel. It is a remarkable achievement for an often
tragic figure so obsessed with those remembrances of things past and tortured by abdominal 'grippe'.

Christoph Willibald Gluck (1714–1787)

As Gluck came to prominence, Italian opera was all but the rule. Driven on by his librettist, Calzabigi, he declared, 'I believe my greatest labour should be devoted to seeking a noble simplicity',[163] which is almost a motto for reform opera, of which *Orphée et Euridice*, *Alceste* and *Iphigénie en Tauride* were shining emblems. Dr Burney described him as a hearty eater and drinker, saying he was 'coarse in figure and in look'.[164] In manners and appearance he bore similarities to Handel, not least a tendency to be bullish as a conductor.

He had married a well-connected lady in 1750, although sadly they remained childless. Croll and Dean delicately describe a disease caught from the singer Gaspera Beccheroni, former mistress of an English diplomat, in 1748.[165] They conclude that this illness may have caused his childlessness. We can only speculate, but gonorrhoea was prevalent, and its effects on the testes can cause infertility. Syphilis is a most unlikely explanation on the available evidence surrounding the succeeding thirty-eight years.

As the 1770s evolved, Gluck's allegiances and ambitions lay in both Paris and Vienna,[166] although there is a suggestion that he retreated from the strife he had unleashed in Paris over 'reform opera'.[167] He produced German and French versions of several operas. Illness kept him away from Paris in the summer of 1775. Howard suggests that developing high blood pressure detained him in Vienna. On 18 May 1779, whilst rehearsing *Echo et Narcisse* in Paris, he had what was generally described as an apoplectic fit, regarded now as being his first stroke, from which recovery was swift,[168] although Howard comments that he now knew his creative career was over. By 1781 he was semi-retired, although he remained busy for several more years with matters of production. One may ask whether his stroke or fit was the beginning of mental deconstruction, or was it perhaps the sick note he desired to let him bow out gracefully after all the musical politics? That was despite a more serious stroke in May 1781 which left him with temporary weakness down his right side.[169] This appears to have resolved quickly, although not fully; he spoke in a letter of 1782 of his 'head being weakened'.[170] Cooper describes Gluck in 1783 as, 'still clear-brained and witty'.[171] He planned travelling (almost escaping) to London in the autumn of 1783, but had to cancel the trip because of a third stroke,[172] before which he had written of 'rheumatism of the head'. By now he was speaking in a word salad of German, French and Italian as he attempted revisions of earlier work.

On 15 November 1787 Mr and Mrs Gluck entertained two old friends from Paris to lunch. His wife slipped out to arrange for a carriage to take them out for an afternoon drive. No sooner had she left the room than Gluck gulped down a glass of something normally forbidden on doctor's orders. He became a little erratic, and half an hour later, when out on his carriage ride, he suffered a seizure, relapsing into a coma from which he never recovered, succumbing the same evening to his final apoplexy or stroke.[173] Gluck died a very rich man, but left only one florin each to the poorhouse and the general hospital, the town hall and the high school.[174] We can intriguingly speculate whether this was because, by the time he made a will, he had become demented. The impact of successive strokes upon composition is readily evident from the dated inventory of his operas, and there seems little reason to disagree with the diagnosis of successive strokes as the cause of death and preceding decline. There were also intervening 'apoplexies' which were most likely to have been mini-strokes (TIAs). In the eight-to ten-year course of this final illness, no significant composition flowed after *Echo et Narcisse* in 1779, whereas from 1741 to 1779 there had been forty-three operas, many of which are still extant.

Charles Gounod (1818–1893)

Gounod, sometimes known as the 'philandering monk',[175] is best known for his opera *Faust*. Even more entertaining was his private life whilst residing for three years at Tavistock House in London with Captain Harry and Mrs Georgina Weldon, characters straight out of Dickens, who himself had resided there earlier. Gounod's many rejected attempts to bed this still attractive woman, encouraged by Harry, are the stuff of Whitehall farce with midnight departures, loaded pistols and lost trousers.[176] Nevertheless, she nursed him through problems with eczema, abdominal colic, dysentery, bronchitis and pulmonary congestion.[177] To these were added in 1874, when Mrs Weldon was in full flow as a self-appointed lawyer and mighty litigant, 'alarming cerebral attacks, with periods of unconsciousness'.[178] The Weldons concluded that 'The old man is off his head again.'[179] This is readily accounted for as a mini-stroke or TIA, although Gounod's survival for another nineteen years could suggest a more benign diagnosis. Extra or dropped heartbeats (extrasystoles), which he may well have had, are usually unthreatening, but can produce unpleasant episodes of light-headedness.

It was Gounod's good fortune that, whilst these medical problems were at their zenith, the formidable Mme Gounod, referred to by Mrs Weldon as the 'little old brown woman',[180] sent M. le Docteur Blanche to England to extricate the great man from 'Chère Mimi' and Whiddles the dog.[181] Back in France, it must be said that his eczema, congested lungs, bowel irregularity and piles all tended to settle, as did his fevered emotions. A renaissance of composition recommenced under his wife's supervision as his daily routine became much more ordered and respectable than it had been amongst the cats, dogs and orphans at Tavistock House. His last ten years were said to be given over to religious reflection and composition, and he continued to compose industriously until the end.[182] This was facilitated by Georgina issuing a writ which made it financially impossible for Gounod to return to England. Thus he reposed with his wife, whose mantra was to only trust a man once he was dead. In 1891 there were features suggesting cerebral decline, with weakness down one side.[183] By 15 October 1893, when he had become old and frail, sometimes struggling to find his words, he was completing a requiem for his grandson. Looking over the score he slumped, clasping a crucifix, and relapsed into a deep coma.[184] A massive stroke was probably correctly diagnosed, and he died two days later. Mercifully, Mrs Weldon was unable to attend the funeral.[185]

We turn now to Felix Mendelssohn, with whom high blood pressure seems very probable, being associated with a congenital abnormality in the circulation at the base of the brain, which was to be his death knell.

✢ FELIX MENDELSSOHN ✢
(1809–1847)

I would gladly give all my works if I had succeeded in writing a piece like the Hebrides Overture

Johannes Brahms, 1890

So what does one say about a very successful composer who was well educated, wealthy, for most of his life healthy, handsome, popular with the ladies and then happily married? Thackeray described him as having the most beautiful face he had ever seen.[186] One could add that he was also a good painter, multilingual, a poet and athletic, being an exceptional swimmer, a good horseman and a gymnast.[187] And, of course, he was a composer crucial in the development of nineteenthcentury Romantic music. Schumann, who suggested his being the Mozart of the nineteenth century,[188] pointed to Mendelssohn's innate modesty and decency. The tragedy was his premature death. Hirschbach and Brockhaus both regarded Mendelssohn's career as easier for him than was the case for other composers.[189]

In modern times some have found his music too facile, too emollient, lacking the inner turmoils of Tchaikovsky and Mahler or the gravitas of Beethoven and Brahms. Mendelssohn was generally a contented man and, of course, he had a lot with which to be contented. Mercer-Taylor believes that with the Octet, composed when he was only seventeen, Mendelssohn evolved a technique and style which would prevail in much subsequent composition.[190] This is what separates Mendelssohn from almost all the other great composers in these pages. His life, until the last few years, was never a struggle and, for all his wealth, composition was generally the holiday job as he pursued an increasingly punishing schedule as virtuoso pianist, conductor and music director.

Into his early thirties Mendelssohn's health was generally good, although during 1829 he injured his right leg in a coach accident on his way back from his first British tour, happily lingering for an extra two months. Although there would not appear to have been any long-term consequences, it is clear from correspondence that a lump of skin and flesh was gouged out.[191] In an era preceding antibiotics and good standards of wound care, there were a number of grave risks that he happily avoided, despite copious blood-letting, such as tetanus (lockjaw) or problems with the wound becoming seriously infected and not healing. Until the Second World War people lost limbs for injuries such as this.

In 1837 he married a calm and reserved girl, Cécile Jeanrenaud, nine years his junior.[192] She was the only love of his life and the marriage was a happy one, bearing five children. Neumayr quotes Mendelssohn's friend Klingemann as saying that, by 1840, doctors noted that complaints of headache had become more frequent,[193] and Mendelssohn was strongly advised to reduce his workload. In 1840 he swam in the invigorating waters of the Rhine near Bingen.[194] He became dizzy and had a nosebleed. Like Robert Schumann, he was rescued from the cold waters by a ferryman;[195] he complained of severe headaches for much of the next fortnight, becoming depressed. 1840 was the year when he wrote to Moscheles's wife that he had become weak and tired.[196] This all suggests hypertension (raised blood pressure).

A shadow was cast when, in 1842, Mendelssohn's mother Leah died of 'apoplexy'; accounts of which by both O'Shea and Cherington would fit well into the clinical picture of a patient succumbing to a subarachnoid brain haemorrhage,[197] of which more soon. Despite this and other possible setbacks, he continued to juggle with his duties between Leipzig and Berlin as well as travel overseas. But by now there were warning signs that his seemingly effortless odyssey through European music was at a price. For a start, he was grossly overworked.

During 1846 he became listless and then restless but weary and even bored, with increasing headaches, although his mastery of the Lower Rhine Festival was a great success during which he seemed to be his old self again. On 19 July 1846, having been told to reduce his work schedule, he gave his final public performance as a pianist.[198] By December 1846 he declared that the concert platform was becoming disagreeable to him.[199] He last conducted at the Leipzig Gewandhaus in April 1847.[200] In Britain again that year he conducted *Elijah* six times in a fortnight, by which he was exhausted, returning home a 'weary, ageing man'.[201] Whilst in Frankfurt, he heard the tragic news that his sister Fanny had died aged only forty-two. She had been playing her brother's *Walpurgis Night* and had complained of nose bleeds when she suddenly lost the use of her hands and quickly relapsed into a coma, dying four hours later.[202] Both parents had died quickly and unexpectedly, their father aged fifty-eight in 1835. Felix's sister Rebecka also succumbed to a stroke in 1858.[203] Mendelssohn's testimony for his beloved sister was his most solemn composition, the String Quartet in F minor Opus 80, also known as 'Requiem for Fanny'. The medical histories of Felix, Fanny and other Mendelssohns were briefly described by Fanny's son Sebastian Hensel.[204] Todd refers to Ward Jones's revelation (published in German in 2000) of Cécile's account of Felix's last month.[205]

After Fanny's death the Mendelssohns, with Fanny's widowed husband, the artist Wilhelm Hensel, went for a prolonged holiday to the Bernese Oberland. Felix's friend the English music critic H. F. Chorley noticed that he seemed sad and looked older than he was as they walked across Wengenalp to reach Grindelwald.[206] After returning to Leipzig, Mendelssohn went on to Berlin and visited Fanny's apartment, by the sight of which again he fell into an inconsolable depression,[207] described by Neumayr as a nervous breakdown.[208]

On 9 October 1847 Mendelssohn went to the house of Livia Frege to play some songs. His friend the violinist Ferdinand David described to the English composer Sterndale-Bennett 'an attack' wherewith Mendelssohn had become delirious for several hours, with cold extremities and an irregular pulse.[209] A doctor was called, who opined that Mendelssohn had become 'overexcited' and experienced 'a disorder of the stomach'.[210] Bed rest and, almost inevitably, leeches were prescribed. By 28 October he felt much better and was able to go for a short walk. On both 19 and 28 October we have it upon the authority of Sterndale-Bennett, whose grandfather had listened to the composer's brother Paul and his wife, Cécile, that up to this point Felix never became unconscious, nor was his speech affected. On 1 November he suddenly collapsed unconscious and became partly paralysed. There was some intermittent, partial recovery.[211] Then, on 3 November, he cried out again with severe headache, and terminally there were shrieks and 'fearful screams'.[212] Then it was all over. The man with the golden spoon in his mouth, who had royalty among his supplicants, was taken away aged only thirty-eight.

Those two redoubtable German musical pathographers Kerner and Franken both believed that the haemorrhage was due to a rupture of a weakness in the wall of an artery at the base of the brain.[213] Cerebral haemorrhage was believed to be the cause of death at the time. These are known as aneurysms, and the weakness often bulges out like a little berry, a condition not described until 1859. It may leak blood, which is known as a cerebral subarachnoid haemorrhage. During the latter half of the twentieth century many patients had their heads opened to place little clips across the neck of these berry aneurysms at the base of the brain. Such surgery is delicate with no margin for error. There can be great difficulties in reaching the berry aneurysm surgically. In the gentlest of skilful surgical hands the aneurysm, which has already leaked, can just give way once more. Recently, non-invasive methods have been adopted whereby a catheter is directed under X-ray control through the circulation to the mouth of the aneurysm and little beads are then placed in it, whereafter the whole thing hopefully will just scar up and seal off.

It is relevant to the Mendelssohn family history that 20% of patients with a subarachnoid haemorrhage because of an aneurysm have at least one similarly afflicted relative.[214] Moreover, someone presenting with a subarachnoid haemorrhage, and the awful headache which goes with it, often reports an earlier lesser, but similar, episode in their recent past. Mendelssohn had an ever-increasing history of severe headaches, probably for several years before his death. The history, with its associated nose-bleeds, increasing weariness and accounts of irregularity of the pulse, does suggest that he also had some cardiovascular disease with hypertension. We cannot know what his blood pressure was when he became ill. The sphygmomanometer, with which blood pressure is measured today, was still decades away. Nevertheless, uncontrolled raised blood pressure can in itself cause severe headaches and can also heighten the risk of a previously silent aneurysm bursting. Moreover hypertension, like aneurysm, may be hereditary.[215]

Mendelssohn thus probably died of uncontrolled high blood pressure and a subsequent subarachnoid haemorrhage from a cerebral aneurysm. The strongly positive family history points to both these conditions, a likelihood first suggested by Hensel. Clearly Mendelssohn's health had been declining for some time before his death, and this is reflected in his pattern of composition during the 1840s. Hans von Bülow commented that Mendelssohn started as a genius and ended as a talent.[216] His last major orchestral works, the 'Scottish' Symphony (1842) and the Violin Concerto (1844), preceded his death by several years. The Sixth String Quartet was possibly the most significant composition in the year of his death. The oratorio *Christus* and opera *Die Lorelei*, upon which he worked during that year, remained incomplete. Despite a premature end and deterioration of his previously good health during the last few years, we behold an unusual composer. He never knew poverty, rejection, humiliation, long-sustained disability or unhappiness in love, nor mental torments, certainly not until Fanny died. Perhaps the one medical aspect which links him with many other composers is a tendency to be downcast after adverse events. Apart from the 'Requiem for Fanny' it is quite hard to trace the reflection of gloom in his music. But then gloom and melancholy were never Mendelssohn's musical accompaniments for long.

Aaron Copland (1900–1990)

Copland is notable because, although it is so common today, his is the only example of Alzheimer's disease in these studies. The onset may be pinpointed to 1972, after which he composed very little, saying at the time that 'it was as if someone had turned off a faucet'.[217] Only a few piano pieces came in his last eighteen years. There appears to have been a degree of dissembling at the time. He said publicly that he composed less because he was having such a good time conducting, expressing surprise that he did not miss it more. Generally with other composers, where there was a conflict between the two, it was the baton, not the pen, which was set aside. Bernstein attributed Copland's falling-off to his having adopted the twelve-tone method in 1970.[218]

He last conducted on 7 December 1982 with the New Haven Symphony Orchestra. The nature of mental fragmentation with early Alzheimer's is exemplified by his conducting *Appalachian Spring* throughout without a hitch, and yet five minutes later having no recollection of having done so.[219] By the early 1980s he became increasingly disorientated and also developed borderline diabetes.[220] In 1985, after having a colostomy, he lived with resident nurses, and it is said that friends visited less and less, but by then he was under very regular medical supervision. Nevertheless, Bernstein visited him in 1988 and, two years later, Copland was able to recollect the visit. Such windows of sanity are very typical in advancing Alzheimer's disease. He died in New York on 2 December 1990 after two strokes and then pneumonia,[221] which was often said to be the friend of the elderly. So passed one of America's first serious symphonists.

✢ **Chapter 8** ✢

Broken Hearts

But his flaw'd heart
Alack, too weak the conflict to support!
                 William Shakespeare, *King Lear*, Act V scene iii, 1606

Introduction

T HE VERY PHRASE 'broken hearts' is a flexible expression for many sources of inner anguish, bereavement or disappointment, and it can also mean what it says. The heart is a mechanical pump, and pumps break. The ancients held that the heart was the seat of the soul, so a broken spirit became a broken heart. This distinction will be vital when we try to comprehend the last years of Gustav Mahler, but first let us consider the workings of this complex organ (see Fig. 3).

The heart is made up of specialised muscle (myocardium). It is divided into two upper, low-pressure and thin-walled chambers (atria) and two lower, thick-walled and high-pressure chambers (ventricles). Huge veins bring stale blood back to the right side of the heart, which then pumps the blood through the lungs, where it is revitalised with oxygen, returning afresh to the left side. The oxygenated blood is then pumped, in systole, through the aorta, whose branches bring oxygen to all other parts of the body. If your blood pressure is 130/70 then the systolic pressure is 130 and the diastolic 70, which is a healthy reading.

The heart is lined internally by a membrane (endocardium) and surrounded by a membranous sack (pericardium). During our embryonic development, parts of the endocardium specialise to form one-way valves between the chambers. For example, the aortic valve controls the exit from the left ventricle. Like any other big muscle the myocardium itself needs a good blood supply, and that is supplied by the coronary arteries. The heart is an electrically activated pump; accordingly a band of electrical conducting nerve tissue traverses the central septum within the heart. If it activates seventy systolic beats a minute, the pulse rate is seventy.

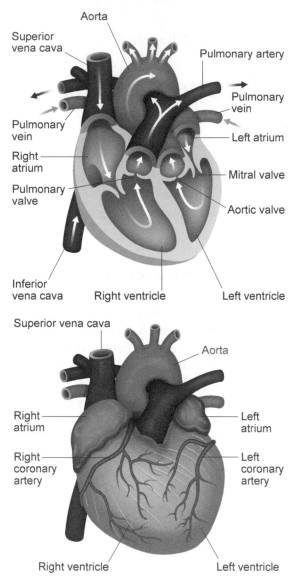

Figs 3 / 4 Diagram of the heart

So what can go wrong with these excellent arrangements? The answer is a lot, of which the following is a very simplified summary.

1 **Endocarditis** is a bacterial infection of the heart's lining, either acute or sub-acute. Previously diseased heart valves may predispose to endocarditis.

Today's treatment: antibiotics.

2 **Valve disease:** Some people have congenitally abnormal valves (e.g. in Marfan's syndrome). Also, diseases such as rheumatic fever can distort the valves, making them too tight (stenosis) so that the blood cannot get out properly, causing inadequate blood supply to the body and harmful back-pressure within the heart itself. Alternatively, the valves may become leaky (incompetence) so that, having been pumped through the aortic valve by the left ventricle, blood partly leaks back. Thus oxygenation of the body's tissues is incomplete and circulation inadequate, leading to breathlessness and heart failure, with peripheral swelling, particularly of the ankles, due to oedema. Minor degrees of valve disease are common and often asymptomatic. They may be first encountered by a doctor hearing a murmur with a stethoscope, whereafter it may be investigated today with an echo machine.

Today's treatment will range from reassurance to open heart surgery, to clear or to replace a diseased valve or valves.

3 **The myocardium:** If the coronary artery supply to this muscle is obstructed gradually, then the patient is likely to experience progressive angina due to myocardial ischaemia, whereas if the obstruction is sudden, a myocardial infarct or MI (aka a 'coronary' or heart attack) will occur.

Today's treatment: Advances over the last four or five decades have been remarkable, originally with open heart surgery to replace the diseased coronary artery and, more recently, with minimally invasive methods to stent and open blockages.

4 **Disorders of conduction** are common, with the pulse too slow (bradycardia), too fast (tachycardia) or irregular (e.g. atrial fibrillation).

Today's treatment: There are many causes and fortunately many good treatments for these disorders, from medication to electrical ablations.

Whether Mozart died of kidney or heart failure or both is discussed in Chapter 1. The final chapter of Bizet's life (Chapter 1) ended with heart failure, as probably did those of Joseph Haydn and Richard Strauss (Chapter 2). Puccini (Chapter 10) probably succumbed to a 'coronary' whilst undergoing treatment for cancer of the larynx. Chopin's lungs (Chapter 9) were so diseased that to make blood pump through them was extremely hard, causing the right side of the heart to fail.

This chapter is set out thematically and not always chronologically.

✣ FRANZ LISZT ✣
(1811–1886)

Love is lame at fifty years
>Thomas Hardy, *The Revisitation*, 1904

Liszt was born two years after the death of Haydn. As an infant he was frail and suffered from febrile convulsions.[1] As he probably never convulsed during adolescence or adulthood, we can conclude that he was not epileptic. Sickly or not, he was soon realised as being a child prodigy and in his teens rose to superstar status amongst the piano virtuosi in Europe. In Vienna he studied with Salieri and Carl Czerny, who described him as pale and sickly and commented on his restless demeanour at the keyboard, concluding, 'He still put a touch of genius into his delivery.'[2] Later, Czerny commented upon his industry and diligence.[3] Throughout his early life Liszt flirted with religion as much as with women, which was to become a lifelong motif. He seems to have lived on his nerves and in the late 1820s, after a government minister ended Liszt's affair with his daughter Caroline de Saint Cricq, he went into a long depression, and may have exhibited catalepsy.[4]

Despite his unpromising beginning, he grew into an aquiline, handsome young man, much admired by ladies. In 1833, he met the attractive Comtesse Marie d'Agoult, with whom he eloped to Switzerland,[5] and later to Italy. There Cosima, the future Frau Wagner, was born. For all the discomforts and dangers of travel Liszt enjoyed 'the tour', especially the adulation, despite sometimes being drunk at a performance's commencement.[6] Watson describes him as an emblem of today's superstar system.[7] On 9 May 1835 Liszt collapsed at the keyboard whilst giving the premiere of *Konzertstück* for two pianos on Mendelssohn's *Songs without Words*.[8] These circumstances suggest a fainting attack rather than an epileptic seizure, or was it part of the performance as O'Shea suggests?[9] Liszt was always a supreme showman, and his motivation may have exceeded his physical capacity.[10] After his relationship with Marie finally broke up bitterly in 1844, a stressful life became increasingly fuelled by brandy and cigars.[11] Berlioz said that Liszt played supremely well with a hangover. Nevertheless, he was the 'first modern pianist', and Walker suggests that he was to piano playing what Euclid was to geometry.[12] Late in Liszt's career Felix Weingartner described him as a confirmed alcoholic.[13]

In Kiev during 1847 Liszt met the immensely wealthy Princess Carolyne

Sayn-Wittgenstein. She was a small, plain, but highly intelligent woman, with teeth stained by heavy cigar smoking.[14] She was also a pious Catholic and a prolix writer. Carolyne left her opulent estate in the Ukraine during 1848 to live with Liszt at Weimar.[15] This was a conservative town, and his living unmarried with a Russian aristocrat who smoked did little to enhance the peaceful retreat which he desired. By his mid-fifties Liszt had become white-haired and stooped, and his once handsome face was disfigured by moles and a shortage of teeth.

The Weimar period had been one of prolific composition, including the *Faust Symphony* and *Dante Symphony*, twelve symphonic poems, seven concertos and much secular and sacred vocal music, as well as pieces for piano and organ. 1857 marked a low point in Liszt's career as a conductor.[16] By 1858, opposition to Liszt and Carolyne in Weimar was increasing, and by 1859 he was sad and disillusioned, having already resigned as Kapellmeister. Although often remote from his children, he was devastated by the death of his son Daniel, probably from TB, in December 1859.[17] He was now motivated to compose *Les morts* in 1860,[18] the year in which Carolyne left Weimar, but not Liszt. Although remaining devoted, they never married, despite twice nearly doing so.

Liszt had been fitted with American dentures in Paris in 1864, but never used them.[19] He became prone to increasing melancholia, was intermittently lonely and drank to excess.[20] In April 1865 he was admitted to minor holy orders, re-emerging with long white hair in a black cassock as the Abbé Liszt. He had retreated to Rome to withdraw from the 'splendour and tinsel' described by the sometimes disapproving Schumanns.[21]

Because of declining eyesight due to cataracts,[22] he adopted a different posture at the keyboard. In 1886 he consulted Alfred Karl Gräfe, a pioneer of modern cataract surgery, which was planned for him in September 1886. His complaints of watery eyes were possibly associated with an eversion of the lower eyelid, known as ectropion.[23] There clearly had been reservations about operating on this frail old man with multiple ailments, and the surgeon was spared possible discomfiture by Liszt's death in July 1886.

Liszt's medical condition when he was in his seventies is well summarised by O'Shea.[24] He complained of severe chest cramps, typical of angina. As a heavy smoker he had developed chronic bronchitis leading to what today is known as chronic obstructive airways disease (COAD) with emphysema. Features of right heart failure are amply described in Liszt's declining years, especially his breathlessness, weariness and gross ankle swelling (oedema).[25] Borodin, who was also a doctor and had been supported by Liszt, noted in 1885 that he was shorter and stouter, that his grey hair was longer and whiter, and that he was out of breath and hard of hearing, with deteriorating eyesight.[26] Similar observations had been made by the famous surgeon Volkmann, who examined him after a fall in July 1881.[27] During March 1886 there was another attack of bronchitis, but he played for the last time in Budapest: a hunched, limping, edentulous old man with white hair and peripheral oedema. He was said to be a ghost from the past who had lost none of his old charisma or technique.[28]

Liszt went in April 1886 to London, where Queen Victoria regarded him as 'a benevolent old priest with white hair and few teeth'.[29] His limp was probably due to osteoarthritis. Jenny Churchill helped him to eat his asparagus and noted 'gouty swellings' on his knuckles.[30] That he required assistance suggests visual problems rather than fingers disabled by arthritis. The nodules may have been due to gout,[31] but it is more probable that they were Heberden's nodes, which are very common in old age, associated with osteoarthritis and usually untroublesome. He had said, 'I sometimes have grave doubts about composing further. Yet I will not give up.'[32]

On 21 July 1886 an ailing Liszt made his way overnight by train to Bayreuth for the festival, which Cosima was supervising.[33] He had to be helped off the train and was accommodated in lodgings near Wagner's home, 'Wahnfried'. He had experienced difficulty with stairs for several years.[34] On arrival he retired to bed with a bad cough and felt very unwell. He slept through much of *Parsifal* on the 23rd and of *Tristan* two days later, apparently wakening only to stifle his cough.[35] The papers of Liszt's student Lina Schmalhausen have recently come to light and are an unrivalled, although probably biased, account of these final days.[36] She infers that Cosima was too preoccupied with the Bayreuth Festival to attend to her father, who perhaps was in the way.[37] However, Liszt had abandoned Cosima after transferring his affections from her mother to Princess Carolyne. Perhaps he reaped as he had sown. The last few days of his life were awful. Dr Landgraf saw him on 25 July, ordered abstinence from brandy and prescribed morphine for his distressing cough.[38] Morphine would have depressed his already compromised respiration, and sudden alcohol withdrawal at that stage could have worsened his confusion. Additionally, and uselessly, foot baths and mustard poultices were administered. He worsened, and giving a second opinion, Professor Fleischer from the University of Erlangen diagnosed a right lobar pneumonia. He told Cosima that nothing further could be done.[39] Despite the Bayreuth Festival, on 27 July Cosima and her daughter claimed to have taken over Liszt's total care until near the end, when a nurse was engaged. Cosima now slept at her father's lodgings, but this was no guarantee of her finding time to actually see him.[40]

On 29 July Liszt again complained of chest pain and spasms, and on the following day he shouted out for air, to the distress of his landlady but not his daughter.[41] On 31 July his dropsy (peripheral oedema) worsened and he became delirious; he received an intracardiac injection probably of camphor, whereupon he convulsed and died fifteen minutes later, without receiving the last rites;[42] Cosima had obstructed the priest. O'Shea believes that his final illness was not lobar pneumonia but the terminal stage of long-standing cardiac failure, probably secondary to COAD.[43] Both are likely and they are not mutually exclusive. We may ask what today's medicine would have achieved. At worst, Liszt's last few days would have been more tranquil and comfortable. Pneumonia is readily treated, and COAD with emphysema at best may be ameliorated, certainly not cured, but his secondary heart failure would have been treated with diuretics and other drugs, with success likely.

Liszt's landlady's husband had to insist that the corpse be removed to 'Wahnfried', as it had started to smell. Cosima then removed the body on a hand cart.[44] The funeral was despatched quickly and with little ceremony, although Bruckner was the organist at a Requiem. The utter bathos was that this towering figure, in a life often adorned by theatrical splendour and intermittently nurtured by religion, died almost alone, almost unmourned and without the final unction which he surely would have desired. Morrison believes Liszt died as a Hungarian, for which turbulent country he became a symbol.[45]

✛ RICHARD WAGNER ✛
(1813–1883)

My mental disharmony is indescribable
                    Richard Wagner, in a letter to Franz Liszt, 1855[46]

With Wagner one fits music between the revolutions, debt, destitution, exile, escape, wives, mistresses and idealistic high culture. He also took himself seriously as a philosopher and writer. After Wagner's flight from the 1848 revolution in Dresden, his health was not good and he was afflicted by an irritating skin condition with rashes, which may have been why he wore silk next to his skin.[47] There have been other (and speculative) explanations for this curiosity, including the suggestion that he was a cross-dresser.[48] The rashes were thought to be erysipelas. They started when he was a puny infant and lasted intermittently all his life. Erysipelas is a skin infection caused by the germ streptococcus. Untreated (before antibiotics) it would have either spontaneously resolved or proceeded to produce further and worse complications. With the mantra of common things being common, this chronic itchy condition was probably a form of eczema. As the rash was often facial and with concurrent symptoms of bowel disorder, rheumatism and both cardiac and respiratory problems, lupus enters the differential diagnosis. This is systemic lupus erythematosus (SLE), a complex auto-immune disease and a distant 'cousin' of rheumatoid arthritis (see Chapter 11). However, there are no known photographs which show the facial ('butterfly') rash characteristic of lupus, with which an onset in infancy would be rare. Then there is the question as to survival for sixty or more years at a time when no effective treatment for lupus was available.

Another chronic affliction throughout his life was alleged migraine. Whether migraine is caused by stress today remains debatable. There is some evidence that sufferers from migraine are most affected during those passages in life that are free from stress. The fact remains that, for much of his adult life, Wagner suffered from severe headaches that were sufficient to make him wretched and unable to work.[49] Descriptions by Cosima of these attacks, with the harbinger of an aura,[50] seem typical of migraine. It was recently suggested that such attacks with 'hammering' pain and cries of 'compulsive plague, pain without end' are depicted in Act I scene i of *Siegfried*, hence a modern production where Mime takes aspirins.[51] Firstly, aspirins are useless for migraine and, secondly, one seriously questions whether the 'German spirit' would have symbolised his own problems in the odious little person of Mime. There are many alternative explanations for chronic headaches, of which eye strain was sensibly suggested by Gould in 1903.[52] This article reviewed Wagner's commentary upon his own health from his correspondence. He clearly had chronic headaches and gastro-intestinal symptoms, and furthermore was cyclothymic. Gould's paper is an inventory of the complaints of an often gloomy and very self-absorbed person.

In 1852 the wealthy businessman Otto Wesendonck generously paid off Wagner's creditors whilst providing him with a salary and a villa. There Wagner is popularly suspected of having seduced Frau Mathilde Wesendonck, which Millington infers, although he questions whether the relationship was consummated,[53] as does Geck.[54] Nevertheless, she became subservient to Wagner's psychological needs, and this was all known to her husband. Wagner even wrote that Mathilde had given him the strength to endure living with his first wife, Minna.[55] From about 1862, when he finally parted from Minna, his complaints of abdominal cramp-like pains increased, with reports of palpitations and chest tightness,[56] probably harbingers of cardiovascular disease. Also in 1862, when he was still inter-mittently on the run financially, he was visited by the leading conductor Hans von Bülow and his wife, Cosima (née Liszt). Thus began one of the most notorious love affairs in the history of music. Whatever the ethi-cal rights and especially wrongs, there can be no doubt of the adoration between these two strange, highly intelligent and overbearing people. In 1866 a halcyon time in their affairs started with marriage and children at a lakeside villa, 'Tribschen', by Lake Lucerne, as musically epitomised by the *Siegfried Idyll*.

These were the days of *Götterdämmerung* and Wagner's realisation that in his cosmic view no existing theatre was fit for the rendition of his music dramas. So in 1871 the Bayreuth project commenced; the theatre opened on 13 August 1876 with *Das Rheingold*.[57] Wagner had by now become even more ill-tempered than usual and increasingly complained of recurrent palpitations and haemoptysis, and also intermittently of tortured depres-sion.[58] Gregor-Dellin's suggestion of Roemheld syndrome is intriguing,[59] but it seems unnecessary to introduce a real rarity when common condi-tions fit the known symptoms quite well. So overbearing is Wagner's pop-ular image that his self-doubt and even feelings of inadequacy are readily forgotten. By 1880 he was inclined to alleviate his problems with a full flow of brandy. Rheumatism and bowel problems were increasingly reported, although he told Nietzsche's doctor in 1877 that he had been cured of erysipelas by hydropathy.[60] The most consistent complaints to derive from

Gould's review of Wagner's letters, mainly to Liszt or Wesendonck,[61] were largely those of anguish, mental torment and depression, relieved only by the six idyllic years at 'Tribschen' (1866–72).

Although he had his first heart attack in March 1882, later that season, during the last performance of *Parsifal* at Bayreuth, Wagner came down to the pit to conduct the conclusion of Act III.[62] However, by then the Wagners were spending more time in Italy, whose weather was more congenial to his declining health. They spent several months in 1882 at their suite in the Palazzo Vendramin in Venice. Nevertheless, on Christmas Eve Wagner seemed in good spirits and recently revived and rehearsed for the family celebrations his youthful Symphony in C major.[63] Wagner left a body of projected and incomplete music throughout his career, including fourteen dramatic works, but wrote nothing significant in his last year, subdued as he was by depression and angina.

On 13 February 1883, according to their daughter Isolde, he arose late and promptly had a blazing row with Cosima.[64] This was provoked by the revelation that one of his flower-maidens, an English soprano named Carrie Pringle, was coming to stay.[65] Cosima was wary of her husband's young flower-maidens. At lunchtime that day he bade them continue lunch without him as he continued in the study writing his essay 'On the Feminine in the Human'.[66] At a little after two o'clock, the maid heard the master cry out and found that he had collapsed. Cosima came at once and panicked, and the doctor was called. Within the hour, aged sixty-nine, Richard Wagner, revolutionary, republican, entrepreneur, philosopher, anti-Semite, writer, animal rights activist,[67] dramatist, adulterer, serial debtor, supreme egoist and the sublime master of musical theatre, was dead. Cosima inconsolably hugged his body for twenty-five hours;[68] then, in an operatic coda, a gondola draped in black velvet took his body down the Grand Canal to the railway station. On arrival at Bayreuth, in a special train sent by King Ludwig, Wagner's body was taken to 'Wahnfried' for a private burial service, and the whole town mourned.

Wagner's physician in Venice, Dr Friedrich Keppler, declared that his primary problems had been with the stomach and intestines,[69] although he did add that other exertions may have strained his heart to precipitate the great man's demise. Perhaps this was dissembling. Richard Wagner had almost assuredly succumbed to at least his second and fatal myocardial infarct. There had been stressful circumstances a few hours earlier due to the imminence of Miss Pringle's arrival, and there had been rumours although, for all the Wagners' wilful ways, Cosima and Richard were devoted to one another. At this sad time, the last thing anyone wanted was a scandal over his death being provoked by a former mistress (if mistress she was) appearing. Whether or not Carrie Pringle had an earlier sexual relationship with Wagner remains a mystery.[70]

Whatever one thinks of Wagner the man, he left an incomparable legacy of music dramas, stimulating some to make decisions about love, life, death, bravery and power. In 1872 a Munich neurologist, Theodor Puschmann, declared Wagner to be an insane megalomaniac.[71] That surely is too facile, although a popular view. He was a man of wild contrasts, being ill-tempered, volatile, selfish and arrogant. But he was also witty and charming and could be sensitive and gentle, just as his music could. It is little wonder that today with the very mention of Wagner, let alone the word *Ring*, box offices are almost instantaneously sold out. Few of those aficionados would agree with Mark Twain's quip that Wagner's music is much better than it sounds.

✣ ANTONÍN DVOŘÁK ✣
(1841–1904)

He is strange, but his heart is in the right place
Johannes Brahms, 1871

Anatomically, it is stretching a point to include Antonín Dvořák in a section on heart disease. The likely cause of his death makes it convenient to settle him into a chapter in which the circulation between heart and lungs has been explained. Dvořák was a man of few words and simple tastes; his hobbies were pigeon-fancying and train-spotting. Initially apprenticed as a butcher, he later went to the organ school in Prague. There he stayed with a cousin who regarded him as a country bumpkin. Dvořák gave music lessons and fell in love with a wealthy pupil, Josefina Čermáková, who did not return his affections. So Dvořák happily married her sister Anna. Most of their eight children died young, although his daughter Otilie married his star pupil, Josef Suk. It has been suggested that Dvořák's purchase of a country retreat at Vysoká was prompted by his unhappiness with crowds and traffic, which may have been due to incipient cerebral arteriosclerosis.[72] To retreat from city hurly-burly to the country is today many people's ideal too, although antipathy to crowds never kept him out of busy railway stations.

Whilst in America during 1892–93 he studied idioms of black music in New York and of native Indian music at Spillville, a Czech settlement in Massachusetts. Dvořák echoed, rather than set, native themes, both Czech and American.[73] Most plangent was the B minor Cello Concerto, which he completed on returning to Europe, lamenting the early death of his sister-in-law Josefina.[74] By that time his friend and great supporter Brahms was himself close to death. For years Dvořák had held at bay Brahms's entreaties that he take a position in Vienna.[75] Here, for all his rustic, taciturn personality, we encounter a man with an independent and determined spirit. He declined a third and remunerative visit to America; Dvořák was a man most contented at Vysoká and just intrinsically Czech.

Steen suggests that, towards the end of his life, Dvořák was increasingly eccentric, stubborn and irritable, and also that his liking for beer was on the increase.[76] In 1903 Grieg said that Dvořák was 'a character, to put it mildly, but he was very likeable'.[77] But were his powers waning? Robertson records that Dvořák's last performance as a conductor on 20 May 1900 was with his own composition *Festival Song*.[78] Dvořák was then increasingly frustrated by his failure to add another great opera to Smetana's output. In April 1900 he procured a score, *Rusalka,* based on a fairy tale by Hans Andersen. By December it had become second only to *The Bartered Bride* in popularity amongst Czech operas. So decisive and swift an achievement is not suggestive of incipient arteriosclerotic senile dementia. On the other hand, study of the catalogue of works points to a drying-up of creativity by about 1900,[79] as summarised below.

The Dates of Dvořák's Last Compositions

Symphonies 1893
Concertos 1895
Other symphonic works 1897
Chamber music 1896
Keyboard works 1903 (only two works after 1900)
Cantatas/oratorios 1900
Other choral music 1885
Songs/duets 1901 (only one work after 1900)(
Operas 1903 (*Rusalka* 1900, *Armida* 1903)

Perhaps it was comfortable contentment at home, along with the respect and honours heaped upon him, which led him to rest more. His remaining drive was to succeed in opera, as he had already done in most other facets of music. The success of *Rusalka* in 1901 was offset by the failure of *Armida* in 1904,[80] during whose preparation Janáček had noted Dvořák to be especially irritable.[81] This is a starting point with his final illness, of which Dr John Stephens gives a full account in Clapham's biography.[82]

On 25 March 1904, Dvořák complained of worsening pain in his left side. His doctor, Professor Jan Hnátek, advised rest, but five days later Dvořák went train-spotting and caught a chill. He returned to bed the next day and, according to his family, consumed 'over his measure of beer'. This worsened his difficulties with passing urine, for which catheters were used. On 31 March, he took to his bed, where he remained until 17 April. Dvořák then went down with 'flu, retreating to bed until 30 April, when Hnatek suggested that he should get up to enjoy the 1 May celebrations. On arising, he was weak and Anna helped him to dress. He then tottered around the dining room and sat down, to take his soup with apparent relish. Suddenly he announced, 'I am feeling rather dizzy; I shall be glad to lie down.' He grew pale, then flushed and tried to speak as he was helped back to bed, where he quickly became unrousable. By the time the doctor came, he was obviously dead.

At the time, very reasonably, he was said to have suffered a major stroke. We cannot say that that, or a massive heart attack, was not the cause of death. Stephens has argued persuasively that here was a man in his seventh decade who possibly had arteriosclerosis and varicose veins.[83] He may have had some pelvic inflammation due to his urinary problems, and he may even have had a degree of kidney failure. Above all else, he had lain in bed for most of a month, and bed is a dangerous place. We have now encountered six risk factors for a deep vein thrombosis (DVT). We know today that sitting on an aeroplane for twelve hours and becoming dehydrated can cause a fatal DVT. The thrombus can break off, passing through the heart and to the lungs, causing a circulatory blockage in the pulmonary artery. Such a pulmonary embolus (PE) may be fatal. With so sudden, quickly fatal and apparently painless a demise, PE is a probable cause of death.[84]

✢ GUSTAV MAHLER ✢
(1860–1911)

I am thrice homeless

Gustav Mahler to Sigmund Freud, 1910

Bruno Walter, who had been Mahler's assistant, tells us that his face was inscribed by sorrow and humour and that gloom was followed by infectious laughter.[85] Thus we see, as we do in most other respects, that he was a man of dramatic contrasts. He was not only a perfectionist, but an intellectual of Renaissance outlook who devoured books.[86] But it was not all books and study. Mahler took physical exercise and recreation just as seriously. Until 1907 he was a tireless walker, climber, a good oarsman, a keen cyclist and a strong swimmer.[87] His friend Alfred Roller, later to be his stage designer, caught a glimpse of Mahler, aged forty, whilst sunbathing, describing a small, virile, lean and muscular man.[88] Although enjoying an occasional beer or cigar, he was ascetic in his habits and tastes and was a creature of habit.

Early Days

Before explaining Mahler's final illness, it is also important to assess his psyche, not least because of the frequency with which it has been impugned. Born to Jewish parents in Bohemia, Mahler was the second of fourteen children, seven of whom survived infancy or childhood.[89] Despite a scholarly inclination which he encouraged in Gustav, his father, Bernhard, was violent towards his own wife.[90] Freud's disciple Marie Bonaparte recalled that Mahler had told Freud of the episode when, as a rather dreamy and bookish boy, he witnessed a violent episode between his parents, whilst a hurdy-gurdy man played some cheerful banality outside.[91] Freud drew Mahler's frequent musical conjunction of levity and tragedy from this episode.[92]

He was noted by many, from childhood onwards, to have a strange gait, which is described by Levy as jerky.[93] Its alleged cause has variously ranged from a mother fixation* to St Vitus's dance.[94] As Mahler was athletic, we should not tarry upon this issue. As an adolescent he studied in Vienna,

* His mother limped.

where he admired Bruckner and Wagner. He earned a meagre living by teaching and playing the piano.[95] Correspondence from the late 1880s and early 1890s reveals that Mahler experienced moods of sadness.[96] In 1880 he turned to conducting, advancing rapidly from lowly jobs in Bad Hall, Ljubljana, Iglau and Olmütz to Kassel. More illustrious appointments came at Prague, Leipzig and Budapest. In 1889 he pronounced his love not only of nature, but of the bucolic village with all its little pageants, sounds and even smells. This was the year when his sister Leopoldine and both his parents died; Mahler had remained loyal and affectionate to them all.[97] As if this was not enough, in 1889 surgery was undertaken for piles,[98] an unusual procedure in a healthy 29-year-old man.

Then in Hamburg, possibly for the first time, Mahler worked with musicians and singers of the first rank. By now he almost certainly had his eye on the top job at the Vienna Opera. Von Bülow's death in 1894 prompted him to complete the Second ('Resurrection') Symphony.[99] This was no conventional requiem, although it is essentially a Christian offering and clearly one acquainted with grief, death and the hereafter. It seems inevitable that, confronted with so much death, including the suicide of his beloved brother Otto in 1895, he should have expressed his intense feelings in music. Mahler clearly realised his own huge and burgeoning talent, as he pushed the size and range of possibilities of the symphony orchestra as never before with this composition. He later told Sibelius that the symphony must be like the world.[100]

Vienna

Shortly after a triumphant debut in Vienna on 11 May 1897 conducting *Lohengrin*, Mahler had to undergo surgery for his tonsils. It is unclear just what that surgery was, but they were not actually removed (tonsillectomy).[101] Despite his robust stamina, he was for many years plagued by probably septic throats, as well as by severe headaches, diagnosed at the time as migraine.[102] Perhaps they were, or perhaps they were due to chronic sinus problems. Had his tonsils been removed then his life might have been different and longer.

At the turn of the century Mahler's routine was one of winters of frantic production and conducting, followed by summers of physical recreation and composition. So far it had been the deaths of so many of those he loved that influenced his music, his own health generally being excellent, piles, headaches and sore throats apart. However, on 24 February 1901 he conducted Bruckner's Fifth Symphony with the Vienna Philharmonic in the afternoon and *The Magic Flute* at the Opera in the evening. During that performance his piles bled so severely that he nearly died, being saved only by emergency treatment starting with 'insertion of a tube' and then elective surgery a week later, probably haemorrhoidectomy.[103] Thereafter he reduced his commitments, resigning from the Vienna Philharmonic, although punishing hikes and swims continued as before at Maiernigg on the Wörthersee in Carinthia, where he had a composition chalet.

On 7 November 1901 fatefully he met Alma Schindler, a musician twenty years his junior and already a femme fatale within the Viennese Secession. A few months later she was pregnant, and there then commenced a stormy marriage.[104] Alma demanded attention, and was accustomed to receiving it. One can understand her frustration as a highly intelligent, good-looking woman married to a workaholic, confronting the 'Do Not Disturb' sign. Prior to marriage he had insisted that she renounce her ambitions as a composer, in deference to his.[105] Also Mahler's potency may not always have risen to Alma's expectations.[106] This was one of Freud's conclusions in Leyden.[107]

Emotional heat came from Alma, who in 1904, with apparent prescience, advised Gustav not to tempt providence with *Kindertotenlieder* (*Songs on the Death of Children*).[108] Although the song cycle was completed in 1904, the first three songs were composed in 1901, before Mahler had met Alma. Kennedy's verdict upon these songs, that they achieve a mood of 'serene acceptance', fits well with a suspicion that Mahler's musical dealings with death were those of spiritual reconciliation.[109] He had always loved children, had seen so many die and, far from wallowing in self-pitying schmaltz, sought a path of comfort that they might finally be at peace with their Maker. It is that probability which suggests that Mahler's accommodation with a Christian church was spiritual, although he was politically clumsy in achieving it. It is suggested that he converted from Judaism to Christianity at least in part to secure his appointment in Vienna;[110] Roller said that Mahler derived no joy from his Jewish origins.[111] Furthermore, he was deeply concerned with redemption and a hereafter. In Judaism there is no afterlife in the conventional Christian sense, a thought which at times must have been unbearable for Mahler. So here, in those early symphonies, were Christian concepts of redemption and resurrection.

The couple's beloved daughter Maria ('Putzi') was born in November 1902, and Anna ('Mutzi'), later to become a sculptor, followed in June 1904. Then in 1907 Mahler's world fell apart. He is popularly supposed to have been hounded out of the Vienna Opera earlier that year. There had been arguments over money and the frequency of his guest performances away from Vienna.[112] That there were spiteful intrigues with a fervently anti-Semitic content cannot be doubted, but it was Mahler who resigned in July 1907, already having secured a lucrative future in New York at the Metropolitan Opera.[113] He said he was leaving of his own accord.[114] *Fidelio* on 15 October was his last appearance at the Opera, and he conducted his final concert with the 'Resurrection' Symphony on 24 November, to a 'hurricane of applause'.[115]

But far worse had already befallen Gustav and Alma for, whilst on holiday, Putzi had died on 5 July 1907, after a gallant fight against scarlet fever and diphtheria. Simple words do no justice to the grief and anguish of both parents. Alma collapsed shortly after the child's funeral and she and Gustav were examined by their general practitioner, Dr Blumenthal, who in January of that year had already found that Mahler had a 'slight heart valve defect'.[116] Now Blumenthal took a more serious view, recommending a second opinion from Professor Kovacs in Vienna.[117] Exactly what was said can now only be a subject of conjecture. Struck down by this dreadful trilogy of events, the three hammer blows,[118] Mahler was down but in no way out. Bruno Walter recalled that within weeks Mahler just shrugged, saying of his new medical regimen that he would soon get used to it.[119] That is flexible and bravely resilient behaviour. With that he packed up, leaving on 9 December 1907. Gustav Klimt said, 'It's over,'[120] but it was Mahler's Vienna which had ended, not Vienna's Mahler. He had weathered the storm but, with his own innate theatricality, further success and disasters still lay ahead, as the curtain rose triumphantly at the Metropolitan on New Year's Day 1908 with *Tristan and Isolde.*[121]

When he conducted the Eighth Symphony in Munich in March 1910, the acclaim was one of adulation from an audience containing Richard Strauss, Thomas Mann, Schoenberg, Webern, Leopold Stokowski, Clemenceau and Lilli Lehmann, who was horrified by how gaunt he had looked and by how much he had aged.[122] Feder quotes Paul Stefan, his first biographer, who said Mahler was tired and sick, and that when he conducted he became exhausted by the work and its passion.[123]

New York, Gropius and Freud

Mahler quickly resigned from the Metropolitan Opera in favour of the New York Philharmonic. His correspondence with Bruno Walter, from the 'saddest summer' of 1908 at Toblach to late 1909, reveals an ascent based upon a love of life, from bitter resignation to creative optimism.[124] He still used a pedometer whilst taking what previously would have been regarded as gentle little walks, often stopping to take his own pulse, although he still enjoyed walking, despite palpitations, and Alma's description of 'torment' was transitory.[125]

His new works, *Das Lied von der Erde* and the Ninth and incomplete Tenth Symphonies, are not cheery, but it would be wrong to regard them as bleak or totally suffused with the gloom of miserable self-engrossment. In keeping with his physical condition, in these last three great works Mahler developed a more economical style of writing and became more philosophical. By the time he was composing *Das Lied von der Erde* and the Ninth and Tenth Symphonies, he reduced the richly romantic tones of the earlier symphonies, paving the way for twentieth-century modernism. This increased asceticism was clearly born in adversity. Garcia observes that throughout his life Mahler turned adversity into creativity.[126] The tragedies of those about him and those he loved, and ultimately the apprehension that his own death might not be far away, greatly influenced his composition. The first movement of the Ninth Symphony carries the inscription 'O vanished days of youth, O scattered love.'[127] Far from being a hysterical neurotic, as Alma sometimes suggested,[128] he was an extraordinarily strong man, physically and spiritually.

Mahler suffered further heartache in the spring of 1910. When the couple returned from New York, Alma was unwell, unhappy and restless. She was advised to attend the spa at Tobeldad, where she met an attractive young architect, Walter Gropius, who later became her second husband.[129] It was a grand passion of the 'can't live without you' type.[130] Scholars will continue to debate whether Gropius addressed his effusive letter of eternal love accidentally or deliberately not to Alma, but to Herr Direktor Mahler.[131] But that was how Mahler, bowed but not bent by anti-Semitism, overwork, his child's death and an ailing heart, discovered his wife to be an adulteress: a chance letter in the post. We have already caught glimpses of Mahler's compassion, as well as his selfishness. So it was that he confronted Alma and Gropius. His reaction to Alma was that it was really all his fault: he had been tyrannical and shown a lack of empathy towards her, but things now would be different, and indeed they were.[132] For her part, Alma realised that she could not desert him now, although her further correspondence and covert meetings with Gropius, if they show anything, demonstrate that she was an unrepentant two-timer. Over those last months Mahler was an attentive, sweet and loving husband, leaving constant messages of tender endearment for his Almschi and at last helping and encouraging her fairly inconsequential compositions. In essence, at the end they maritally reversed roles. She is said to have cast this aside as a 'sham' once Mahler was dead,[133] although she also said she had loved Gustav and only Gustav.[134]

In the fateful summer of 1910, Mahler had started work on his Tenth Symphony, with its anguished and autobiographical annotations and declarations of adoration for Alma: 'You alone Alma know what this means' 'To live for you! To die for you! Almschi!'[135] Perhaps by 1910 it had all mentally overwhelmed him, although correspondence and first-hand accounts by no means support that. He had bravely survived so much; Mahler was amazingly resilient. The Ninth and Tenth Symphonies show the signs of his precise and meticulous approach to composition.[136] The Tenth has been completed by Deryck Cooke,[137] who, like Colin Matthews,[138] clearly rejects the thesis of failing powers due to declining health inferred by Redlich,[139] saying that any imperfections in its realisation are dwarfed into insignificance by its strength and beauty. Cooke himself believes the Tenth is about love, not death.[140] Mahler was also practical, and arranged an appointment to consult Sigmund Freud.[141] The two men met in Leyden, the Netherlands, where Freud was on holiday, during late August 1910. They walked and talked for four hours, which informs us about Mahler's cardiovascular fitness even then. Seckerson has questioned whether his needing to seek advice in itself reveals more about his mental fitness.[142] Freud's views, in a letter to his colleague Theodor Reik, were succinct, almost prosaic: 'The visit had appeared necessary to him, because his wife at the time had rebelled against the fact that he withdrew his libido from her.'[143] Freud also identified Mahler as having a mother fixation,[144] not to mention Alma's father complex.[145]

The session appears to have been truly useful. Mahler's libido possibly improved, and for him and Alma the few months left to them were more loving and possibly even happier. Alma realised that she could not leave him;[146] if she did, he would die.[147] She had protested that she was married to an abstraction, not a human being.[148] Nevertheless, that did not stem the flow of love letters between Alma and Gropius, which she sometimes signed 'your wife',[149] although she was unstinting in her care of Mahler for the rest of his life.[150] Shortly after Leyden, Mahler had his tonsils cauterised (not removed) in Vienna.[151] That on returning to New York in November 1910 he felt overwhelmed suggests a mental, if not physical, decline. Like many others, Mahler found that rich, cultured New York Music Committee ladies can be very demanding, and after his death there followed a newspaper debate as to how much American demands and pressures had hastened his early and tragic end.[152] He had promised his friend Gustav Adler that he would not return to the USA.[153] By now he was in covert discussions for a return to the Vienna Opera. They had done less well without him than he had without them.

The End

On 21 February 1911, despite a bad throat with fever, Mahler insisted on conducting out of loyalty to his friend Busoni, whose *Berceuse élégiaque* he premiered.[154] He never conducted again. The following day he deteriorated and called in his physician, Dr Fraenkel, who referred him to Dr Libman,[155] then the leading authority on bacterial endocarditis (septic heart valve), whose diagnosis relied upon an assessment of the patient and blood cultures, a technique he himself had pioneered. These are tests whereby blood is taken from a patient and mixed with a broth which encourages bacterial growth, allowing the causative organism to be isolated and identified microscopically. Libman was not surprised to find a heavy growth of the germ streptococcus viridans. Levy believes that by then Mahler's case was hopeless,[156] and he disputes Kennedy's view that penicillin thirty years on probably would have saved Mahler,[157] regarding Kennedy's opinion as 'purely speculative'. Kennedy is probably correct, because today patients at the same clinical stage as Mahler was then can be saved by antibiotics. This is academic because there were no antibiotics then, although in Paris, at the Pasteur Institute, an antiserum was being developed. This was a possible reason for the Mahlers urgently leaving New York for Paris via Cherbourg, accompanied by Busoni. On the journey they were befriended by Stephan Zweig, who later wrote, 'Boundless sadness was in his look, but also something transfigured with greatness, something that faded away into sublimity, like music.'[158] This resonates well with Alban Berg's verdict on the first movement of Mahler's Ninth Symphony:

> The first movement is the most heavenly thing Mahler ever wrote. It is the expression of an exceptional fondness for this earth, the longing to live in peace on it, to enjoy nature to its depths, before death comes, for he comes irresistibly. The whole movement is permeated by premonition of death.[159]

Only a year earlier Mahler had written to Bruno Walter, 'I am thirstier than ever for life.'[160]

At Cherbourg, Zweig watched as Mahler was carried off the ship:

> He lay there deathly pale, motionless, his eyelids shut. The wind had
> blown his greying hair to one side, his rounded brows stood out clear and
> bold and beneath them the hard chin, showing the vigour of his will. The
> skeletal hands lay folded wearily on the blanket. For the first time I saw
> him, the pillar of fire in his frailty.[161]

Dramatic contrast persisted to the end. In Paris, Dr Chantemesse, an eminent microbiologist, became over-excited by virulent streptococci, cultured from Mahler, looking like chains of seaweed down his microscope.[162]
In his enthusiasm he overlooked that they were killing one of the greatest
of all symphonists, still a relatively young man, whose wife was clearly
distressed. The transfusion of antiserum was unsuccessful, and Professor
Chvostek was summoned from Vienna.[163] By the time he arrived in Paris,
Mahler had deteriorated further. Chvostek recommended an immediate
transfer to Vienna. Whether this was because it was believed that Vienna
was the top medical centre, or more probably that Mahler wished to be
buried next to Putzi, remains uncertain.[164]

In Vienna he was taken to Dr Loew's sanatorium, where he was intermittently delirious, calling out 'Mozart' and asking, 'Who would care for
Schoenberg now?'[165] He was toxic, wasted, fevered and confused. He was
given oxygen and digitalis as well as caffeine and radium compresses to his
painful swollen joints.[166] On 18 May 1911, this bold visionary finally passed
away, like Beethoven, during a thunderstorm.[167] The cause of death was
recorded as being bacterial endocarditis.[168] Two days later the *New York
Times* reported that, upon his dying instructions, a needle was passed into
his heart to ensure that he really was dead.[169]

Mahler withstood pressure and tragedy which would have crushed
almost anyone else, but he was always a realist. Close to his end he said,
'My time will yet come, I have time on my side, living or dead, that is
indifferent, I can wait.'[170] As Franklin judges, there is little evidence of
him being obsessed with premonitions of death.[171] A neurotic megalomaniac, as Alma implied, despot or tyrant would have directed that his
tomb become a mausoleum, a place of future pilgrimage. Instead, upon
his directions, his simple headstone just says 'Gustav Mahler' for, as he
remarked, 'Any who come to look for me will know who I was and the
rest do not need to know.'[172] His was a life of triumph in adversity upon a
scale as epic as his great symphonies.

✢ CARL NIELSEN ✢
(1865–1931)

Music is life and, as such, inextinguishable
Carl Nielsen's personal motto

During a recent radio concert it was suggested that the Danish composer Nielsen was so unwell with heart disease in his last years that he gave up composition and conducting. Schonberg wrote that 'Whilst conducting a programme of his own music in 1926, he had a heart attack and lingered a very sick man until his death in October 1931.'[173] Biography by those who have studied Nielsen in depth and from the Danish reveals a different story.[174] In 1928, for example, whilst skiing with his wife in Norway, he fell, breaking two ribs, which is not exactly a picture of crippling heart disease.[175] We can comment similarly upon his response to more serious injuries in 1930. But heart disease he certainly had, and probably for many years.

Nielsen was a practical, usually cheerful and direct type of man, unswayed by convention. He and his wife, Anne-Marie, before their marriage in 1891, had lived happily in Bohemian Paris. When in 1893 they moved flats in Copenhagen, the piano slipped and got stuck on the stairs. In restraining it, Nielsen developed some chest pain, which was subsequently regarded as the start of his angina.[176] It is an easy assumption to make, but probably incorrect, especially as shortly after the piano episode he was treated for 'catarrh' (possibly gastritis) with a stomach pump.[177] Any benefits from such a ghastly treatment remain elusive, although young men with chest pain usually have indigestion from a stomach ulcer, despite believing that they have heart trouble. However, this young man probably had broken ribs. Had Nielsen experienced acute angina in 1893, his survival for thirty-eight more years would have been unlikely. In the autumn of 1905 he described symptoms possibly suggestive of myocardial ischaemia (angina).[178] Previously that year he had been snubbed by the Royal Theatre Orchestra and briefly became dejected,[179] which was overcome as he quickly composed his successful comic opera *Maskarade*. In June 1907 Nielsen went walking in Norway.[180] A year later, he and his wife were hill walking again in Switzerland. Accordingly, one is very guarded as to the severity of angina, even in the first decade of the twentieth century.

When Anne-Marie departed to work in Germany, Nielsen missed her and consequently engrossed himself creatively. Grieg's widow looked after

him at Troldhaugen, where he worked on his Violin Concerto in the composing hut.[181] The first unqualified major success came after this with the
Third Symphony, 'Sinfonia espansiva'.[182] Then in 1914 Anne-Marie left
him, citing previous infidelities, which included at least two illegitimate
children.[183] But now Nielsen was effectively thrown out and lonely. During
and immediately after the Great War he worked in Gothenburg as deputy
to Stenhammar.[184] The ebullient and optimistic Fourth Symphony, 'The
Inextinguishable', was premiered in January 1916; its very title enshrined
Nielsen's mantra that music is life and as such inextinguishable.[185] A brief
period of depression was followed by composition of the Fifth Symphony,
which was very different from the ebullient and optimistic Fourth. By the
time of this work and the Wind Quintet (1922), which quickly followed,
he was engrossed, saying that despite starting work at 10a.m. and retiring
to bed at 5a.m. the following morning, there was no sense of fatigue.[186]
Such is the power of creative adrenalin, and it is hardly typical of a cardiac
cripple. However, the payback probably came in the spring of 1922 with a
serious attack of angina. For a few months his normal cheerfulness again
deserted him but, on the day he finished composing the Fifth, Nielsen and
his wife were happily reunited, and they remained so until his death.[187]
Schoustoe regards them as having been mutually supportive.[188]

In 1924 his health had deteriorated and he was advised to give up
horse-riding, whereafter came his first car;[189] this enabled him to get away
easily from Copenhagen to compose in rural solitude in his seaside cottage at Skagen, whence came *Aladdin*. There he started his sixth and final
symphony, the 'Sinfonia semplice'. In the first movement Nielsen's theme
is the fruitless search for childlike joy;[190] with shades of Mahler and Britten
here. In the final movement he strove for jollity.[191] The Sixth Symphony
may betray a greater apprehension of cardiac disease.[192] Further illness followed with a fever during the summer of 1926 whilst he was on holiday
with his daughter in Italy. This time Anne-Marie came to his bedside.[193]
In October they went on to Paris for an all-Nielsen concert, including his
new and acclaimed Flute Concerto. He was to conduct, but his health
then led him to delegate most of that task to his Hungarian son-in-law
and close friend Emil Telmányi.[194] Nielsen was not the man he had been.

In 1927 his family persuaded him to resign as conductor of the
Copenhagen Philharmonic but, instead of the restful summer the doctors had prescribed, he devoted his time to writing his rural memoir *My
Childhood in Fyn*.[195] As is so often the case, a creative urge became irresistible. Nielsen still felt well enough for the ski trip in 1928 and then went
to work on his Clarinet Concerto.[196] In November, against the advice of

his cardiologist, he went to Gothenburg to conduct a revival of *Saul and David*.[197] Now he realised, perhaps at last, that he was still living too much in the fast lane. With memoirs now despatched, six symphonies increasingly acclaimed and much else, he instead turned his last three years into a project to combine ancient polyphony with his personal version of modern tonality.[198]

In October 1930, on a misty day in Copenhagen, he was knocked down by a tram, dislocating the joint between the shoulder and collar bone, and he was concussed.[199] Within a month he was back at work, and 1931 was ushered in by his becoming a director of the Copenhagen Conservatory.[200] But he was white-haired, losing his youthful appearance and worrying about his musical legacy. As usual he was told to rest in the summer of 1931. By the late summer he had become totally absorbed with a revival in Copenhagen of *Maskarade*. On 22 September he was helping to move scenery. It was one move too many and he suffered his most serious attack of myocardial ischaemia – a coronary attack by any other name. His other son-in-law, a doctor, insisted that he go into hospital. and for once he concurred. On 1 October he listened to a performance of his Violin Concerto on the radio.[201] During the next day he drifted into a coma, re-emerging briefly on 3 October as his family rather awkwardly gathered around his bed in a wake, and then he quietly slipped away. Today it is likely that, with the onset of angina, X-rays of the coronary arteries (angiograms) would have revealed blockage(s). These in turn would then have been stented, extending his life productively for at least another decade.

It is unusual for coronary artery disease to start so early, but not unheard of. If the chest pain caused by the piano in 1893 was due to a cracked rib or muscular strain, which is probable, then the likely first episode of angina was when he was in his forties, which is reasonable speculation. However, he could have had other forms of heart disease, perhaps a defective valve. The setback in Italy in 1926 followed a fever although, on balance, the story is one of intermittent episodes over many years and not the inexorable decline due to a septic heart valve which we saw with Mahler, or even the progressive heart failure we are about to see with Britten. His last three years were full of a renewed intellectual vigour for absolute music and a burst of further creative and very original composition. His theatrical death is fitting for a man whose greatness was recognised by Sibelius, who observed, 'I don't even reach your ankles.'[202]

✠ BENJAMIN BRITTEN ✠
(1913–1976)

The Heart of the Matter
Graham Greene, 1948

Peter Ackroyd, in his review of the English imagination, *Albion*, concluded that England's musical roots lie with folksong and religious music.[203] Britten's output often reflects just that. Also he was both generous and practical, for he consciously wrote for people, whether it was friends like Rostropovich, a school choir or the Festival of Britain. He was adept at adjusting his scale. Sir Arthur Bliss reckoned that no English composer for five hundred years had been endowed with such innate musical gifts.[204] Most impressive of all is the range of those musical gifts. Not least of them was as an impresario. When on 19 June 1969 his music theatre, The Maltings, at Snape burned down only two years after its opening, it was Britten's immense drive and energy which rapidly created the theatrical phoenix which is today's wonderful new theatre.

Born of middle-class parents in Suffolk and educated in Norfolk, Britten appears to have had a happy, very English childhood.[205] Oliver has suggested that in some of his music there is an unfulfilled striving for the idyll of a past blissful childhood.[206] That he was a musical prodigy was realised by the time he was five or six years old; as a young teenager he became the only pupil of Frank Bridge, who, with his wife Effie, was childless, and the personable Ben must have been a compensation for them. Neither was he a totally musical swot. At school he boxed and played cricket and other sports.[207] Enthusiasm for badminton, tennis and swimming continued into middle age, and he expected to win. It is said that he was skiing in Austria in 1952 when he first conceived *Gloriana*;[208] it was dedicated a year later to Queen Elizabeth II for her coronation in 1953, when he was made a Companion of Honour. Much of his life was thus a complete contrast to an image sometimes found today of a sickly, reclusive man.

Earlier his patriotism and courage had been severely criticised because, shortly before the outbreak of the Second World War, he and the singer Peter Pears, whom he had first met in 1937, went to live on the east coast of the USA. Whilst he was staying in 1940 at Amityville, New York, with a medical family, the Mayers, Britten was taken seriously ill.[209] The known facts are that he had a severe septic throat, with a very high temperature of up to 107°F. He felt and looked ill and experienced 'rheumatic' aches and pains with a skin eruption. His host, Dr Mayer, regarded this as strepto-coccal infection, and he was treated with sulphonamide.[210]

In 1942 Britten and Pears returned to England on a Swedish cargo boat, then to register as conscientious objectors.[211] During this voyage he com-posed his *Ceremony of Carols*. Inevitably, Britten and Pears's relationship has always elicited mixed reports, as has Britten's fascination with children. John Bridcut's *Britten's Children* relates Britten's alleged infatuation with the young actor David Hemmings,[212] although Britten was unquestionably loyally loving to Pears over four decades, and he abhorred promiscuity.[213] For the rest of the war he worked on *Peter Grimes*, a masterpiece whose triumphant premiere in 1945 heralded a new era of English music.

By the early 1970s his prodigious energy had declined. He was prob-ably exhausted by his own triumphant response to the Maltings burning down in 1969.[214] Like Elgar and Wordsworth, Britten composed in his head whilst on country walks, which now became less frequent. Kennedy has recalled seeing Britten becoming breathless on stairs during the 1972 Aldeburgh Festival.[215] Before that he had been fit, still playing tennis and swimming regularly. He admitted to having had pain down the left arm 'for several years', especially whilst conducting. Whereas it is now supposed that the left arm pain was due to angina, he had previously experienced two episodes of frozen shoulder,[216] which is a painful condition, often causing pain down the arm. Presumably the recovery was satisfactory, for otherwise swimming, conducting, playing tennis or the piano would have become difficult, if not impossible.

Britten's general practitioner, Ian Tait, was becoming increasingly con-cerned regarding evidence of progressive heart failure and had wanted him to consult a cardiologist earlier to advise on the need for surgery.[217] Britten delayed, saying he would complete *Death in Venice* first and 'then be ill';[218] he realised that this would be the final opportunity to create a starring role for his beloved and ageing Peter Pears.[219] At last in March 1973 he saw Dr Graham Hayward, who advised him to delay surgery no further,[220] and on 7 May he was admitted to the National Heart Hospital for surgery. When he came round post-operatively, it was clear that he had suffered a stroke,[221] a well-recognised surgical risk, though more so then than now. His speech was only temporarily affected, but the weakness of his right arm and leg never fully recovered. Sometimes patients' perceptions of disability after a stroke, despite apparently recovering well, may leave sufferers with what they regard as a persistent disability. The cause for this cannot always be objectively identified. Three weeks after surgery, Britten went to convalesce and Rita Thomson, who had first met him as a nurse at the National Heart Hospital, joined his family team.

An early concern was that Pears had now lost his piano accompanist, and Britten had been a wonderful pianist. The immediate response was the introduction of the young Murray Perahia to accompany Pears.[222] Britten's conducting also became a thing of the past. The more pressing difficulty was with composition, and he had always said that his prime purpose in life was to compose.[223] Initially he probably had a degree of dysmusia, that is, a disability in getting the music out, as we saw with Ravel. Later Britten admitted that, apart from problems in using his right hand, he had inhibitions with his musical self-confidence: as he put it, his 'powers of selection'.[224] Rita Thomson becoming his full-time carer and family friend seems to have boosted his self-confidence.[225]

By the time of his sixtieth birthday in late November 1973, Britten had already attended a semi-private pre-Covent Garden run of *Death in Venice* at the Maltings.[226] It was a triumph, although old friends were horrified by how ill he still looked. Never good at taking criticism, he was hurt by the various rumours as to where he was, ranging from his having gone 'gaga' to a Tolstoyan retreat into rural Suffolk.[227] Happily, by Easter 1974, although far from truly well, he became involved with recording *Death in Venice* at the Maltings.[228] Then he returned to composition during July 1974 with *Canticle V*, based on T. S. Eliot's poem, although he complained of difficulty in physically reaching the top right area of the manuscript paper. This could have been due to an old problem with the shoulder or an aftermath of his stroke.[229] Britten then went back to Hardy with a *Suite on English Folk Tunes*, subtitled 'A Time There Was', using material he had previously drawn upon in 1953. *Sacred and Profane* (also based on poems), *Phaedra* for Janet Baker in 1975 and *Welcome Ode* in 1976 all displayed his fertile imagination and showed his drive to compose to still be very much intact.[230]

On 12 June 1976 Britten received a peerage, but he knew he would never take his seat in the House of Lords.[231] He was seen less frequently, and then often in a wheelchair. In November there was good news regarding the security of the financial future for Aldeburgh and he told Pears, 'I don't need to fight anymore.'[232] Barnett has described this time.[233] Britten said he was not afraid of death, although he would be sad to leave his friends. He wanted to die before Peter Pears, saying he did not know what he would do without him. Early in the morning of 4 December, with Rita Thomson as ever in attendance, he died in Peter Pears's arms.[234] All Aldeburgh and many far beyond mourned. Three days later he was buried at Aldeburgh.

During the following year, with a magnificent service, a memorial stone to him was unveiled in Westminster Abbey. So there passed an extraordinary man, and one very much for his time. He was surely one of the great musical polymaths of not just England, but the twentieth century: composer, soloist, conductor, innovator and musical impresario. He was also an educator, and there the matter would have rested until, in the year of the centenary of his birth, controversy re-emerged.

Controversy in 2013

That Britten died of progressive heart failure three years after surgery is certain.[235] In February 2013 the cause of that failure then became a matter of much-publicised controversy. The immediate reason was that, on 20 January 2013, an article appeared in the *Sunday Telegraph*: 'Benjamin Britten: Death in Aldeburgh', being 'the words of Paul Kildea'.[236] This was an abstract of approximately seven pages from Kildea's recent Britten biography, a splendid book of 666 pages. Subsequently, I studied both article and book and additionally talked with Paul Kildea, an open and friendly scholar. I also spoke at length with Dr Michael Petch, a consultant cardiologist who, as a senior registrar in 1973 at the National Heart Hospital, had conducted the thorough pre-operative assessment on Britten.[237] He later became his cardiologist and a friend. Colin Matthews, composer and Britten trustee, also advised me.[238] Dr Nick Clark, Librarian at The Red House at Aldeburgh, graciously gave me full access to all Britten's medical records.[239] Lastly, in 2012 and early in 2013 I spoke with Dr Ian Tait, for many years Britten's general practitioner.[240] Sadly, two days after our last conversation he himself died.

Fortified by such counsel, the following summarises the key facts. The notably athletic Britten was said to have had a heart murmur early in the 1960s, if not before.[241] So do many people, and such murmurs can remain untroublesome. In the spring of 1968 he was treated with antibiotics in Ipswich for bacterial endocarditis, with a good recovery.[242] Without them his end might have resembled that of Mahler. When in the early 1970s his energies waned, Britten initially postponed surgical treatment until March 1973, although Tait was already treating heart failure.[243] Also the heart was enlarged, not least at the point where the aorta emerges from the heart's left ventricle. The X-ray showed that, but no calcification – of which more below.[244] Two weeks later cardiac catheterisation with angiograms, undertaken by Dr Petch, displayed the heart's malfunction. There was incompetence of the leaking aortic valve, although the left ventricle contracted 'vigorously'. Petch's conclusion was 'Moderately severe aortic regurgitation (leakage or incompetence of the aortic valve) with a slight dilatation of the aorta.'

Two weeks later Donald Ross, an eminent heart surgeon, operated to insert a new aortic valve, using a tissue graft rather than a mechanical valve. This was done with Britten on a bypass machine which enables the surgeon to operate on an isolated, temporarily still heart, whilst the machine deputises for the patient's own heart in ensuring that oxygenated blood reaches all around the body. Britten was on bypass for an hour and forty minutes,[245] although Kildea describes the 'surgery and mop-up' as having taken six hours.[246] That Britten was intensively nursed in the operating suite recovery area for several hours is not surprising. As Kildea says, there were difficulties in getting his already weakened heart to resume its normal functions. Ross recorded in his operation note that the aortic valve showed some congenital abnormality, but no evidence of previous infective endocarditis.[247] But he was 'perplexed' and took numerous biopsy samples of tissue for laboratory analysis. These showed no evidence of any previous infection.[248] Ross later speculated whether this might have been an example of mild Marfan's syndrome.* A doctor and family friend of Britten's advised me that there is a family history of Marfan's.[249] At surgery Ross had commented on the heart wall feeling flabby, and in a letter a month later, he expressed surprise at the heart's size, although this partly diminished after surgery,[250] as it should. Ross, who was one of the giants of post-war British surgery, died in July 2014. He had been very frail for several years, during which time those interested in Britten's case were advised that he would be unable to discuss it.[251]

There was a suggestion that neither Ross nor Hayward fully recognised the gravity of Britten's stroke,[252] so critical an issue for a musician. That may be fair, and there are several reasons. As recoveries from strokes go, Britten's was good. Secondly, not all cardiologists are as subtle as neurologists in assessing the sequelae of stroke. Of course, the reverse sometimes holds; it is called specialisation. Furthermore, standards of assessment of neurological impairment are possibly better today than they were forty years ago. The key is Britten's complaint that he felt as if his right hand

---

* Marfan's is an inherited disorder with many features which include abnormalities of the aorta, hernias and dislocation of eye lenses, with short sight. The skeletal system is affected, the sufferer often being tall, and thin with unusually long fingers and toes, as well as spinal curvature.

was in a glove.[253] Standard clinical testing of sensation does not always convey the patient's own perception of his own body part, or even its exact position in space.

We may ask: where did the controversy emerge? Kildea's account firstly claims that 'Ross had found that the aorta was riddled with tertiary syphilis', that 'It was almost impossible to make the new valve fit' and that this was, suddenly, 'the wrong procedure'.[254] He states, 'They had to make do with what was at hand', the implication possibly being that a mechanical valve might have been better. Kildea suggested that the cross-stitching which Ross used to insert the valve was a valiant attempt to make a misfit fit.[255] The explanation in fact is more prosaic: it was used to prevent the exit of the aorta stretching further, and was described as being in a 'conventional manner'.[256] It is a time-honoured strengthening technique in needlework, as sailors and seamsters will confirm.

So where did Kildea's diagnosis of syphilis come from? In the late 1990s, when Kildea himself was working in Aldeburgh, he had met a cardiologist from North America, Dr Hywel Davies, who had known Ross, Hayward and Petch in London. Davies, who was not involved with Britten's treatment, had been reminiscing socially with Ross in the late 1980s and, by his account, the surgeon had unburdened the view that Britten's basic aortic diagnosis had been tertiary cardiovascular syphilis.[257] Davies believed this information should be in the public domain. In principle that makes sense, provided that the case is sustainable on a balance of probabilities. So what are the available facts?

1   There are no WR test reports filed in the remaining case notes, but that which is preserved, as is customary with archived records, consists of typewritten correspondence which quotes operative reports and case summaries. There is no mention of syphilis.

2   Kildea believes that the high fever and septic throat in America may have been an early stage of syphilis, except that with syphilis one would have expected a fever of 100° or 101°F, not 107°F. The story then was one of a streptococcal infection. Neither is there any contemporaneous nor subsequent clinical entry to raise a suspicion of syphilis. Although syphilitic manifestations were not rare in ENT clinics in the 1940s, that does not infer that everyone with a high temperature and sore throat had early-stage syphilis. The lingering stigma of having been infected with syphilis is WR tests remaining positive for life. His own general practitioner told Petch and me that several WR tests were taken much later on and all were negative.[258]

3   The surgical problems were in getting Britten's rather flabby enlarged heart working again off the bypass machine. Obviously it did, and it is interesting that an anaesthetist working on the case, Dr Edward Sumner, has recently stated that he was present, vigilant and remembers the case vividly: 'There was no suggestion of any syphilitic involvement. The whole thing is ludicrous.'[259]

4   The inference that doing WR tests in the early 1970s was not current practice is misleading. There was still quite a lot of untreated syphilis about at that time, giving rise to all sorts of surprises. As surgeons we were all cautious about surgical stab injuries to ourselves. Kildea is also concerned about confidentiality during surgery. His assumption is that, if Ross had felt any concern regarding syphilis during surgery, he would not have mentioned it in the operating theatre for fear of subsequent indiscreet revelations from other members of the theatre team. The medico-legal situation is clear. Firstly, if Ross or any other member of his medical team had been concerned as to the possibility of syphilis, the immediate obligation would have been to request appropriate blood tests and then refer the patient to a specialist in venereology (now called genito-urinary medicine). That did not occur. Moreover, the second legal point is that the duty of confidentiality rests upon *all* members of the operating team, from senior surgeon to junior scrub nurse. Throughout my consultant career I was involved with the surgical treatment of many well-known people from sport and the arts, so Kildea's concerns resonate with me. One was careful as to what was said, but that duty of discretion did not extend to a deliberate obfuscation of critical clinical data.

5   Dr Petch, whilst excluding syphilis from his own clinical assessment, also rejects any suggestion that the surgeons were doing the wrong operation.[260] The case was clear pre-operatively, and a graft of appropriate size and nature was used, with a range of choice in the operating theatre anyway. It was secured with appropriate stitching. Even with the benefit of hindsight the clinical picture was not one of syphilitic aortitis, although Petch recalls Ross having reflected on just such a case, upon whom he had operated at about the same time as Britten.[261] There was no chalk formation in the aorta on X-ray, as is typical with syphilis, and the biopsy material was strangely unenlightening with no indication of syphilis.[*]

---

[*] The pathologist Professor Tony Freemont attests that there being no microscopic evidence of syphilis is not absolutely exclusive of syphilitic aortitis.

6   Ross had considerable experience of operating on patients with syph-
    ilitic aortic regurgitation, although none of the fifteen anonymised
    cases he reported in 1976 bear any resemblance to Britten's clinical
    details.[262]

7   Kildea implies that if Britten, who was monogamous, a bit of a prude
    and later celibate, did have syphilis then he would have acquired it
    from Peter Pears, who was neither. Speculations as to what Pears did
    on dreary Sunday afternoons play only a peripheral part in judging
    whether Britten was syphilitic. The Pears link is one easier to proffer
    than to sustain or refute.

8   Conspiracy theories regarding doctors hiding the details clearly must
    not extend to operation notes or case summaries including false
    information or deliberately excluding crucial information. Such acts
    would then, as now, have been condemned by the Medical Defence
    Union and the General Medical Council, opening the responsible
    clinician to risk of serious censure.

9   The historian is dependent on the facts and, outside her or his own
    particular area, needs the advice of experts. Kildea has spoken with
    doctors, Hywel Davies in particular, just as I have with musicolo-
    gists and cardiologists. When we spoke Kildea was understandably
    anxious to safeguard the integrity of his book. Others have com-
    mented that, with 666 pages, it is a shame that so much of the public
    interest has been upon this one issue.[263] That it was abstracted into
    a respected Sunday newspaper surely made that inevitable.[264] The
    basis for Kildea's diagnosis is Dr Hywel Davies, to whom I have
    been unable to speak. Like most of the people who actually did
    treat Britten, he has for some years been retired, although he pub-
    lished his views in the *New Statesman*.[265] Kildea's otherwise excellent
    biography has excited interest, concern and perhaps anger, and that
    hangs largely upon Davies's recollections of a conversation at least
    twenty-five years ago regarding an operation with which he was
    unassociated and whose fortieth anniversary had recently passed. In
    a court of law today, the balance of probabilities would probably
    weigh against Davies's remembrance of things past evoking this egre-
    gious diagnosis.

10 The syphilitic controversy so active in 2013 would not go away
    in 2014 when Petch presented his essay 'The Heart of Benjamin
    Britten' in a respected peer-reviewed medical journal.[266] Having
    talked many times with Dr Petch, I was unsurprised by his argu-
    ments, but impressed by their objective and balanced presentation.

In conclusion he presented 'the most persuasive evidence to rebut tertiary syphilis'. This was the degenerative changes seen in the microscopic biopsy samples in 1973 and not well understood then: 'Ross was puzzled.' Petch quoted a recent American study of 268 patients operated upon for aortic incompetence. Although none had syphilitic aortitis, fifteen (6%) had some evidence from biopsy of Marfan's syndrome.[267] Also striking was his emphasis that Hayward, Ross, Tait and he himself were all openly familiar with the possibility of syphilis in aortic disease and that testing for it was part of their routine preoperative protocol. Petch concluded by raising the issue, resonant with much of this book, of the ethical probity and responsibility of doctors caring for famous people.

Recurrent themes in much of Britten's output are innocence, virtue and their loss, which is why clarification of the syphilitic issue is important. They are themes coursing strongly through *Peter Grimes*, *The Turn of the Screw*, *Billy Budd* and *Death in Venice*. Britten's friend Donald Mitchell summarised this most eloquently:

> At the centre of his music there is an intensely solitary and private spirit, a troubled, sometimes despairing visionary, an artist much haunted by nocturnal imagery, by sleep, by presentiments of mortality, a creator preternaturally aware of the destructive appetite that feeds on innocence, virtue and grace.[268]

The reason Ross's operation failed was that it had been delayed at Britten's own insistence, enabling him to complete *Death in Venice* for Peter Pears. Such selfless generosity is a more appropriate and medically sustainable emblem of this great man's life than syphilitic aortitis.

Alexander Borodin (1833–1887)

Borodin was a multi-talented man, one of the famous 'Mighty Handful'.* These five fervently nationalistic composers were followers of Glinka and were led by Mily Balakirev. All five had daytime jobs. Borodin distinguished himself as both a chemist and a physician in St Petersburg, but also whilst working in Germany and in Italy, where he made significant contributions to organic chemistry.[269] He described himself as only a Sunday composer.[270] The illegitimate son of an aristocrat, he was given a good education and upbringing, and became happily married.[271] In 1878, at Borodin's instigation, the medical faculty in St Petersburg started courses in medicine for women.[272] By 1963, 70% of Soviet doctors were women and, had the far-sighted Borodin not broken down prejudice and barriers, there would have been an even greater shortage of medical personnel during the two world wars. So Borodin's legacy is immense, but today he is now best remembered for his compositions, especially the incomplete *Prince Igor*, three symphonies (the third completed by Glazunov) and the Second String Quartet in D.

In 1885, the year in which he survived cholera, he wrote to his wife that he was finding it very demanding to wear so many professional hats. At the beginning of 1887 he was again working on the conclusion of his great opera *Prince Igor*. Ominously he started complaining of chest pains.[273] He was a kindly, philanthropic and sociable man, and on 14 February 1887, after working on the Third Symphony in A minor, he attended the Academy of Physicians ball, wearing Russian national dress. As he always did, Borodin entered into the spirit of the evening, Cossack boots and all. At about midnight he jumped up to enjoy one more energetic dance and, falling to the floor, died instantly. He was only fifty-four. O'Neill states that an autopsy showed a 'burst artery of the heart'.[274] This is unlikely to have been a ruptured coronary artery, as they block rather than burst. An alternative interpretation is that he had a dissecting or ruptured aneurysm of the aorta, which is the great artery emerging from the heart, for which today emergency surgery can sometimes save patients, restoring them to full vigour. The alternative diagnosis is that a blocked coronary artery caused a massive heart attack. This is consistent with the earlier complaint of what was probably angina. Limited as his output was,[275] he contributed to the Russian catalogue of symphonies, opera, song and chamber music,

---

* César Cui, Rimsky-Korsakov, Borodin, Musorgsky and Balakirev.

whilst altering European medical practice, contributing to chemistry and caring for an invalid wife.

Nikolai Rimsky-Korsakov (1844–1908)

Rimsky-Korsakov is probably the most popular of the 'Mighty Handful'. Like all five members of the group he was a weekend composer, for professionally he was a naval officer who later obtained a sinecure as Inspector of Naval Bands.[276] He even composed whilst afloat, completing his First Symphony in E flat minor in Gravesend. Substantially self-taught, but with rigorously high standards, he revised early works in mid- and late career. When he was elevated in his second career as a musical academic, there came self-doubt. Accordingly, his psychological health, as well as his final illness, is considered here. During 1881–88 there was some 'creative paralysis',[277] when he found it easier to work with his friend Glazunov, who was similarly afflicted, on the work of others. So came their final realisation of Borodin's Third Symphony and *Prince Igor*, work which was started before Borodin's death.[278] as well as of Musorgsky's *Khovanshchina*. Rimsky laboured intermittently, even agonised, for many years on his own incomplete Fourth Symphony. His *Sinfonietta on Russian Themes*, as well as two string quartets, did not suggest a recrudescence of future fluent composition,[279] although by 1887–88 a renewed inclination was found to write *Scheherazade*, *Spanish Caprice* and the *Russian Easter Festival Overture*, the works by which he is best known.

In 1890 he returned from Brussels to find his wife dangerously ill with diphtheria. There was another lapse in composition in the early 1890s, after the deaths of his mother and two of his children.[280] Rimsky suffered intermittent bouts of depression associated with 'alarming physical symptoms', which included rushes of blood to the head, confusion, memory loss and unpleasant preoccupations leading to obsessive-compulsive behaviour. Additionally, he was asthmatic. The diagnosis given at the time was neurasthenia,[281] today a generally meaningless term. Whatever the cause it was non-progressive, although for a time he considered relinquishing composition altogether.[282] At this time Rimsky described his feelings for his opera *Mlada* as being 'cold like ice'.[283] They recuperated in Switzerland, where he said, 'While I was abroad it seemed to me that music didn't grip and satisfy me.'[284] Headaches and dizziness were reported at this time.[285] In the summer of 1893 he and his wife, Nadezhda, took their child Masha to the Crimea, where Rimsky read, swam, enjoyed long walks and hardly touched a piano. Then little Masha died and her father's creative zeal became stale and subdued.[286] He complained then of torpor, weariness and memory lapses, again with a disinclination to compose, instead turning to write his *Record of My Musical Life*'.[287] Strangely, after Tchaikovsky's death in 1893, there came a creative renewal with the composition of eleven operas in the fifteen years until his death in 1908.

Rimsky remained an active man until his sixty-fourth birthday in March 1908, when he became breathless with chest pain (angina pectoris),[288] for which oxygen and morphia were given. But he would not rest, suffering a second heart attack five days later. Now strict rest was enforced with alterations in his diet and withdrawal of coffee and tobacco. For a week there was no composing and no visitors. Work on *The Golden Cockerel* then resumed. It was his last composition, and one where a fight with the censors and publishers may have provoked his end.[289] In May he was well enough to travel to Lyubensk, where, on arrival, there was another attack of angina followed by a quick recovery.[290] Returning home he acquiesced to a quiet regimen, pottering in the garden, reading and receiving only a few friends, but not composing. Rimsky was not well enough to attend his daughter's wedding,[291] shortly whereafter came another attack of angina. He died on 21 June 1908 of what almost certainly was a final heart attack, having described complaints of suffocation and 'asthma'.[292] This is consistent with a diagnosis of heart failure subsequent to angina, and earlier symptoms which suggest hypertension. He had died leaving sketches for two operas, of which *Heaven and Earth* was based on Byron's poem.

Francis Poulenc (1899–1963)

Poulenc was an heir to the Rhône-Poulenc pharmaceutical giant, and so, unlike most other composers, he never worried about money. There were early notable compositions such as *Rapsodie nègre* in 1917 and the ballet *Les biches*, commissioned by Diaghilev in 1924. In 1936, after the deaths of several friends, he visited the shrine at Rocamadour and experienced a religious reawakening, which he commemorated in *Litanies à la Vierge Noire*,[293] then a mass, and in 1950 the *Stabat mater* followed. Poulenc became depressed after the death of Raymonde Linossier, at the age of only thirty-two and shortly after he proposed marriage to her.[294] In June 1954 he experienced symptoms of declining mental and physical well-being, confessing himself to be 'in terrible fear',[295] which was regarded then as a nervous breakdown. Hypochondria is at least a partial explanation, for he admitted to 'cancerophobia'.[296] Benjamin Ivry suggests that Poulenc was over-medicated with psychotropic drugs for years.[297] In 1961 came *Gloria*, from a man now probably affected by heart failure. After experiencing severe angina, just before boarding a plane in August 1962, he was given penicillin![298] His death in January 1963, from an acute heart attack, was sudden and, Ivry suggests, not totally unexpected by Poulenc.[299] No work was left incomplete, but there had been final notes to friends. He had sent flowers with a prescient note to his old friend Denise Duval: 'My Denise, it is to you I owe my last joy. Your poor Francis.'[300] His output and composition were fairly constant until his death, in spite of his advancing heart disease, although Ivry implies that his composition mirrored Poulenc's compliance with his medication.[301] Had he survived into the 1970s, his life could well have been improved and extended by stenting or coronary artery bypass surgery.

✣ Chapter 9 ✣

Breathless:
Respiratory Diseases

As tho' to breathe is life
Alfred, Lord Tennyson, 'Ulysses',1842

Introduction

AFTER HEART FAILURE, we pass to the other common causes of breathlessness and weakness, namely bronchial and lung conditions. There is a popular image of the tragic composer coughing his last in an impoverished attic. Although it is almost a cliché, there have been examples, with some raising the question of how composition occurred at all.

Respiratory disease affects either the airways to the lungs or the lungs themselves. The airways convey inspired air through the larynx (voice-box) to the trachea (windpipe) and thence to the bronchi and their smaller multiple divisions, the bronchioles. The action of the chest is to expand, thereby creating a negative pressure in the pleural cavity, which is the membranous sack surrounding a lung. That in turn causes the sponge-like lung to expand, sucking the fresh air in during inspiration. The basic lung mechanism is an exchange membrane, wherewith oxygen in the inspired air is transferred to the blood. Then, as the chest pressures reverse, the lung shrinks as we expire and exhale carbon dioxide.

There are several broad groups of lung disease:

1 **Pulmonary embolus** (PE), which we encountered in Chapter 8, involves a circulating blood clot, usually from a deep veino thrombosis (DVT), obstructing the pulmonary artery, the main blood vessel through which stale blood is pumped to the lungs, in order to be refreshed with oxygen and relieved of carbon dioxide. Sadly a PE can be fatal.

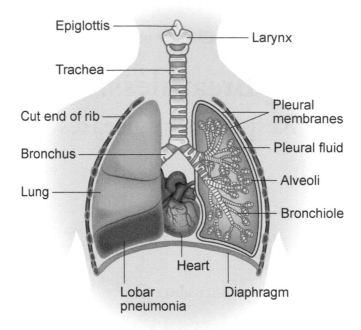

Epiglottis

Larynx

Trachea

Cut end of rib

Pleural membranes

Bronchus

Pleural fluid

Alveoli

Lung

Bronchiole

Heart

Lobar pneumonia

Diaphragm

Fig. 5 Diagram of the lungs

2   **Lung cancer** is usually (but not always) a malignant tumour of the lining of the bronchi. Although a very serious condition, it carries a better prognosis with modern treatment than it did twenty-five years ago.

3   **Chronic obstructive airways disease** (COAD) is a group of diseases wherewith there is partial obstruction to air being exhaled. This causes back-pressure, one result of which is that the actual lung tissue becomes distended (emphysema); that, in turn, causes the chest to apparently enlarge (barrel chest). There are several classic causes of COAD:

   a   **Asthma** – because of spasm in the walls of the bronchioles, which narrows them, making it more difficult to exhale.

   b   **Chronic bronchitis** – again because of chronic partial obstruction.

   c   **Cystic fibrosis** will be explained in the section regarding Chopin. Suffice it to say here that those bronchiolar tubes become blocked with abnormally sticky mucus. (It can also affect the pancreas and liver.)

d **Bronchiectasis** occurs when a bronchial tube dilates and becomes infected, usually chronically so.

4 **Infection, bronchitis and pneumonia** may take various forms, as follows.

a **Bronchitis**, which may be acute or chronic, is an infection of the bronchial tree.

b **Pneumonia** is an infection of the lung tissue itself. This may be associated with bronchial infection – hence bronchopneumonia, or just of one lobe (lobar pneumonia). Before antibiotics, pneumonia could often be fatal, even in previously fit people. The next great challenge is likely to be antibiotic resistance, which is already ominously on the increase.

c **Tuberculosis** (aka TB or consumption) is a chronic infection of the lungs' sponge-like substance, ultimately destroying it and eroding into blood vessels, so that the sufferer coughs up blood (haemoptysis).

One last point is that, if the right side of the heart has to work overtime to pump blood through diseased lungs then, ultimately, it fails, a condition known as cor pulmonale.

✢ CARL MARIA VON WEBER ✢
(1786–1826)

I see it is better to sell music than to write it

Carl Maria von Weber, 1826

Weber's story is valuable in understanding much of the accepted legend of tragic young composers. He was small, his appearance frail and latterly sickly. At the end of his life he went to London to work at the Royal Opera House, Covent Garden, with Charles Kemble, whose daughter Fanny described Weber as 'Very ugly … high cheek bones, long hooked nose with spectacles … his hollow, sallow, sickly face bore an expression of habitual suffering and ill-health.'[1]

Weber was born into a travelling theatrical family,[2] whose modus vivendi never seems to have left him, as exemplified by his sad ending. He was nearly always on the move. In contrast to Chopin, that the cause of his ill health was TB seems incontrovertible and was confirmed by autopsy, the report of which now reposes in the British Library.[3] It is hard to decide whether Weber regarded performance or composition as his priority. For much of his life he was seriously preoccupied with money, for which perhaps he paid the ultimate price. The period 1807 to 1810 in a then rather uncultured Stuttgart, as secretary to Duke Ludwig of Württemberg, was one of scarce composition,[4] but we cannot obviously blame Weber's health for this. In 1809 his elderly and unscrupulous father joined him and led him unwittingly into financial scandal.[5] This resulted in his immediate imprisonment and then unceremonious expulsion from Stuttgart to Mannheim. Yet three days before this ignominy he completed his opera *Silvana*, an early example of German Romantic opera foreshadowing *Der Freischütz*.[6]

During 1811, after a concert in Zurich, Weber took a four-day walking trip with a friend. He loved the Swiss Bernese Oberland, but walked with a limp.[7] In view of both his suspect hip and his reduced respiratory reserve, it clearly was not the obvious holiday choice. At about the age of eight Weber had complained of a sore hip, which steadily worsened during his remaining thirty-one years.[8] This may be ascribed to TB, as he was known to be consumptive, but neither Weber nor his associates recorded features suggestive of TB until 1813, when he was twenty-seven. O'Shea's suspicion that Weber had Perthe's disease, in which the hip bone softens, is sound.[9] With an incidence in North America and Europe of one in two thousand,

Perthe's is not a rarity, and it most commonly presents in boys between the ages of four and nine. To conclude the issue of Weber's hip, it is sensible to reflect that not everyone who limps has pain, although when he was older he complained of both.

After Switzerland he was quickly on the road again. It is fascinating, when reading diary entries by Weber and other composers, to realise what not being salaried meant to many of them. Weber would often describe the evening's success, not by commenting on how much the audience had liked the opera, but by stating what his fee or the takings at the door had been. It was a hand-to-mouth existence.[10] In early 1813 Weber had been ill, complaining of chest pains and cough, probably the first early features of consumption.[11] He also had throat complaints, which were often regarded in the nineteenth century as being due to tuberculous laryngitis. But again the picture is a little cloudy because, in 1806, Weber had drunk from a wine bottle into which his father had decanted engraving acid, after which he had been ill for two months, ending what might have been a promising career as a singer.[12] At the end of 1813, he met an attractive young singer, Caroline Brandt.[13] Initially it was like so many of Weber's entangled love affairs. Both his love life and his directorship of the Prague Opera became increasingly hectic during the 1814–15 season, and his by then frail health again deteriorated. Later in 1816 Weber bounced back and became betrothed to Caroline. At Christmas he accepted the post of Royal Saxon Kapellmeister in Dresden.[14] The next year his respiratory symptoms became accompanied by gastrointestinal symptoms, especially diarrhoea. There is no obvious reason to assume that this was not due to TB, although he also had that condition to afflict many composers: bleeding piles.[15] Less than two years later his health relapsed again, although he was working frantically, a period culminating with the triumphant premiere of *Der Freischütz* in Berlin during June 1821. But this was the year of his first coughing up blood.[16]

From Jahn's catalogue of all 308 works,[17] it is clear that considering major orchestral works, with or without soloist, as well as sacred, chamber or other stage works, *Euryanthe* written during 1822–23 and *Oberon* during 1825–26 were his only late major compositions. The three clarinet concertos were all composed in 1811, and the two piano concertos either side of them. He composed only two symphonies, both in 1807. The only chamber work after 1816 was a trio in 1819. From this it seems likely that, with declining health and constant money worries, the job of conducting took precedence over any urge for spare-time composition. Weber's pupil Julius Benedict observed in 1823 that although Weber 'stuck to his official duties as before, his creative powers were at a complete standstill'.[18] Weber often composed whilst overshadowed by fears of penury, rather than from divine inspiration. His case assuredly shows that, far from TB producing toxins to fuel composition, the opposite was dismally the case.

After his marriage in 1817 he became even more concerned about his family's long-term financial security. His own health had taken further turns for the worse in 1818, 1821 and 1823. By 1824–25 he was at last persuaded to rest more, and he even took 'the cure' at the spa of Ems.[19] The dilemma which this poor man faced came to a head in March 1824. He was coughing more and had become increasingly breathless and there was further haemoptysis, as well as creditors at the door. In spite of this, and probably because of it, he needed projects which paid well. So it was that Charles Kemble, Manager of the Royal Opera House, Covent Garden, solicited an opera. Weber agreed to a moderately lucrative contract which included producing his last opera, almost his last composition, *Oberon*.[20] In addition there were to be concert performances. The duality of his concerns is exemplified by his consulting Dr Hedenus as to how long he might live and then his starting to take English lessons. Ultimately he took 153, although he never really mastered English grammar or syntax.[21] By this time he had intermittently become indifferent to music. Hedenus predicted that, were he to seek his fortune in Italy, he was likely to survive a few more years, whereas if he went to England he might live for only a few more weeks.[22] How perspicacious that was. But Weber knew exactly what he was doing. Warrack quotes Weber's letter to his friend Frederick Göbitz: 'I shall earn a great deal of money in England – I owe it to my own family. I am going to London to die. Be silent – I know it.'[23]

When Caroline bade him farewell on his last and long journey to London, she closed the coach door sobbing that she had closed the coffin lid.[24] Weber withstood the journey to England reasonably well, and wrote upbeat letters to Caroline. As the coach crossed Kent, he was obviously enchanted by an English spring. In London people were kind to him and his companion, Fürstenau. Sir George Smart, he Managing Director of the Royal Opera, invited Weber to stay at his own home in Great Portland Street, where every comfort was afforded. In turn, Weber tried to conceal the severity of his condition, but it is said that people were struck by his sad, fragile appearance. He was homesick and his haemoptysis worsened. On one such occasion Smart had to carry him upstairs after a haemorrhage in his carriage.[25]

In spite of all this, he fulfilled his commitments and people were pleased. On the evening of 4 June 1826 Weber dined with Smart, being a little ungracious about the wine and taking instead two or three glasses of port.[26] He could talk and probably think of little other than his imminent return to Germany, Caroline and their children, which had been planned for two days later. At about 10p.m. he retired to bed. In the morning his personal effects and financial affairs were found all neatly sorted out. Weber himself was stone cold dead.[27]

An almost immediate autopsy took place, and of that we know that the larynx was ulcerated and the lungs showed all the classic features of gross tuberculosis.[28] Frustratingly, post mortem details regarding either his bowels or his bad hip are elusive. He was interred in a sealed casket, and the coffin was taken to the cemetery at Moorfields. It was not until the end of 1844 that Carl Maria von Weber's mortal remains were returned to Dresden.[29] His successor there, Richard Wagner, had much to do with the arrangements and later recorded, 'This second funeral was an event that stirred me to the very depth of my being.'[30] For sure, Weber had paved the way for a more modern conducting technique and for the music dramas of the man who later claimed to be the 'German spirit'.

✤ FRÉDÉRIC CHOPIN ✤
(1810–1849)

He is a sickroom talent

John Field, 1832[31]

On 28 August 1848, before a crowded concert hall in Manchester, a small, frail, fair-haired man of asthenic bearing made his way to the piano. Most agreed that he played beautifully, but his lightness of touch created insufficient sound to satisfy the full audience of 1,200 people.[32] The soloist, Frédéric Chopin, looked gravely ill and so he was, having only another year to live. Moreover, he had always eschewed large concert halls, developing a legendary reputation as a salon recitalist, particularly in Paris, which he had made his home in 1831. Whether this was due to nervousness (stage fright) in a large auditorium or to his light touch remains unanswered. Perhaps the latter led to the former. He himself had said that he was 'embarrassed by many strange faces'.[33] Similarly, the question remains unresolved as to whether his light touch was born of his almost ethereal grace and elegant delicate charm or was a direct consequence of his frailty. Either way, he all but retired from the concert platform in 1835, telling Liszt he was not cut out for it.[34] Whether that frailty was due to tuberculosis will be discussed at this section's conclusion.

Both Liszt and George Sand said Chopin had been sickly since before puberty, although they did not meet him until he was in his twenties.[35] That he was frail, meaning small, pale and skinny, does not mean he was necessarily an unhealthy child, and there are accounts of his love of skating and frolicking in adolescence.[36] That he seldom played much above mezzo forte did not turn him into an early invalid, but simply highlighted a delicately idiosyncratic style; as von Lenz observed, he made Beethoven sound 'small'.[37] Chopin made it clear that he strove for a perfection of form, not muscular noisy brilliance. Neumayr comments on little ill health beyond coughs, colds and sneezes until he was sixteen.[38] Then in 1826 Chopin was ill for several months with headaches, lethargy and 'swollen glands' (enlarged lymph nodes) in his neck;[39] the family went to the spa at Bad Reinerz, where the treatment consisted principally of bracing country walks and drinking spa water and whey.[40] Chopin's health and weight improved and he became bored, even of climbing hills.[41] It is believed that, by this time, his younger sister Emilia was mortally ill with open TB. She died in 1827, aged only fourteen.[42] It seems that the final manner of Emilia's passing was a massive haemorrhage from the stomach (haematemesis) rather than from the lungs (haemoptysis), as would be typical of TB.[43]

In 1830, on his way to Paris via Vienna, Chopin's friend and former teacher Würfel was gravely ill with open TB.[44] It was also at this time that Chopin showed strong signs of a developing melancholia.[45] Of particular interest are his diary entries from when he was in Stuttgart. He had written, 'You see death is the best thing there is.'[46] How much this was due to his anger over Russian depredations in Poland, where his father advised him not to return, or whether it was just a constitutional melancholy, is hard to say. It is difficult to correlate declines in his mood with those in his general health, although it is popularly supposed that the 'Revolutionary' Study was an expression of anger, an association refuted by Brown.[47] Hedley suggests that the early Nocturne in C sharp minor and those of Opus 9 and Opus 15, as well as the E minor Piano Concerto, reflected his mood in 1830.[48] Neumayr describes clinical features of depression expressed in melancholy.[49] But there is no history of true suicidal attempt or even of gesture. Thus Neumayr rejects a diagnosis of serious depression (inferring psychosis). He then cites imputations that Chopin had pseudo-schizophrenia, for which the evidence is hard to sustain. Some psychiatrists have suggested that Chopin had a personality disorder. He variously was a paradox, seeming to be the archetypal romantic, an ascription which he rejected, just as he was melancholic but not seriously depressed.

In 1829 Chopin had fallen for an attractive and prosperous singer, Konstancja Gladkowska, but he was shy in coming forward. She later confessed that she had not appreciated the strength of Chopin's feelings for her. Jordan believes that the slow movement of the F minor Piano Concerto was an outlet for these feelings.[50] Or did it perhaps just reflect Chopin generally? In 1831 he had haemoptysis and this was treated by bed rest, with a surprisingly quick recovery, although he had developed a chronic cough for which he took opium on sugar.[51]

Chopin's health once more impinged upon his romances. He had been friendly with the Wodzińskis, a Polish family, since childhood. He now met them during 1835.[52] Maria Wodzińska and Chopin became engaged the following year,[53] whereupon her mother gave Chopin constant reminders to look after his health.[54] The year of 1836 started with rumours that Chopin had actually died.[55] He was very ill again early in 1837, and by the summer of that year he looked pale, thin and tired. Inevitably he was rejected by Maria and, whilst recovering from this misfortune, he met a swarthy woman with long hair, a cigar, trousers and an allure. On

Chopin's first meeting with George Sand, as by then she was known, he said, 'What an unprepossessing woman La Sand is. Is she really a woman?'[56] However, there quickly followed one of the most remarkable musical love affairs of the nineteenth century. Sand was an unconventional and fiercely independent woman, as well as being generous to a fault. By her earlier marriage she had two children. Her son, Maurice, came to hate Chopin, and her manipulative daughter, Solange, possibly loved him. Sand was attracted not just by his musical genius, but also by his frailty.[57]

Chopin always dreaded the winter. He and Sand heard that the weather in Majorca during autumn and winter could be lovely. So off they went in October 1838. Sand left an account of this whole episode.[58] Despite difficulty with lodgings, which were primitive, they were happy for the first few weeks,[59] as Chopin managed to enjoy some long walks under blue skies. Then the weather broke, and one day they returned walking into a gale force wind, by which Chopin was totally exhausted.[60] Worse was to come, for it became persistently cold and wet, the very conditions from which they had taken refuge. This was probably his turning point, after which illness relentlessly consumed him.[61] Chopin developed a severe cough, which was productive of sputum with haemoptysis. The three best doctors on the island were called. Neither Sand nor Chopin respected them, and he wisely refused to be bled.[62] After this, word spread in Majorca that Chopin was consumptive. People had a very different view of TB in Majorca from that prevalent in northern Europe, where the possibility of infective spread was still not appreciated,[63] and Chopin quickly became very unwelcome. The couple's landlord evicted them, instructing them by post to burn all drapery and furniture and, of course, to cause it to be replaced later at their own expense.[64] By Christmas 1839 they were lodged in a cold monastery, but with a piano (of sorts). More calm temporarily prevailed, Chopin's health stabilised for a period and many compositions such as the Preludes Opus 28, numbers 2 and 4, the Mazurka in E minor Opus 41 followed.[65] The 'Raindrop' Prelude's origins from rain on Majorcan window panes have probably been fancifully exaggerated.[66]

By early 1839 Chopin and Sand loathed Majorca, and in February they undertook a horrible sea journey to Barcelona accompanied by, amongst others, many stinking pigs.[67] The lethargy, weakness, cough and haemoptysis all recurred, although they possibly had never fully subsided. Chopin and Sand went on to Marseilles, where he was well looked after by naval doctors. By the end of March, he wrote to his old friend Grzymala that he was 'feeling much better'.[68] There ensued one of the best and musically most productive periods. Chopin went to stay at George Sand's old family home in Nohant, in the peaceful Indre countryside. Their friend Eugène Delacroix has left us an account of this rural idyll, indicating that from 1839 to 1846 Chopin was financially secure and that, over a five-year period, his health possibly stabilised.[69] During this time he was 'never actually ill, never quite well', according to Sand.[70] His surroundings were warm, comfortable and sunny. She nursed him and set his daily routines. Most importantly, she revered him as a musician and had him examined by her friend the local general practitioner, Gustav Papet. The doctor, possibly correctly, declared there to be no evidence of TB, but sensibly prescribed rest and fresh air.[71] So Chopin ate and slept well, retiring to bed when the children did, rather than with their mother. By now, for all its closeness, Chopin's association with George Sand was, as she had said, that of child and mother.[72] The key to this remarkable relationship was Sand's statement 'I have to be able to suffer for someone. I have to nourish in myself this motherly care which likes to watch over a suffering, weak creature.' She later exclaimed that the act of sex became one which she feared might kill him, writing to Grzymala that for seven years she had lived like a virgin,[73] hardly a view supported by Chopin's letter to Delphina Potocka in late 1842.[74]

Each autumn they returned to their adjacent Parisian apartments. The period 1840–46 was prolific for composition. Impromptus, mazurkas and nocturnes flowed. By March 1846 Sand had written to Chopin's sister Louisa that she was hoping to take Frédéric to the south of France for the winters, if she could earn sufficient funds.[75] However, there were soon to be other demands upon her generous purse. Maurice and Solange had grown up. Solange made an unhappy marriage to a man called Clésinger.[76] Their apartment, originally paid for by Sand, was later appropriated by the bailiffs, for which Solange blamed her mother. Chopin sympathised with Solange, to Sand's indignation. As with many family feuds, the *coup de grâce* was in itself a relatively minor episode: Chopin lent Solange his coach, and Sand wrote Chopin a crucial letter which effectively ended their relationship. This letter is believed to no longer exist, but Chopin read it to Delacroix, who declared it to be 'an atrocious letter', revealing 'bitter passions'.[77] Thus George Sand separated not only from Chopin but also from her daughter. Chopin and Sand met just once more on a staircase, and it was from him that she learned that she had recently become a grandmother. But if it was a turning point for her, it was much more so for Chopin, and the road was thenceforth unremittingly downhill.

Back in Paris during 1847 his health declined further, composing occasionally and resting for much of the time. Of seventy-four opus numbers, only four were composed after the separation. Chopin gave lessons, often for big fees, sometimes whilst reposing upon the chaise longue, and sometimes he was too ill for that. He performed little, and then usually privately. He lived alone, attended only by his personal servant, Daniel, who by 1848 had to carry his master up the stairs and help him to bed.[78] And now he was often troubled by persistent diarrhoea. For many years he had avoided fatty food, favouring carbohydrates, fish and chicken. Procuring food which did not disagree with him was, for Chopin and Sand, an additional problem in Majorca.[79] He suffered frequently from headaches, sometimes referred to as neuralgia.

During the 1848 revolution in Paris, Chopin withdrew to Britain, where we have encountered him playing in Manchester. By now he had found another benefactress, Jane Stirling, or more probably she found him. Jane was a well-connected, wealthy and kindly Scottish lady, often in attendance with her sister Mrs Erskine.[80] Moreover, Jane may have been in love with Chopin. Once more his finances were precarious, and some of Miss Stirling's munificence became discreetly and generously anonymous. Chopin commented that Miss Stirling should not marry a corpse.[81] His gallows humour caused him to tell Grzymala in 1847 that he was closer to a coffin than to a marriage bed.[82]

Chopin felt oppressed in Scotland by both the hospitality and the weather. His diary for this time reveals a sick, tired and rather bored man.[83] After further recitals he fled the Scottish mist, but only for the fog of London, where he gave a charity concert for wounded Polish soldiers. He returned to Paris on 23 November 1848, almost impecunious and feeling so weak that he declared in a letter to Grzymala that he could not compose.[84] Teaching too had almost become a thing of the past. By now he was obviously dying, although his mind remained clear. His friend the singer Pauline Viardot probably gave the key to his state of health in a letter of 15 February 1849.[85] She reflected that he had good and bad days, perhaps driving out in his carriage on Tuesday and being in bed coughing until he choked on Wednesday. She also continued to inform Sand of Chopin's health.[86] Most significantly, she noted gross ankle swelling,[87] a sure sign of heart failure. What was constant and consistent is that, by early 1849, Chopin had given up all hope of longer life. He was still energised at the piano stool, whilst often too weak to sit upon it, just as he had to be carried into dinner parties. In a brief respite he even sketched two mazurkas (Opus 67 No. 2 in G minor and Opus 68 No. 4 in F minor).[88] His departure from Sand and Nohant had marked all but the end of composition, and clearly there is no evidence that worsening illness inspired anything beyond an increasing, despairing silence.

Accounts vary as to who was with him when he died on 17 October 1849; Solange and Louisa were, but George Sand was absent.[89] That passing was accompanied by convulsions with murmurings about his mother. Chopin's funeral at the Madeleine, followed by four thousand people, was two weeks later. Meanwhile, at his own direction, a post mortem was carried out by the eminent French TB specialist Professor Jean Cruveilhier, Chopin's own physician. Frustratingly, we do not have the autopsy report. It disappeared, allegedly in a Paris fire, in 1871.[90] Nevertheless, Jane Stirling's letter to Liszt recorded Cruveilhier as declaring that 'The lungs were less affected than the heart.'[91] Cruveilhier told Louisa that the heart was enlarged, a view also communicated to Chopin's sister.[92] This is consistent with his having cor pulmonale. During his dying weeks, Chopin was waterlogged by the oedema of heart failure. His heart was embalmed and returned to the church of the Holy Cross in Warsaw, where it has lain ever since.

The Cause of Death

Upon a balance of probabilities, it seems likely that Chopin died of TB. His illness lasted over twenty years, possibly a long course in untreated TB. The seminal sign of onset was the illness in 1826 involving lymph nodes in his neck. That in turn implied a previous primary infection, and, with his sister Emilia or early friends such as Wilhelm Würfel or Jan Matuszynski, there were several likely candidates from whom he may have originally contracted the disease. The three cornerstones in diagnosing TB are X-rays, laboratory tests for the causative germ and examination of the patient. Only the third was available in Chopin's time, and then competence with Laennec's recently invented stethoscope varied enormously.

More important and striking is the link between Chopin's well-being and his ability to perform and especially to compose. The conclusion of his affair with Maria Wodzińska, the shambles in Majorca, the folly of visiting Scotland and, most especially, the end of his relationship with George Sand were all attended by medical, and parallel musical, deterioration. Hedley reasonably postulates that, had Solange not provoked the ultimate separation of Chopin from the generosity and care of George Sand, then he might have spent several more tranquil summers at Nohant composing further works of incomparable beauty, before TB finally and inevitably caught up with him and blew him away. Well, perhaps.

O'Shea, a dissenter from the diagnosis of TB, very reasonably suggests that Chopin suffered from a hereditary condition, cystic fibrosis (CF), also known as mucoviscidosis.[93] However, TB was enormously prevalent throughout the nineteenth century and the first half of the twentieth. In 1876 12% of all deaths in Germany were due to 'the white death',[94] and it has been estimated that in the first half of the nineteenth century half the population of Great Britain had some form of TB, as many as a third dying from it.[95] Indeed, storm clouds are once more on the horizon as today new strains of TB emerge that are resistant to all known antibiotics.

In CF mucous secretions are viscid (sticky) and, in affected organs such as the lungs, pancreas or liver, the small ducts become blocked by them, leading to destructive changes with cyst formation and fibrosis (scar tissue formation). Today modern treatment including physiotherapy, antibiotics and, where necessary, hormone or enzyme replacement, allied to an encouragement of a very active lifestyle, is changing the outlook enormously.[96] Even in 1950 80% of sufferers died in early childhood. O'Shea puts considerable weight upon photographs showing Chopin to be barrel-chested,[97] a more typical feature with CF than with TB. Although these photographs are not convincing, features consistent with O'Shea's views are Chopin's poor growth, haematemesis and the heart failure which was almost certainly his ultimate primary cause of death. As well as having presumed infertility he did complain when he was twenty-two, 'I have one side whisker – the other won't simply grow.'[98] That too fits well with CF, as do Chopin's long-standing diarrhoea and intolerance of fatty foods,[99] which strongly imply a gastrointestinal problem, something less likely with TB, but typical of enzyme deficiency seen in CF. Our vestigial knowledge of the autopsy reports is consistent with heart failure, but it is Cruveilhier's surprise at there not being obvious cavities in the lung at autopsy which makes the diagnosis of TB most open to challenge.[100] Both Frédéric and Emilia Chopin suffered haematemesis (vomiting up blood), which is less probable with TB than with CF. Nearly two hundred years later we must accept that the distinction between coughing up blood and haematemesis may have been vague.

O'Shea's theory in favour of CF may weaken in the light of survival from that condition. For Chopin's epoch there are no data; CF probably was not recognised then anyway. However, we do know that in the era preceding the introduction of antibiotics it was a sad sentence of death in infancy. This makes the argument in favour of CF, that Chopin survived too long for TB to have been the diagnosis, very questionable. People did survive into their twenties and thirties with TB in the first half of the nineteenth century but were extremely unlikely to do so with CF. Since then CF survival rates in the Western world have steadily improved, with useful life persisting into middle age in many cases.[101] That this has been due to increasingly effective regimens of care, in which antibiotics are central, cannot be contested. There probably is an additional reason for this improvement, which is that increasing awareness of CF has resulted in the recognition and diagnosis of milder cases, such as Chopin's may just have been. There is just a small point of strength opposing CF: people in that epoch were inveterate diarists, and nowhere is there any reference to Chopin's skin tasting salty. Had it done so, surely Sand or Chopin himself would have commented upon this common feature of CF and recorded the fact.[102] Nevertheless, it is well documented that he tended to sweat excessively, and this is another point in favour of CF, as is his family history.[103]

Kubba and Young have introduced an alternative diagnosis, the Alpha-1 antitrypsin deficiency syndrome (α1AT), which correlates well with the medical history of the Chopin family.[104] This is an inherited disorder with an imbalance in the role of the digestive enzyme trypsin. Although the respiratory features of this disease concur with what we know of Chopin, the usual cause of death given, liver failure, does not resonate at all with his demise, although it could with Emilia's. Alpha-1 deficiency syndrome can be a cause of bronchiectasis, which is characterised by susceptibility to respiratory infections. Ultimately wasting, weakness, cough and haemoptysis may all supervene. But because it was so common, TB would remain the probable diagnosis to accept were it not for the alleged absence of tuberculous features in the lungs at autopsy. Chopin's oedematous state shortly before death and the brief details we know regarding that autopsy make clear that, whatever the primary lung condition was, he died in heart failure. Today in the UK, TB is usually successfully treated with antibiotics, and we may again speculate as to what the sixty-year-old Chopin might have left us. But his illness was as intrinsic to him as he was to the music. Balzac described him as a soul expressing itself in lyricism.[105] We cannot know what he might have composed aged sixty, but it is highly probable that such a degree of survival would have influenced his psyche and demeanour in his thirties and so probably also his compositions.

✥ EDVARD GRIEG ✥
(1843–1907)

Bonbons wrapped in snow
           Claude Debussy, 1883

The Rev. W. A. Gray met Grieg at a hotel in Jotunheim in about 1889, describing a small man with a shock of white hair and a cigar. He was dressed in an ulster with gaiters and a hat.[106] Gray observed that he was generally splattered by both the weather and the heather. Tchaikovsky gave a charming account of Edvard and his wife, Nina, but described him as looking sickly. He wrote that his blue eyes were irresistibly fascinating, reminding him of the gaze of a charming child.[107]

Grieg was not always an easy person, but clearly he was popular and had the advantage of a contented marriage. Although a nervous person, he was outspoken, quick-tempered and quick-witted. His early mentor, the Norwegian violinist Ole Bull, persuaded him to enter the Leipzig Conservatoire, with the staff of which Grieg then quarrelled,[108] although they quickly became amicably reconciled. Whilst in Leipzig during 1860 he became severely ill with fever, chest pain and pleurisy.[109] There was damage to one lung, which collapsed.[110] After this, and in spite of it, he became a dedicated mountaineer until his last few years. His diaries and the reports of his doctor Klauss Hanssen are quoted in translation by O'Shea and Monrad-Johansen,[111] and reveal that, for all the mountain walking, he experienced problems with energy and breathlessness.[112] In 1896 he admitted that in 1891 he had left the *Peace Oratorio* unfinished, partly because of a deterioration in his health, but there is also evidence of some indifference to the project.[113] The lung remained permanently collapsed, and the cause was confirmed as TB at autopsy in 1907.[114] Tuberculosis causes a collapsed lung through air getting into the pleural cavity (pneumothorax), which normally works under a negative pressure. Asthma can also cause pneumothorax, and there is evidence that Grieg was also asthmatic, a condition not helped by his fondness for cigars.

He was subject to mood swings and melancholy as is evident in *Ballade in the Form of Variations on a Norwegian Folk Song*, composed in Bergen after the deaths in 1875 of both his parents.[115] Composition sometimes became the weekend and holiday job, as with many other composers. He was a renowned pianist, especially of the Romantic repertory, as well as being a good conductor, a music critic and a journalist. Ironically, in 1874 he had been musically unenthusiastic about the *Peer Gynt* project,[116] but he retired to Lofthus to compose once more. There followed a barren period which he attributed to travel, concert-giving and indifferent health. To this the Norwegian historian Keilhau adds Grieg's highly self-critical approach to composition.[117]

His most arduous tour was in 1887, when he wintered in Leipzig, befriending Delius and a less well-known Dutch composer, Julius Roentgen, who recorded mountain expeditions into the early 1890s.[118] In 1888–89 he had success in England, followed by a mixed reception in Paris. He must have withstood the London fog and smog quite well. Until the last three years his health was very variable, although Monrad-Johansen marvels at his stamina on the concert tour after 1900[119] and reports Grieg's enthusiasm in the mountains again during 1900.[120] There is probably truth in both views. Furthermore, there were numerous events and achievements which are both well recorded and do not sit well with the picture of permanent invalidism. In late 1891 festivities to celebrate his twenty-five years as conductor and pianist took place in Christiania (now Oslo).[121] The following year there was a big party at his villa at Troldhaugen, above the fjord outside Bergen, to celebrate his and Nina's silver wedding anniversary, which he marked by writing 'Wedding Day at Troldhaugen' for Nina. In 1893 Grieg informed Cambridge University that he was too ill to go over in order to accept an honorary degree along with Tchaikovsky. He went to Cambridge the following year, an occasion about which he was somewhat scathing.[122] In 1894 he spent six months in Copenhagen but, because of pneumonia, was insufficiently well to go on to Berlin. He wrote that his major achievements were sluggishness, weakness and shortage of breath.[123] Two years later in Stockholm he wrote that he was healthier than he had been for years.[124]

In 1898 he flung waning energies into the first Bergen Festival, at which much Norwegian music was performed. Afterwards he retreated to mountain huts.[125] In 1899 he turned down an invitation to Paris on account of his strong disapproval of the notorious Dreyfus case.[126] He subsequently published a strong letter to the *Frankfurter Zeitung* as a condition of his accepting an invitation to conduct in Paris,[127] which he did in April 1903, to a very mixed reception. Composition declined after 1900, although *Lyric Pieces* came in 1901 followed by *Norwegian Peasant Dances* in 1902 and *Four Moods* in 1905. Opus 74 (*Four Psalms*) was his swansong in 1906. By then there had been a substantial oeuvre for an alleged 'miniaturist', as even today some regard him. There are piano, orchestral, chamber, stage and vocal works, some still not well known today outside Norway.

Late in life he complained of 'wretched rheumatism' when he noticed swelling and deformity of finger joints and the wrist.[128] Photographs taken around 1900 show bulbous swelling of the fingernails, often called finger clubbing. This is commonly associated with lung disease, which can also evoke arthritis in more peripheral joints, such as those of the hand. In 1900 he was admitted to a sanatorium in Christiania, greatly weakened by early respiratory failure.[129] He is said to have taken chloral hydrate to help him sleep, and it may have been that or just shortage of oxygen which caused him to hallucinate.[130] Nevertheless, he enjoyed his sixtieth birthday celebrations,[131] and in 1903 he was still on the road. Monrad-Johansen suggests that it was nervous excitement that carried him through performances. By 1906 his ankles were very swollen, probably because of heart failure. In the summer of 1907 the Griegs entertained family and friends at Troldhaugen, and Roentgen found him in better health than he had expected.[132] When he left, however, Grieg told him that his 'strength was spent' and that they 'would not meet again'. Then, perhaps typically, in 1907 he was again planning a trip, travelling on 2 September to Bergen in order to sail to England, where he was to play in Leeds. He stayed overnight in a hotel, but the following morning he felt much worse and went to the hospital rather than to the boat. On admission he commented, 'This must be the end of me.'[133] After a restless night he relapsed into a coma, and he died on the morning of 4 September 1907.[134] The night nurse, just before his passing, recalled that he had sat up in bed and seemed to make a respectful bow of farewell.[135] Adolph Brodsky estimated that between forty and fifty thousand people watched his funeral.[136] Like Verdi in Italy, Grieg was more than a composer; he had become a symbol of a newly independent nation.

Dr P. H. Lie undertook an autopsy and gave the primary cause of death as congestive heart failure secondary to lung disease.[137] The left lung was collapsed of old, causing the failed heart to shift its position. There was evidence of TB, and of emphysema in the right lung. Thus Grieg had multiple pathology in his lungs with secondary cardiac complications. Also the chest was said to be deformed. In a footnote O'Shea suggests this could have been due to possible 'concurrent rickets and TB'.[138] In northern climates rickets should be considered, but Grieg's childhood was not deprived, and his history was that of a man sound of limb if not of wind. Importantly in countering rickets, he was often out of doors; in particular, his knees were not rickety. Chest deformity can follow a collapsed lung, which, on a balance of probabilities, appears to have been its cause. Rickets seems very improbable.

Relating Grieg's health to his career as a composer, we see that part of creativity was an innate drive, up to a point of tolerance. So it was that Grieg simultaneously led a very active life, probably of mind over matter. Towards the end there is then little to support a notion of increasing sickliness driving on an inspiration to compose. Clearly, after 1900 he found life increasingly exhausting, and became dejected as the rate of composition declined. There seems little cause to believe that his ill health spurred him on, which would be very different from his deliberately ignoring earlier disability. He clearly decided to get on, in spite of his lack of respiratory reserve, with obvious stoicism and courage. Today his pneumothorax and collapsed lung would be treated by placing a drainage needle into the pleural cavity, allowing the lung to re-expand. Asthma and TB also would be amenable to treatment. We might anticipate survival for another ten to fifteen years, and one suspects that Grieg would have continued composing in much the same way as he always had.

✢ IGOR STRAVINSKY ✢
(1882–1971)

All his life, wherever he might be, he always managed to surround himself
with his own atmosphere

Theodore Stravinsky (the composer's son), 1973[139]

Possibly the most extraordinary aspect of Stravinsky's history is that he
lived to be almost ninety. He was said to have been a delicate child.[140] How
much this attribution stemmed from real disease and pathology or from
his relatively diminutive appearance and bookishness remains unclear. His
survival through long chapters of serious ill health was of titanic proportions and in particular not redolent of frailty. Stravinsky's influence on
twentieth-century music was enormous.

As pro- and anti-Stravinsky factions gathered in 1913, he became very
ill in Neuilly for six weeks with typhoid.[141] During the First World War
he lived in Switzerland. It was in 1916 during her fourth pregnancy that
his cousin and wife, Katya, was found to have TB.[142] They had planned a
return to Russia, but the 1917 October Revolution put an end to that. In
1918 Stravinsky survived Spanish 'flu.[143]

Stravinsky moved from Nice to Voreppe, close to Grenoble, in 1931,
and three years later became a French citizen. Throughout his life he
remained restless and constantly on the move, which made his medical
management increasingly difficult, often with polypharmacy from multiple doctors.[144] No sooner had he become a Frenchman than the lure of
the USA was beguiling him, probably for financial reasons, but he was
apprehensive about the European situation in the mid-1930s. Events then
overtook him as, by 1936, two of his daughters had joined their mother in
a TB sanatorium near Geneva,[145] and Stravinsky moved to be near them,
and then he too succumbed to tuberculosis. As he approached composition of *Dumbarton Oaks*, in 1937 he developed a peptic ulcer,[146] and there
was a lull in composition. A strict diet was prescribed, and probably was
ignored.[147] In the autumn of 1938 his daughter Ludmilla died, and Katya
finally slipped away in March 1939. By now he was still badly affected by
TB and sought treatment in the USA. By September 1939 Stravinsky was
well enough to undertake a series of lectures at Harvard.[148] He married a
previous mistress, Vera de Bosset, in March 1940,[149] and the couple 'emigrated' to Hollywood, which at that time was a cultural mecca, being
inhabited by some of the musical cream of European Jewry. At the end

of 1945 this adoptive Frenchman and his Russian wife became American citizens. By the late 1940s Stravinksy was helped increasingly by a young American music student, Robert Craft. His two sons led their own lives and, for the remainder of Stravinsky's life, Craft became a surrogate son.[150]

Health issues became more frequent during the late 1940s. In July 1949 composition had been inhibited by 'neuritis' in his right arm, probably due to osteoarthritis in his neck. He said he could not compose, attributing that to his being unable to play the piano.[151] Then, on his way to Italy, he developed pneumonia.[152] Presumed colitis was a problem from the early 1950s onwards, although it had probably started in 1937.[153] Ulcerative colitis seems unlikely, and the descriptions are those which would resonate more readily with a diagnosis of diverticulitis (see Berlioz in Chapter 7), to which his biographer Walsh later inclines.[154] Like many elderly men, Stravinsky also developed enlargement of the prostate, which was removed in July 1951, after which he was slow to recover, also having pneumonia later that year.[155] His first real decline may be traced back to this time, with an increasing dependence upon Craft, who became as much an amanuensis as a secretary or personal assistant.[156] In a man so amazingly resilient to illness, we should perhaps not attribute any creative block or even diminution in composition to his precarious health. The early 1950s were, for Stravinsky, a time of musical soul-searching, such as his 'crisis' when driven to the Mojave Desert. There he is said to have wept whilst realising that he had until then wrongly eschewed Schoenberg and serialism.[157] As the 1950s passed, so his musical activities were increasingly interrupted by illness, often respiratory and not helped by his accidentally gargling with formaldehyde in 1954.[158]

In early October 1956 Stravinsky was in Berlin to conduct his Symphony in C. Craft had been obliged to undertake the rehearsals, but during the performance Stravinsky's right arm suddenly dropped and stayed down.[159] The orchestra continued without him, but then he felt numbness down the right side of his body, which became accompanied by a slurring of his speech.[160] He had suffered a stroke, which Craft curiously barely mentions in his *Chronicle of a Friendship*.[161] On 10 October he was admitted to the Red Cross Hospital in Munich, where he stayed for five weeks.[162] His medical bills became alarmingly large and recurrent.

On 7 December Stravinsky consulted the eminent neurologist Sir Charles Symonds in London; he diagnosed stenosis of the basilar artery,[163] which ascends through foramina (holes) in the neck bones to supply blood to the base of the brain. More importantly, Symonds found that he also had polycythaemia vera (PCV). This is the opposite of anaemia, being a condition where the blood haemoglobin level is too high because of an excess of red blood cells which thicken the blood. One of its treacherous side effects is an increased proclivity to blood clotting, in other words thrombosis, itself a potent cause of strokes. He was advised to reduce his conducting schedule, a solution his usually friable financial affairs hardly encouraged. Symonds told him that he had a 'fair chance of survival'. Another mini-stroke seems to have occurred whilst he was visiting Italy in October 1959.[164] Throughout his life Stravinsky was seldom in the same place for long. When he was in London again, shortly thereafter, Symonds proclaimed him to be much better,[165] despite indigestion and heartburn that were presumably due to his peptic ulcer.

A momentous trip took place in the late summer of 1962 when he returned to his native Russia, setting foot there for the first time in half a century. In describing that return, Figes suggests that the wound of his separation from the country of his birth never fully healed.[166] Only when he and Vera arrived in Moscow in 1962 did Stravinsky realise how much Russia meant to him. He even told the press that he thought in Russian.[167] But despite an obvious continued vigour with and for music he was slowing down, limping and using a stick and sometimes a wheelchair. He was well enough to celebrate his eightieth birthday in Hamburg, and on 18 January 1962 to dine with John and Jackie Kennedy.[168] By JFK's assassination a year later, and the death of Aldous Huxley, he was greatly saddened.[169] During 1963 Igor and Vera were at home in Hollywood for only five months. Another great highlight followed when, in August of 1964, he conducted his *Abraham and Isaac* in Jerusalem.[170] After this, almost his last significant composition was *Requiem Canticles*. Like Mozart, he conjectured that he might be writing his own requiem,[171] and he was a man devout in his own Christian faith. For all his frailties, and now in his eighty-fifth year, he conducted in Paris, Athens and Lisbon during 1966.[172] By now Craft was standing in for him increasingly often on the podium, not just at rehearsals. Defying the odds again, he was said to have conducted *The Soldier's Tale* in Seattle shortly after that 'with a vigour which belied his years'.[173] Then on 17 May 1967 he conducted *Pulcinella* in Toronto, for the first time sitting to do so. This proved to be his last appearance on the conductor's rostrum,[174] and reports suggested that Stravinsky had by then lost the plot.[175] His undoubted decline was physical and not mental.[176]

In August 1967 he vomited blood from his peptic ulcer. Simultaneously he developed both anaemia and alleged gout. In November he noticed that his left hand had become purple, which was due to a thrombosis of his subclavian vein;[177] this is the principal deep vein, draining blood from the arm into the chest and thence to the heart. Deep vein thrombosis is much less common in the upper than in the lower limb, but should not be confused with gout. Walsh reports that over these tribulations he severed professional relations with his previously devoted, but allegedly not wholly competent, physician, Dr Max Edel.[178] In December he suffered a further stroke, becoming drowsy and immobile with his speech unclear.[179] Thereafter he had little appetite for composing. He revised earlier works and occasionally set pieces by others.

In 1968 he 'dislocated a vertebra' in his back. This was treated by four weeks' bed rest, an unwise step in someone obviously predisposed to thrombosis. Then a corset was prescribed, which he ripped off.[180] It is extremely unlikely that he had a dislocation. More probably he had osteoarthritis in his lumbar spine (low back), as he had experienced it earlier in the neck. One bone may have slipped (not dislocated) upon another, a condition known as spondylolisthesis. Painful episodes of nerves trapping may be caused by such degenerative changes.

The most remarkable aspect of these declining years was Stravinsky's ability to fight back, despite shortness of breath. Although very frail and almost completely dependent by then on others, he was working on his Bach transcriptions in April 1967. Walsh, however, implies that this was more occupational therapy than serious composition. On 27 April 1969 he attended a 'Homage to Stravinsky' concert at New York State University. Two days later he was admitted to hospital for removal of emboli (plugs of clotted blood) from the main arteries to his legs.[181] If emboli are not promptly removed, gangrene and amputation may quickly ensue. Stravinsky again developed post-operative pneumonia. His recovery was neither fully assured nor necessarily expected, and yet a month later he flew home to Los Angeles from New York.[182]

Matters were not eased then by increasing factions and tensions within his own immediate family, including Robert Craft, over the various trusts and schemes for tax reduction and inheritance. In most families such issues usually bring out the best or worst in people. Anyway, much of Stravinsky's wealth had gone on enormous medical bills, not to mention his often lavish lifestyle. Vera demonstrated her affection for Craft, which Walsh believes may explain Stravinsky's two faces at the time.[183] With his family he had become the frail, weary, rather senile old man, saying little and apparently losing mental faculties. This may have excused him from toil and strife with those near and dearest to him. Alternatively with lawyers, colleagues and particularly newspaper editors, he had lost none of his speed of thought and was fired by a feisty Russian temperament and a weakness for teasing people.[184] We are back with Sir George Pickering's 'creative malady' (see Schumann in Chapter 6). When his son Theodore visited Stravinksy in the spring of 1969, he reported that his father's legs were completely paralysed and he could not walk, standing only with assistance.[185] Theodore said that he hardly spoke but his mind was clear, despite a failing memory. The word 'paralysed' probably implies a severe reduction of mobility due to a combination of factors. That he had lost motor function in his legs and become truly paralysed is very doubtful.

By the autumn of 1969 he had improved and was receiving visitors, dining with friends and family and being driven out and about. Then on 6 April 1970 he was rushed into intensive care with pneumonia and heart failure, further complicated by uraemia suggesting a degree of kidney failure too.[186] It was a miracle of medicine that by the month's end he was planning a final trip to Europe. So it was that on 12 June 1970 the Stravinskys checked into the Hôtel Royal at Évian-les-Bains. Having initially expressed some indifference to being there by Lake Geneva, he started to discuss revisiting Russia.[187] Once more we see a formidable resolve and ability to overcome medical conditions which would have killed many a lesser mortal. In March 1971 he was seated at a piano apparently trying to compose.[188] Griffiths believes that it was a "creative desertion" in Stravinsky's last four and a half years, more than physical frailty, which would make him miserable.[189] He and Vera had moved into a new flat with beautiful views of Central Park in New York City. A couple of weeks later he was back in hospital with congestive heart failure. During the night of 5/6 April 1971 this giant of twentieth-century music and defier of medical odds died quietly in his sleep.[190] Ten days later his body, by now at the cemetery of San Michele in his beloved Venice, was interred, close to the grave of his great friend and champion Diaghilev; the cultural wheel had come full circle.

We now turn to the composer who Stravinsky is supposed to have said composed 'The 700 Seasons'.

Antonio Vivaldi (1678–1741)

Vivaldi's red hair certainly underlay the soubriquet 'the Red Priest',[191] and it is a clinical associate of asthma. Pietro Berri in 1942 identified bronchial asthma as his lifelong illness,[192] a view confirmed in 1982 by Travers.[193] But was he truly a martyr to his respiratory condition? As an ordained priest he claimed to be physically unable to administer Communion. Nevertheless, he was able to become the unofficial *Maestro de Concerti* at the Ospedale della Pietà in Venice.[194] He did complain of chest pain ('strettezza di petto'),[195] and angina has been suggested, as, inevitably, has syphilis,[196] the latter without any apparent validity. In retrospect, his musical energies confound the alleged respiratory disability. Not only did Vivaldi become a famous composer of operas from 1714, ultimately claiming to have written ninety-four,[197] although only fifty are extant, but he also pursued a dual career as composer of sacred music, becoming, for a time, very successful, not least financially.[198] It is the ease and speed of composition as Vivaldi commuted between various European courts that arouses scepticism regarding serious respiratory disease, let alone angina. As he aged, his popularity waned; perhaps the 'Vivaldi brand' failed to keep abreast of changing musical fashions. He fell into relative poverty,[199] but his drive to compose (he ultimately produced at least 770 works) continued relentlessly. He was described by de Brosse in 1739 as 'an old man with a mania for composing'.[200]

Then posterity loses track of Vivaldi until 1741, when he was found living at a saddler's shop in Vienna, where he suddenly died. His cause of death was given as 'innerlicher brand' (internal inflammation).[201] Its sudden brevity is not suggestive of an exacerbation of any respiratory disease, although acute pneumonia is possible and was often fatal until seventy years ago. What we call an acute abdomen is more probable: perhaps a burst appendix or bowel, or even a perforated stomach ulcer.

Arnold Schoenberg (1874–1951)

Schoenberg remains as a composer to arouse controversy, although he was no firebrand in the manner of Scriabin or even Stravinsky. When a young man in Vienna, he attracted admiration and sympathy from both Brahms and Mahler, literally on their deathbeds. Schoenberg's achievements, which may be summarised as atonality and serialism, are intellectual.

Falliers recounts his belief that a system such as twelve-tone writing was a 'psychological necessity' for Schoenberg.[202]

Schoenberg's early years were hard and often impoverished.[203] By 1908 he had abandoned tonality with his first truly dissonant piece, *Das Buch der hängenden Gärten*. In 1910–11 he orchestrated his masterpiece *Gurrelieder*.[204] With the advent of the First World War, he was rejected by the army because of a goitre.[205] Indeed, there are photographs and a self-portrait which suggest he may have been exophthalmic (a sign of an overactive thyroid, possibly presenting with a goitrous neck swelling). Six months later he was signed up for one year, only to be discharged in October 1916 because of asthma.[206] After the death of his first wife and then remarriage, his professional fortunes improved with prolific composition, and in 1926 a return to Berlin gave him sufficient time and money to devote himself to more composition, as well as teaching, to which he was always dedicated.

In the winter of 1930–31, the climate of Berlin affected him so badly that he went to Barcelona.[207] By 1933 it was not just northern winters but anti-Semitism by which he was overshadowed. His response to the latter was to re-convert from Lutheranism to Judaism whilst in France on his way to the USA.[208] The USA was to be Schoenberg's home for his remaining eighteen years. The winter of early 1934 in Boston affected his asthma even more severely, and thus he finally emigrated to Hollywood, taking up a professorship at the University of California at Los Angeles.[209] The weather there was sufficiently invigorating for him to become George Gershwin's tennis partner. However, his music failed to find much of an audience, which depressed him, but, significantly, he then started to compose more.

In 1944, when he considered emigrating again, Schoenberg developed diabetes, and he had to resign his professorship by his seventieth birthday. He is then said to have sustained a cardiac arrest, from which he was resuscitated only by an intracardiac injection.[210] This story is suspect. Had he been anywhere but in an intensive care unit (something which hardly existed in 1946 anyway and was thus unlikely), then the time window of about three minutes in which to get his heart started again (or at least to commence external cardiac massage) without subsequent brain damage would have been too short to prepare and immediately introduce a cardiac needle. Today, as then, cardiac arrest is over-diagnosed, usually because of failure to feel a weak pulse or to hurriedly hear heart sounds with a stethoscope. Accordingly, cardiac arrest can be unequivocally confirmed only by an electrocardiograph (ECG).

The importance of this episode is that it was a brush with death to be reflected in his String Trio.[211] Although composition was sparse in Schoenberg's last four years, his music was often short and of a religious nature, as with *Psalmen, Gebete und Gespräche mit und über Gott*, which was to be his swansong. So there passed a man of enormous drive and integrity, who became for many the apotheosis of twentieth-century modernism.

Several other composers died of pneumonia after a short illness, including Johann Strauss II and Janáček. With others pneumonia was probably the ultimate cause of death, concluding other fatal conditions, Mozart and Beethoven being the best-known examples.

✣ Chapter 10 ✣

Cancer

As quick a growth to meet decay
Robert Herrick, Hesperides, 1648

Introduction

S O STARK A CHAPTER TITLE befits the subject. Even today, with
the outlook for many malignancies dramatically improved, the word
'cancer' can strike fear into many hearts. Any attempt to over-simplify the
subject would be facile, but there are a few basic rules. Cancer implies a
malignant growth or tumour, although the word 'tumour' actually means
a swelling or lump, and many tumours are benign, the majority (but not
all) remaining so. For a tumour to be malignant (cancerous) its method of
cell division and replication becomes disordered and goes out of control, a
cellular *Sorcerer's Apprentice*. Human tissues are living and shed old cells to
replace them with new ones but in an orderly, even pre-ordained, fashion.
Two definitive features of cancer are, firstly, that it invades neighbouring
tissues and structures and, secondly, that it spreads to remote organs by the
blood or the lymphatic systems to cause secondary deposits (metastases).
 The detailed classification of malignant tumours is complex. It is reasonable to simplify it. Malignant tumours arising from lining surfaces are
carcinomas, and those from connective tissues such as fat or bone are
sarcomas. To subdivide again, lining tissues are the epithelium (e.g. skin,
mouth, gullet) and endothelium, including the lining of the gastrointestinal tract from stomach to rectum. Then there are cancers arising from
more specialised tissues, particularly the nervous system. A survival rate is
the percentage of patients still alive years after treatment for that growth.
Achieving these benchmarks often reassures patients enormously. There
are sarcomas for which a survival of two years after therapy almost behoves
a cure. For other tumours that may be achieved within five.
 Treatment can readily be classified. Surgery may involve just a local

excision, or removal of part or all of an organ and lastly of the total structure, plus a more extensive dissection, removing surrounding tissues. Modern scanning techniques (e.g. CT, MRI and PET) now enable doctors to accurately define the edges of a growth and plan treatment accordingly. Surgery is often supplemented or even supplanted by radiation (radiotherapy) and/or by anti-cancer drugs (chemotherapy). These are sometimes given in conjunction with one another. The specialty of caring for cancer is oncology, now an encouraging and forward-looking discipline; in a way Dukas's Sorcerer. Fifty years ago we often talked of 10–50% five-year survivals. Today oncologists are energised by many 80–95% five-year survival rates and some permanent cures.

We have encountered several composers in other sections. Gershwin (Chapter 3) died of a malignant brain tumour (glioblastoma). Elgar (Chapter 2) may be added to those in this chapter who died of carcinoma of the rectum, Rossini and Debussy. Vaughan Williams (Chapter 2) died with, but not of, carcinoma of the prostate gland. Shostakovich (Chapter 7) had many things wrong with him, of which one was lung cancer.

✢ GIOACHINO ROSSINI ✢
(1792–1868)

Buffoon and poet, lover and sensualist;
A deal of Ariel, just a streak of Puck.

W. E. Henley, *In Hospital,* xxv, 'Apparition', c.1900

Henley's verse later reads, 'Most vain, most generous, sternly critical.' He might have been describing Rossini, but wasn't. So there we have it, a man of contrasts and one whose public persona often belied the real man. Several biographies of Rossini raise uncertainty as to who the true man was, and whether Rossini himself knew.[1] His enormous girth, variety of wigs and witty epithets, often tinged with self-deprecation, give us the buffoon who said, 'Give me a laundry list and I will set it to music.'[2] Then there was the sharp, occasionally cruel, critic. The stark contrasts are also there in the opinion of others. Donizetti was just one who laughingly said Rossini was lazy.[3] But sloth sits uncomfortably with writing thirty-nine operas, many before he reached the age of thirty. There is the crux, because this effortless master of melody and bel canto had almost totally retired from the composition of opera by the time he was forty and wrote little beyond two major and a few lesser religious works during his last thirty years. The great question is why, and the answer, if only in part, leads us to consider his very variable mental and physical health. His early years were mainly unremarkable apart from the early realisation of his prodigious and effortless talent. His first near-brush with anything surgical was when his mother stopped an uncle, a butcher by trade, from making her son a castrato.[4] In fact Rossini's life might have been easier had the butcher prevailed.

His first success, *The Italian Girl in Algiers,* came when he was just twenty-one. His greatest triumph, *The Barber of Seville,* followed in 1816. Six years later he married Isabella Colbran, seven years his senior and one of the greatest sopranos of her day.[5] Their match was hardly a grand passion, and yet until 1823 most of his composition was for her. Most of Rossini's adult life was blighted by probable gonorrhoea; whether he contracted it before or during the marriage is unclear. O'Shea suggests that he contracted the condition from a prostitute in 1832.[6] Osborne describes it becoming serious in the 1840s, partly because of stricture, which is a late complication.[7] The marriage was childless, and in his old age Rossini tended to adopt young people as his own surrogate offspring. He wrote in 1865 to Michael Costa* as 'My dearest son', signing the letter as his 'Father'.[8] Untreated gonorrhoea can cause sterility, quite apart from sometimes creating indispositions which may make the very mechanics of fertilisation very difficult. This is of considerable importance in considering Rossini's 'mid-life crisis' and his tendency to severe depression. But before we piece that together, other keystones in his story are important.

Rossini's father said that Gioachino had promised to retire at thirty – 'He has toiled long and wearily enough'[9] – and Rossini himself talked of this. Perhaps even more perspicacious was a note by an early English musicologist, the Earl of Mount Edgcumbe, who said, 'His musical imagination seems already to be nearly drained.'[10] Perhaps Rossini had established the Rossini brand, but by the mid-nineteenth century music had moved on dramatically, leaving the brand, if not Rossini himself, behind.

In November 1823 the Rossinis visited Paris, where at a grand dinner he first met Olympe Pélissier, a courtesan and at the time the painter Vernet's mistress,[11] of whom more later. By now Isabella Colbran's career was in decline as Rossini's triumphed. So they came to live apart, although when many years later Colbran, aged sixty and by then impoverished by gambling, was close to death, she asked to see Rossini. He went at once, departing in tearful distress.[12] On 3 August 1829 Paris saw the triumphant premiere of his last and thirty-ninth operatic masterpiece, *William Tell*. Ten days later the Rossinis hastily left Paris for Bologna, and Francis Toye marks 1830 as the year of Rossini's 'great renunciation';[13] this was subsequently psychoanalysed by Schwartz, with the conclusion that it was brought on by his mother's death two years earlier.[14] Accepting Freudian mother fixation seems far-fetched, when his dreadful physical and mental health, his not always serious approach to music and his having become financially rich all seem sensible, if prosaic, explanations. Richard Osborne has rejected Toye's theory, and he also reminds us that Rossini's 'retirement' during his last thirty years was not absolute. Neither does he accept Schwartz's theory.[15]

It is strange that in 1831 Rossini commenced composition of what subsequently was to become his late masterpiece, the *Stabat mater*. Once started, it was cast aside to be sub-contracted, for completion, to a little-known composer, Tadolini. Weinstock attributes this to Rossini being confined to bed with lumbago.[16] There is little evidence at this stage of a mid-life crisis, although by now his health was indifferent, with worse to

---

* Costa, later Sir Michael Costa, was of Italian birth, but as a naturalised Englishman was an imposing figure in mid- to late nineteenth-century music as both composer and conductor.

come. He was grossly overweight, chesty and possibly by then carrying problems with his urethra, that is, the passage from the bladder through the prostate that ultimately emerges at the tip of the penis, hopefully with a good flow of urine. Ultimately, unpleasant yellow and green discharges emerged from Rossini's urethra, and the chronic inflammation (urethritis) caused the urethra to narrow (stricture) so that passing urine was not only painful (dysuria) but mechanically difficult, sometimes impossible. This could lead to what he feared most, which was an acute and total inability to pass urine (retention), despite a very full bladder. There are few more distressing surgical emergencies than retention of urine. All this was compounded by his cyclothymic mood swings. In these he veered from a witty, entertaining, 'fat, jolly-looking person', described at the court of George IV,[17] to someone seemingly detached from much around him and saying, during his time in Florence, that he had lacked the courage to take his own life.[18] For all this there were no histrionic or tragic gestures. That may have been due to Olympe Pélissier, by now his constant companion. Clearly Pélissier was an impressive woman with fading good looks, but superficially cold. She remains a controversial figure, but what is certain is that she cared faithfully and diligently for Rossini during the remainder of his life.

As early as 1836 Rossini was subject to morbid introspection as to his condition, but this was tempered by what Osborne describes as his intelligent self-awareness.[19] Osborne summarises the venereal condition, much of which derives from a medical report given in 1842 to Olympe and appearing in Appendix B of Weinstock's biography.[20] The problem was coyly said to start when Rossini 'abused Venus from his earliest youth', whence gonorrhoea developed. By 1836 he was inclined to reduce his sexual activity. He probably had little choice in the matter by then. By 1842 the situation had become much more critical, probably owing to stricture, although Rossini became adept at daily self-catheterisation so as to relieve himself from 1835. That is some achievement because, with the rigid metal instruments then available, one hard push too many could cause awful complications. Even today the instruments can occasionally challenge a urologist.

By the early 1840s the full nastiness of Rossini's chronic gonorrhoeal urethritis was increasingly apparent. Furthermore, all manner of potions were introduced via the catheter, including almond oil, cream of tartar and flowers of sulphur.[21] By this time he was also bothered by haemorrhoids as well as rashes and secondary infections of the scrotum. The latter has been labelled psoriasis.[22] As other more common manifestations of that condition have not been recorded, psoriasis seems unlikely. Problems in his nether regions did not stop there, for he had leeches applied to his haemorrhoids, whilst also suffering from chronic diarrhoea.

Much of this was probably sufficient to elicit a desire to retire in his early thirties. Whether that was the only reason is more doubtful. In 1837 Liszt had described Rossini as 'rich, idle and illustrious'.[23] This is overstated as Rossini was not inactive, for he often travelled, becoming involved with production and promotion of his own works and those of protégés such as Bellini, and there were still minor compositions. Perhaps it was just too demanding, not least because he no longer needed the money. He had sufficient to sustain an indefinite life of luxury. We have already seen many composers driving on, often in awful adversity, but Rossini was different. Firstly, he succeeded both professionally and financially before he was thirty. Secondly, he was without doubt a master of wit and melody, but almost his entire output consists of delightfully crafted and tuneful works which befitted the era in which his success evolved. There are within it few signs of anything profound, as we saw with the suffering Beethoven. Mahler's view of the symphonic world would, one suspects, have been dismissed by Rossini with a witty epithet. Shostakovich, Tchaikovsky and Beethoven composed 'potboilers' to pay the rent, but those were consciously pragmatic acts. There is only sparse evidence of Rossini writing from spiritual conviction, as Bach or Handel did. The paradox is that the *Stabat mater*, initially cast carelessly aside whilst still incomplete, was then dusted off ten years later and completed as a 100% pure Rossini work.[24] This is not to discard him entirely as superficial or irreligious, although he invited such suspicion by saying that he was inspired to write the *Stabat mater* whilst sampling cheese.[25] When he was close to death his priest helped him prepare to meet his Maker, and he said to the Abbé Gallet de St Roch in 1865, 'Would I have been able to write the *Stabat mater* and the *Messe* if I had no faith?'[26] However, this is to overtake the main story.

In May 1843 Olympe took him to see the foremost urologist of his day in Paris, Jean Civiale. Before either anaesthesia or Listerian asepsis Civiale had ushered in many newer and enlightened techniques. Ever the pragmatist, Rossini received a prescription from Civiale for a more settled life and an austere regimen, probably excessively so.[27] Olympe Pélissier, whom he married in 1846 after Colbran's death, was just the woman to ruthlessly supervise such a course.

From 1848 to 1850 he composed almost nothing and seemed in poor health and very indifferent spirits. His obsession with minutiae in legal and domestic matters consumed him; Frank Walker, quoted by Osborne, refers to 'everything from horses to inkpots'.[28] Four years in Florence were marked by extreme nervousness of everything, especially gas appliances and railway trains.[29] Walker also describes an epistolary buffo style with his correspondence, betraying themes suggestive of manic depression and obsessive-compulsive disorder (OCD). The cyclothymic had, for a long time, been evident.[30] That he was obsessional, not least meticulously neat and tidy in his habits, is clear from the descriptions of those visiting him at that time, such as the painter De Sanctis, to whom he observed that order was wealth.[31] Whether a contemporary psychiatrist would diagnose him as truly having OCD remains very questionable. That he was depressive for long periods is clear; it may account for his retirement from composition (the 'great renunciation') after *William Tell*, and is a more probable cause than his mother's death as suggested by Schwartz.[32] Moreover, the rigid daily ritual had been ordered by Professor Civiale and imposed by Olympe. Indeed, it may be argued that his own acquiescence with these arrangements betrayed a strong core of sanity and orderly common sense. At a physical level he did have rheumatism, and probably arthritis. Many very obese people do. By 1865 just walking was difficult and he became a great patron of sedan chairs; otherwise he was almost housebound. O'Shea postulates very reasonably that this may have been due to arteriosclerosis.[33]

Fun, a Rossinian hallmark, re-emerged in his last decade. He had picked up wonderfully when Olympe took him back to Paris in 1853. By 1858 the Rossinis were enjoying their place at the heart of Parisian music. Their 'samedi soirs' were attended by the great and good from all the arts.[34] Olympe presided and Rossini programmed the evenings, sometimes playing the piano, and superbly so. His health for a few years seemed more cheerfully robust, although in 1863–64 he confessed to being unsettled whilst composing his last major work, the *Petite messe solennelle*,[35] which was completed only in the year before he died.

In December 1866 he suffered a stroke, from which he recovered by February 1867 in time to fully enjoy his seventy-fifth birthday.[36] In September 1868 he developed what Dr Bonata thought was a rectal fistula.[37] This is where a false passage develops between the rectum and the skin close to the anus. Further progression of the problem revealed that the real disease was cancer of the rectum. Great fears were expressed about subjecting such an obese and frail old man to more than five minutes of chloroform anaesthesia.[38] He was by then bedridden. Thus a decision was made by Professor Nelaton, called in by Bonata, to remove the bulk of the tumour piecemeal through the anus.[39] In 1868 there may have been some logic to it; today such a procedure would defy all criteria of accepted practice.

Today many rectal carcinomas are successfully treated by removing the diseased area of bowel (colectomy). If the bowel cannot be stitched back together the patient has to have a colostomy bag, with which endless patients manage well. Thus it is unfortunate that Osborne ended an excellent biography as recently as 1986 with a judgement beyond his own expertise: 'Nowadays doctors would no doubt administer a massive sedative and wait for the end',[40] which seems to have been Elgar's fate. Even patients with advanced rectal cancer can be actively helped, made comfortable and not bumped off, and that was already the case in the 1980s. Unsurprisingly in Rossini's case the procedure had to be repeated a few days later. From there on it went from bad to worse as infection set in.[41] Whereas his surgeon had used anaesthesia, it is less clear whether aseptic surgical technique was also applied. It is unlikely, in that Lister's first and initially rejected paper regarding surgical asepsis was not published until 1867.[42] The infection, or erysipelas, ultimately involved the whole of Rossini's ample body from the waist down, despite all of Olympe's attention to his daily dressings. Even today infections of that type can sometimes be devastating, even leading to widespread gangrene of soft tissues. Rossini was probably right in paying tribute to Olympe, for she had cared for him in his 'excessively long and terrible illness'. Toye suggests that early in the 1850s he was mad. In 1854, Professor Mordani had declared him to be 'almost out of his mind'.[43]

Ten days after Dr Nélaton's first operation Rossini, having received extreme unction, died on 13 November 1868.[44] Now his remains lie with Olympe's in the exquisitely beautiful Florentine church of Santa Croce. One irony is that it was Nelaton who introduced the first flexible rubber catheter, which has been the subsequent bastion of so much successful surgical practice ever since. Its earlier introduction would have made Rossini's life much more comfortable.

Like Verdi after him, Rossini died a very rich man and left generous provision for the establishment and maintenance of a home for retired opera singers, the 'Maison de Retraite Rossini'. He was both a gracious and a good-natured man, undeserving of G. B. Shaw's silly verdict that he was 'one of the greatest masters of clap-trap that ever lived'.[45] The German poet Heine writing of the *Stabat mater*, spoke of Rossini's 'eternal grace' and 'irresistible tenderness'. To that let us add warm humour.

✝ CLAUDE DEBUSSY ✝
(1862–1918)

The musicians of my generation and myself owe the most to Debussy
Igor Stravinsky, 1959[46]

The scholar Roy Howat believes that Debussy was self-engrossed rather than frankly selfish.[47] Others have described him as grumpy and a 'bear', as he described himself to Proust.[48] This strange, stocky man with his oddly shaped head and constant cigarette nevertheless wrote delicate, serene music.[49] He inspired devotion from a number of women, to not all of whom was he very nice. To launch at once into character analysis in a discourse upon medicine and music opens the author to criticism, but it is a dangerously limited doctor who does not observe and attempt to analyse medical problems without considering other qualities. They are part of the clinical picture, particularly if diagnoses such as depression are given, and especially when we consider a patient's response to disease. Both are germane in a consideration of Debussy.

He also stretched with apparent disregard the social mores of his day. His friend Paul Vidal wrote that he was morally underdeveloped.[50] He was certainly a shameless scrounger. As a young man he became close to Marie Vasnier, a fellow music pupil and wife of a successful lawyer. Whilst Debussy, probably unbeknown to her husband, carried on with Mme Vasnier, who was fourteen years his senior, he also depended on M. Vasnier for help and advice over a five-year period.[51] He dedicated much of his earlier work to Marie.[52]

Later he lived for six years with the alluring Gaby Dupont, nevertheless writing at the time of his 'plodding on dismally'.[53] In the early 1890s he had been depressed by his lack of success and his inability to 'run his own show'. Nichols affirms Debussy's dissatisfaction with his own work.[54] Whether this caused his sometimes morose mood or vice versa is hard to tell. Whilst still living with Gaby, he became engaged to a singer, Térèse Roger.[55] The engagement didn't last long, but *Prélude à l'après-midi d'un faune* was at last a success in 1894, and by then he was crafting Maeterlinck's play *Pelléas et Mélisande* into an opera, which did not reach the stage of the Opéra-Comique until 1902. Although successful, it typified Debussy that conflict over who should sing Mélisande caused sufficient controversy to lead to a legal case.[56]

When Gaby left him, a possible source of his sometimes morose disposition became apparent, as he wrote to his close friend Pierre Louÿs to say that he was afraid of 'losing that little which has ever been good about me'.[57] Here is clear evidence of both self-engrossment and self-critical candour. He probably had no illusions about himself. When his patron, Georges Hartmann, died in 1900, drying up Debussy's regular stipend,[58] money became even more of a problem for the remainder of his life. Between 1895 and 1902 he experienced much misery and soul-searching and, it is suggested, even considered suicide,[59] composing little. Then in 1903 came *La mer*. Debussy caustically rejected the idea of great artists producing through their tears. He said that he saw music which was 'a dream from which the veils have been lifted'.[60]

In April 1899 he met a pretty, naïve and gentle milliner's assistant and mannequin, Lilly Texier. Debussy's correspondence reveals a very physical and rather sweet attraction to Lilly.[61] They married, and in the following year Lilly was hospitalised with TB, needing to have an abortion.[62] The happiness was short-lived. It is clear from Debussy's later correspondence that he was seldom contented and believed that the world was against him;[63] perhaps it was sometimes. Even his friends shunned him when he started an affair with Fauré's former mistress, Emma Bardac, who was now married.[64] He deserted the not very intellectual Lilly, who then shot herself beneath the left breast.[65] Fortunately, she survived until 1932. We can see the state of Debussy's mind in his sketch book for *La mer*, which is reported by Nichols. Written amongst the notes for this great work are his thoughts as to how he might successfully divorce Lilly, who was still his wife, because Emma by now had become pregnant.[66] Debussy's claims against Lilly make dismal reading. In October 1905 Claude-Emma (aka Chou-chou) was born.[67] He clearly adored the child. By now both Emma and Claude had divorced and were free to marry, finally doing so in January 1908.[68] But he saw shadows and threats where many people's lives are illuminated by kindness and sunshine. His stepdaughter, Hélène Bardac (Fauré's 'Dolly'), said that beneath the ursine exterior was a gentle, sensitive man, always young at heart,[69] which resonates with his music.

Whilst in England during early 1909, he passed blood from his rectum, which was diagnosed then as due to piles (haemorrhoids). Nichols implies that this was the first sign of rectal carcinoma, which is good speculation, although doubt must remain.[70] Although rectal carcinoma is a slowly growing tumour, it was not for another six years that the diagnosis became all too clear. Had the bleeding in 1909 been the onset, then survival for another nine years, most of them untreated, would have been improbable. It may be argued that his feeling unwell for some time after the haemorrhage suggests that the diagnosis was more serious than piles. The practical fact is that many unpleasant tumours until very late in their evolution remain symptomless, whereas severe bleeding from any cause, piles included, is very enervating, given that the patient may remain anaemic for weeks. Yet 1909 was when he started work on the first book of *Préludes*, including the disturbing *La Cathédrale engloutie*. Then Debussy became quiet and dejected when his father died in October 1910. A year later he turned his attention to making two Edgar Allan Poe stories into operas. At the end of 1911 he abandoned this project, saying that everything was 'as dull as a hole in the ground'.[71] So was the failure of *The Fall of the House of Usher* to reach a full score, let alone an opera house, due to composer's block or depression, or did he just lose the inclination for it in favour of one to write again for the piano? There he was probably at his best, which possibly answers this riddle.

Reading of the period from 1912 until the outbreak of the Great War is also dismal. Money worries were worsened by a sometimes unreasonable and increasingly demanding wife. He was snubbed at the opera house. Grumbles persisted. Roberts reports that early in 1913 he had an operation,[72] which is today still a little cloaked in mystery. Debussy wrote to a friend about a 'cyst' which had been removed from his bowel and which had 'wanted to keep on growing. A pair of sharp scissors have cut it off in its prime.' There are different levels at which this can be interpreted. The 'cyst' suggests doctors being economical with the truth, or Debussy himself concealing it from his friends or even from himself. The 'wanted to keep on growing' implies cancer. That it was 'cut off in its prime' suggests surgical optimism. Shortly after this he came close to bankruptcy, writing now that were it not for Chou-chou he would consider blowing his brains out.[73] Instead, he drove himself on to exhausting but profitable tours, to Moscow and later to Rome, Amsterdam and London. From these travels he wrote home to Emma in gallant and romantic terms laced with bluntness and irony.

In the autumn of 1915, his 'piles worsened' and he went in for surgery.[74] On 7 December 1915 the surgeon found and removed extensive rectal carcinoma and wisely fashioned a colostomy, whereby the bowel above the tumour is transected and brought out and stitched to a hole in the abdominal wall,* thereafter to discharge permanently into a colostomy

---

* It may alternatively be that in only the second decade of the twentieth century the terminal bowel was brought out through the hole where his anus had been, now without the continent properties of an anal sphincter muscle. Such a procedure was quite popular a hundred years ago in France, but it made the application of any bag, made as they often were then of animal skin, difficult, dirty and uncomfortable. Which procedure Debussy had remains uncertain.

bag.[75] Debussy was an early recipient of both this procedure and post-op-erative radiotherapy, surviving for more than two years, but at what price? Friends were received, especially Erik Satie, but Debussy required con-siderable quantities of morphine.[76] He had little energy, was miserable and lost weight. In June 1916 he wrote, 'I wonder whether this illness isn't curable. I might as well be told at once.'[77] Later he said, 'Dressing is like one of the labours of Hercules.' Writing to Durand, he went on to say that he had to fight against illness and against himself, concluding that he felt a nuisance. For comfort he sat on a rubber ring. People were struck by his limp, waxy appearance and by an almost vacant look which was probably due to his drugs.[78]

To some extent the changing medical culture in dealing with advanced cancer is revealed here. Presumably Debussy suspected that he had a fatal disease and wasn't long for this world, but he probably was not told so. In the 1960s it was almost forbidden to be so unkind as to tell patients the truth. There were several well-intentioned euphemisms, and some patients preferred not to know anyway. Today doctors are (or should be) honest, open and explicit with their patients. The road ahead is mapped out with the patient and his or her family, and the remaining days ahead are made as comfortable and positive as possible. Poor Debussy wrote at Christmas 1916 that he no longer took his 'tattered body' for walks in case he 'fright-ened little children and tram conductors'.[79] He still wrote lovingly to Emma and Chou-chou at New Year, as he always had. A year later he was almost bed-bound, and he listened to the distant pounding of Paris by the German Big Bertha guns as he died on 25 March 1918.[80] In his last days, greatly weakened, now unable to walk and increasingly sleepy between the episodes of pain, that final protracted passing of a gruff, determined man was truly dreadful. His consolation had been Chou-chou, who tragically died sixteen months later of diphtheria.

Debussy was a deeply complex man. Did the vicissitudes of his health match a pattern with that of composition? Probably not. He was with-drawn and moody, and sometimes his own worst enemy. His music, so utterly free of pretension or even grandeur, is both sensuous and astringent. Clearly his tendency was to be morose, unlike much of his music. But he enjoyed wine, good food, attractive women and intelligent conversation and, as with many composers, he seems to have been long-suffering and brave, as well as resigned in his final, truly terrible illness. For the rest he probably composed when he felt like it, and didn't bother when he didn't.

Accurate scholarship by Nichols, Roberts and Jensen reveals in his final illness a courageous, resigned stoicism, but little evidence of composition during his last twenty-seven months. The Sonata for violin and piano was completed in April 1917; his last public performance was of this a month later.[81] That year he had again dabbled with *The Fall of the House of Usher* and even contemplated setting *As You Like It* with the writer Toulet, although this was originally proposed fifteen years earlier.[82] His legacy is an immense influence on twentieth-century music, from the labyrinths of Russia to the bars of New Orleans, and taking composition from Massenet to Messiaen. His unusual genius and unique legacy is that he was at the same time innovative and intellectual, but he was no self-conscious revolutionary. Howat believes that it was his musical integrity, his lack of money and above all his poor health which led to what was in many ways an awful life, especially at the end.[83] That perhaps we don't know the man as well as we might like to is probably what he would have wanted.

Today, how would Rossini, Debussy, Field (Chapter 5) or Elgar (Chapter 2) be treated? Firstly, and most importantly, the diagnosis would almost certainly have been made years earlier. In all cases the affected area of bowel would be removed. The level at which this was possible would determine whether the bowel could be reconnected or a permanent colostomy bag would be necessary. Today, even in more advanced cases, radiotherapy and/or chemotherapy may substantially extend life expectancy.

✢ JOHANNES BRAHMS ✢
(1833–1897)

Whoever comes after him will not continue him;
He must begin anew;
For his predecessor left off only where art leaves off.
Franz Grillparzer, funeral oration for Beethoven, 1827[84]

And there we have one of the three principal problems to afflict the life of the short, but metaphorically titanic, figure of Brahms. He was born in near-poverty in Hamburg only six years after Beethoven's death.[85] From the time of Robert Schumann proclaiming, almost messianically, the then twenty-year-old to be the 'new way',[86] Brahms became aware of the mantle of Beethoven which would descend upon him. When years later Hans von Bülow described Brahms's First Symphony as Beethoven's Tenth, Brahms spoke of 'constantly hearing a giant tramping behind me'.[87] That great symphony was fourteen years in the ferment of its creation, and here we see that first problem, which was the insecurity that had left him a self-critical perfectionist: perhaps why he destroyed twenty string quartets and possibly much else.[88] That insecurity derived from his childhood, some of the ghosts of which never leave us. He needed company, but only at the edges of his existence. That Brahms changed his whole appearance, from gilded youth to bearded sage, in his early forties as his fame grew may have been the adoption of a disguise of anonymity.[89]

One of the last scores he read before he died was that of Arnold Schoenberg's early String Quartet in D. Brahms, always a generous man, so admired what he saw that he is said to have offered money to forward the young composer's cause.[90] Schoenberg greatly admired Brahms,[91] regarding him as a progressive, not a conservative. Across this monumental bridge from Beethoven to Schoenberg strode the usually single-minded Brahms; beneath flowed the symphonic poems of Liszt and Berlioz, whose forms he rejected.

With Clara Schumann we encounter Brahms's second problem, which, like the first, was to assail his mental health: his relationship with women. The women problem was perhaps revealed when Brahms told the Schumanns' daughter Eugenie that he had seen things in his childhood 'that cast a dark shadow over my soul'.[92] The origin of this oft-repeated and bleak reference was that, as little more than a child, he was sent out by his father to earn a few coins playing in piano bars on the Hamburg dockside. Swafford and MacDonald tell of Brahms mixing with vice, nudity and prostitution in brothels, where he himself may have been sexually molested.[93] Recently Swafford's charge has been repudiated by both Avins and Hoffman.[94] The weight of circumstantial evidence that the small, beautiful child and later adolescent was disturbed by the bars and bordellos must remain hard to contest. Anyway, Brahms thought he had been and, although he could be jolly when older, he often referred to his melancholic side, which, he told the conductor Vinzenz Lachner, was clearly expressed in the opening movement of his Second Symphony.[95] But the introduction to lust stuck with him. Like many people with disturbed childhoods, later in life he could nostalgically reminisce about joyous summers in the countryside,[96] only to then bark about 'a man cursed with a childhood like mine'.[97] The two positions are not mutually exclusive. Brahms probably developed a Madonna/prostitute complex in that he could not sleep with the women he loved and he certainly did not love the women with whom he slept. He was a visitor to the bar-brothel scene in Vienna.[98] It is possible that the closest the complex came to resolution was with Clara Schumann. His love for her and hers for him, like so much of his music, were passionate. Whether that passion was ever consummated we shall probably never know. Perhaps the problem was that neither resolved the question of whether Clara was a mother substitute or a potential wife, let alone a lover. Perhaps this was why in old age they still bickered. Lest we over-simplify, we should remember that he also had a strong urge to remain private, and thus single and untied. 'I cannot wear fetters', he said on breaking his 'engagement' to Agathe von Siebold,[99] one of many attractive women whom he befriended. Or was Clara the problem itself? Later in 1874 he fell in and out of love with Baroness Elisabeth von Stockhausen; this episode was followed by the Piano Quartet Opus 60, which according to his biographer Max Kalbeck reflected his covert love for Clara.[100]

The apparent conflict between the views of Swafford and those of Avins has become another of the causes célèbres of musical pathography. In many ways both are correct, with a dedication to historical primacy of sources. Their two classic papers both contain references to old original sources, such as Kalbeck, May, Heuberger or Schauffler.[101] The differences are with interpretation. Avins argues from paintings, photographs and household accounts that Brahms's family were not slum dwellers on the breadline; they were petty bourgeois, although impecunity has no respect for class or circumstances. That his parents paid for music lessons and a decent primary education did not exempt them from encouraging their son to contribute to the family finances by bar work in the evenings. Avins has been assiduous in her research, as exemplified by reading Dr Lippert's 'Account of Prostitution in Hamburg in 1858'. There were restrictions on who did what with whom in bars, not least in relation to the age of the participants, which merely reiterated what the law had said, rather than what actually happened. Similarly, much weight has been put on the condition of the Gängeviertel district of Hamburg. But then Brahms's youthful residence there and inspection by authorities such as Florence May, his first English biographer, were separated by decades. Anyone familiar with cities as diverse as New York or Edinburgh would testify that last year's doss-house area may become next year's chic place to eat or live. Avins rightly emphasises that in old age Brahms reminisced 'with pleasure and satisfaction' about the 'jolly circumstances of his youth, playing dance music'.[102] But this should not detract us from May's report that at sixteen, 'he played amid the sordid surroundings of the Hamburg dancing salons'.[103] These two apparently conflicting statements merely reflect differences in attitude and reminiscence at separate times. May's source material came from contemporary accounts of what the Brahms she once knew personally had said. So Swafford's sensible conclusion is that to ignore the recorded dark reminiscences of Brahms's childhood is to ignore Brahms himself,[104] who was a famously honest and outspoken man. It is a typical example of Occam's razor. This is not conflict or even confusion; it is an insight into the state of Brahms's mind and thus mental health. There were days when he recalled the bucolic and jocund in his youth, just as there had been darker events by which he always remained overshadowed. Similarly there were prostitutes and Madonnas, probably conceptually as well as physically. These issues were never resolved, especially as Brahms and Clara Schumann in 1886 agreed to destroy much of their very personal correspondence.[105] Eugenie Schumann recalled how much Brahms hated being talked or written about.[106] But that is not to take the music itself into account, which is why the dichotomy is important for us today.

The compositions of Johannes Brahms have a gravity, sometimes solemnity. As well as always being beautiful they are sometimes fearful, seldom maudlin and always uplifting. They were frequently slow in gestation and are often reflective; throughout they have the hallmark of absolute musical integrity. It was with music that Brahms resolved his own inner demons, neither destroying his heritage nor leaving a legacy open to great controversy. That is probably why, when he was dying, Brahms made sure to leave an empty desk.

In seeking to rationalise Brahms's sometimes torrid psychology we

turn to his mother's death in 1865, which he lamented in the E flat Horn
Trio Opus 40. That death is customarily related to *Ein deutsches Requiem*,
whose premiere he conducted on Good Friday 1868 in Bremen.[107] Its origins return to another event by which he was saddened and disturbed:
Robert Schumann's tragic death in 1856. Religious affiliations within this
and other works, such as the *Alto Rhapsody* dedicated to Julie Schumann or
the *Four Serious Songs*, and especially the Opus 122 Chorale Preludes, have
always been controversial. The Bremen music director Karl Reinthaler and
Brahms's Roman Catholic friend Dvořák said that Brahms had a great
soul yet did not believe.[108] On his bedside table reposed a well-thumbed
Bible, and also the Koran with passages underlined which chastened and
reproved women.[109] The first line of the *German Requiem* (which Brahms
considered naming a Human Requiem) is 'Blessed are they that mourn for
they shall be comforted', which is possibly a declaration of belief in a God,
for who else might bless us in our bereavement? It was probably about the
church's slavish conventions that he was sceptical. We can only speculate
how much religion bothered him. Probably it was an important facet of
his psychological make-up.

Brahms's middle age had a comfortable bourgeois veneer to it. This
once slim, handsome, quite small young man became stout, bearded and
grizzled. He ate out, enjoyed food (usually in large quantities), beer and
wine and admired pretty women. He also lived on a high intellectual plane
with politics, physics, philosophy and medicine amongst his interests. He
had a wicked sense of humour and was notoriously scruffy.[110] One of his
long-standing and closest friends was the Professor of Surgery in Vienna,
Theodor Billroth.[111] The two men, who had met in Zürich in 1865, were
dissimilar in many ways. Unlike Brahms, Billroth was sociable, elegant
and urbane. He was also a seriously good musician, as well as being one of
the giants who developed modern surgery in the late nineteenth century.
The first successful removal of the voice-box (laryngectomy) for cancer
and partial removal of the stomach were his best-known innovations. But
he became anguished over surgical failures and complications. Music for
Brahms was his consummation; for Billroth it was refuge and consolation.
In turn Brahms, the younger man, frequently showed new compositions
to Billroth privately before performance or publication, and was often
encouraged by him. He dedicated his Opus 51 String Quartets in C minor
and A minor to Billroth, and they were known as Billroth 1 and Billroth 2,
as are the two stomach operations which bear his name.[112]

Billroth and von Bülow died in 1894 within a few weeks of one another.
Brahms had already lost his sister Elise, thereby outliving all his relatives and

other friends, including his once beloved Elisabeth von Herzogenberg.[113] Even before all this in 1890 he had completed the G major String Quintet Opus 111, saying it would be his last work.[114] His last full year, 1896, opened with him conducting for the last time, in Berlin.[115] In March he heard that Clara had suffered a stroke. She had become increasingly deaf with tinnitus and said she was 'befuddled'. There was even a wheelchair.[116] He moved near to her and composed the *Four Serious Songs*, a profound statement of last things,[117] but he did not visit; he hated illness in others. Then he heard that she had suffered a second, and soon to be fatal, stroke on 20 May.[118] He hurried to her funeral, but missed a crucial train. The service was even held back, and he was able to sprinkle earth in the grave and retreated in tears.[119] Although Clara had borne eight children, he still regarded her as maidenly. If nothing else, it is a reminder of how much sexual relations are conceptual as well as physical. He had said to Richard Heuberger, 'Apart from Frau Schumann, I am not attached to anybody with my whole soul.'[120] Back in Ischl he composed the Eleven Chorale Preludes, described by MacDonald as 'meditations on endings',[121] which marked the onset of his final decline. By now his friends noticed that he had lost weight and developed a yellow tinge. He protested that it was an 'ordinary jaundice' and pointed to his excellent appetite, which lasted into the autumn,[122] as did freedom from pain. And so we come to Brahms's third and final problem: cancer.

When, later that summer, he and Gustav Mahler walked by the Traunsee, Brahms's mood was fatalistic.[123] Mahler's last glimpse of him was later in that holiday: through a window he saw an old and solitary man making himself a sausage sandwich.[124] Brahms consulted Dr Hertzka in Ischl and then Dr Grünberger, who diagnosed malignant enlargement of the liver.[125] Professor Schrötter came from Vienna to examine Brahms and removed all the doctorish restrictions under which Brahms had been placed, which suggests that by then the diagnosis of cancer had been made. That summer Brahms 'took the cure' at Karlsbad. Schrötter said, 'Poor devil, poor devil. For Brahms's disease there is no Karlsbad. It does not make a bit of difference where Brahms goes to spend his money.'[126] Still there was no pain, his appetite remained excellent, and he said he had just a 'bourgeois jaundice'. His usual prodigious energy was in decline, and friends were appalled by his wasted and sallow appearance. He walked more slowly and became increasingly testy, whilst his discreet and kind housekeeper, Frau Truxa, secretly took in the waistbands of this previously stout man's clothes. So Brahms triumphantly declared it was obvious that he wasn't wasting because his clothes still fitted. But over his swansong, the Opus 122 Chorale Preludes, he had written, 'Oh world I must leave you.'[127]

He had been late for Bruckner's funeral on 11 October and went away muttering, 'Soon my coffin', despite reassuring his friend Heuberger that he was as fit as a fiddle.[128] Most ominously, in December 1896 he first complained of back pain.[129] He spent his last Christmas with friends and clearly did not want to be alone. In January Professor Engelmann and his son-in-law Professor Narath from Utrecht were consulted.[130] A diagnosis of gallstones was suggested, and surgery considered and then rejected. They must have quickly concluded that obstructive jaundice caused by gallstones has almost invariably an acute and very painful onset, the very antitheses of the insidious and painless course in Brahms's case. The jaundice deepened typically with an itchy skin. His friend Max Friedlander tried to cheer him up by discussing a trip to Italy in the spring. Brahms responded that he would soon be going on a much longer journey.[131] By now his months of public obfuscation and self-denial were ended. He just did not want sympathy or to be a burden.

In late February 1897 he developed a paralysis on one side of his face. As there was a concurrent difficulty with speech, this was probably a stroke, as stated by Swafford,[132] and not a Bell's palsy, as suggested by Neumayr.[133] On 7 March 1897 he attended a performance of his Fourth Symphony under Richter.[134] The Viennese audience drew the now frail, ill old man to his feet to tearfully acknowledge their immense applause. After the performance he tottered home, helped by friends. By now the appetite had gone. He felt sick, and there was blood-stained vomit on several occasions. By March he became partly bedridden, lying in his frugal bedroom with a bust of Bismarck. Before he finally became permanently bedridden, friends found him by his stove, which was full of the ashes of papers, perhaps letters, perhaps from Clara or incomplete compositions, probably both.[135] Brahms was finally and sadly covering his tracks.

On the morning of 3 April 1897 Frau Truxa relieved the young Dr Robert Breuer of his vigil. Brahms opened his eyes. His hands and those of the good housekeeper met; he tried to speak and could not. He sobbed a few tears and was no more.[136] Robert's father, Dr Joseph Breuer, who had superintended the final days, wisely professed that he was not sorry that it had all been so brief. He also thought that from quite early in his illness Brahms knew what was amiss.[137] There was no autopsy. A few days later the Viennese poured onto the streets as the cortege passed on its final journey. In the docks of Hamburg flags on the boats flew at half-mast.[138] An era had closed. The century of musical modernism and military madness was about to start. There was Mahler and the young Richard Strauss. Then there would be Schöenberg and serialism, which Brahms had been early to apprehend.

The Cause of Death

It is almost beyond all reasonable doubt that the cause of death was neither gallstones nor cancer of the liver. A case of painless jaundice later accompanied by back pain, wasting and a good appetite is all but a cast-iron diagnosis of carcinoma of the head of the pancreas. The diagram (Fig. 6) shows how the pancreas fits into the curvature of the duodenum, which connects the stomach to the upper bowel (small intestine). The pancreas produces many digestive enzymes which flow in the pancreatic duct to meet the common bile duct from the liver and the gall bladder in the duodenum. If the bile duct is blocked by pancreatic cancer, then the back-pressure of bile causes jaundice. The pancreas produces insulin, which is normally discharged into the bloodstream. Cancer of the pancreas can result in its excessive production, causing an abnormally low blood sugar, which stimulates the appetite. Even at Christmas 1896 Brahms told Heuberger that he still ate and slept well.

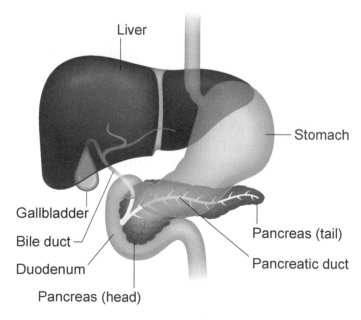

Fig. 6 Diagram of the pancreas

The late occurrence of vomiting blood (haematemesis) in Brahms's case has led to Kerner's suggestion that he died of alcoholic cirrhosis of the liver.[139] This cannot be sustained as a cause of his death. Haematemesis is certainly a feature of the alcoholic close to death, but other explanations are more readily to hand. Projectile vomiting occurs late in the development of pancreatic cancer. The basis for the suggestion of alcoholic cirrhosis, as with other composers we have encountered, is that Brahms enjoyed beer and wine, both of which he could drink in considerable quantities. He also enjoyed rising early in the morning, something almost unheard of amongst alcoholics. In alcoholic cirrhosis the liver is initially enlarged, as was Brahms's but, as the disease progresses, the liver shrinks (fibrosis), which his did not. Severe jaundice is not an early presenting sign. The patient dying of alcoholic cirrhosis must have a history of excess alcohol dependency with drunkenness, poor diet and mental disorientation, as with those famous metaphorical pink elephants, which were all conspicuously absent. We rarely hear of Brahms truly drunk or of any embarrassing accumulation of empties being tidied up by Frau Truxa. At a time when Brahms was still eating heartily, although jaundiced, Professor Schrötter had clearly assessed the situation and realised that removing Brahms's regular and enjoyable libations would achieve nothing beyond depriving a dying man of a comfortable pleasure. Had there been the typical appearance of alcoholic cirrhosis then Schrötter's first duty would have been to advise Brahms to refrain from taking wine and beer, counsel which in an alcoholic could even be life-saving. The curious feature in February 1897 of the left side of his face becoming weak or even paralysed is best explained by Brahms having suffered a stroke, due to thrombosis. Disorders of blood clotting are common with liver disturbances.

Several biographies have given cancer of the liver, of which Brahms's father died, or of the gall bladder as the cause or possible cause of death.[140] Hepatocellular carcinoma (HCC), to give it the modern description, is in many ways a modern disease in that most cases are secondary to previous infection with hepatitis B or C, which reached epidemic proportions in the late twentieth century and of which cirrhosis may be an intermediate stage. Typically HCCs are localised tumours and as such they present as a discrete swelling *in* rather than an enlargement *of* the entire liver. Anorexia is a common early feature, as is abdominal pain; both were conspicuously absent in the first four or five months of Brahms's final illness.

What might be done for a patient like Brahms today? Sadly, carcinoma of the pancreas is still an awful diagnosis. A surgical cure is possible only in 10–15% of cases, although five-year survival rates are higher now with aggressive chemotherapy. Otherwise the only contribution the surgeon can make is with procedures to bypass the enlarging growth and to provide alternative drainage for both the pancreatic duct and the bile duct, as explained in Fig. 6. Even by today's standards Dr Joseph Breuer's comment, that the brevity of the illness had been a mercy, was apposite. It is also tantalising to speculate, if Brahms had lived on into his mid-seventies, what else we might have heard from him: the 'if only' question. However, Brahms had occasionally declared his intention of ceasing composition initially after a bout of 'flu or pneumonia, his first real illness, in 1889.[141] Conspicuously, after the Double Concerto's mixed reception in 1888 his output tailed off, although it never totally ceased, there being a late acquaintance with the clarinet. Until his final illness he was robust and energetic and could often be sociable and fun. His musical standards had always been set remorselessly high. Perhaps as old age approached he just enjoyed his success, his holidays and his friends. Some great professionals continue to the last gasp; others retire if only in stages, like his friend Dvořák.

Clearly Brahms could be a testy difficult fellow, but anyone who had sufficient humorous self-awareness to discard collars, ties and socks, or to leave a party shouting that if there was anyone there to whom he had *not* been rude then he apologised, must have been an engaging companion. Eugenie Schumann described him as warm-hearted but usually hiding his passionate nature under an appearance of ruggedness.[142] He was generous and humane, although very few conflated power and pathos with the unswerving but unsentimental assurance of Johannes Brahms.

✢ GIACOMO PUCCINI ✢
(1858–1924)

Is the devil to have all the passions as well as all the good tunes?
                    G. B. Shaw, *Man and Superman*, 1903

Puccini always claimed that a melancholy often hung over him.[143] Whilst wrestling with *Turandot* at the end of his life he said, 'The Almighty touched me with his little finger and said, "Write for the theatre – mind, only for the theatre."'[144] For the fusion of passion, sensuality and tenderness, pathos and despair, he is almost unrivalled. Puccini seems effortless in respecting the theatrical classical unities of action, time and place, but he was a slow and meticulous worker. Carner infers that he stimulates the tear glands more than the cerebrum. Late in life he wrestled with psychological problems, which probably adumbrated his music more than physical problems had done or would do.

Born into a musical family, in his teens he walked from Lucca to Pisa to hear Verdi's *Aida*, whereafter there was no going back. His first successful opera was on the subject of *Manon Lescaut* and was his first collaboration with the librettists Illica and Giacosa.[145] After this success *La bohème*, *Tosca* and *Madama Butterfly* followed. They did so with a repeated pattern of critical condemnation and public adulation, not that he should have worried; he was by then peerless and very rich.

In early 1903 whilst working on *Butterfly*, he had been out to dinner with his son and future wife and was returning, chauffeur-driven, in his latest expensive motor car. The car cornered too fast on an icy road, leaving the road, with Puccini trapped beneath.[146] The fumes nearly killed him and, when extricated by a local doctor, he was found to have suffered a fracture of his tibia (shin bone). It took many months of immobility and plaster casts for the fracture to heal; moreover, it was not set straight.[147] Although it was later reset, he always limped, walking with a stick for two years afterwards.[148]

Shortly after his accident, the husband of his long-term mistress, Elvira Gemignani, died, and in January 1904 they were at last married.[149] Unlike wives such as Cosima Wagner or Giuseppina Verdi, Elvira was always on the periphery of her husband's musical world and his high living. As Carner says, she was her own worst enemy.[150] There is no doubt that Puccini had a roving eye. Whilst recovering he was found to be diabetic,[151] and later he went to Vienna for the new insulin treatment. A much greater trauma of medical relevance came in late 1908 when the perpetually jealous Elvira came downstairs to find her husband happily chatting with a pretty teenage maid, Doria Manfredi, originally engaged to help nurse Puccini after his accident.[152] Elvira immediately concluded that a good deal more than a cheery conversation had occurred and persecuted the poor girl viciously and relentlessly.[153] Doria retreated, feeling that her reputation was sullied in the village, where she was then refused communion, and thereafter refused to eat. Ultimately she took poison and died painfully.[154] The autopsy revealed that she had remained a virgin.[155]

It was then the turn of Doria's family to become vindictive, and they sued Elvira Puccini, who was sentenced to five months' imprisonment for libel, defamation and endangering life and limb.[156] Italy was scandalised, after which Puccini compensated the Manfredi family financially to prevent his wife's imprisonment. Jackson believes that despite their problems and his infidelities Giacomo and Elvira were a curiously inseparable couple, a view not supported by Phillips-Matz.[157] He remained scarred by this episode. In the early 1920s the often prosaic and sometimes ridiculous aspects of Puccini's life came to the fore, not least his morbid dread of senescence.[158] He dyed his hair and investigated possibilities for surgical rejuvenation. Seven months before he died he investigated having an operation whereby an ape's manly organs might be incorporated with his own.[159] Typically in an ageing man with diabetes, problems of impotence were likely.

In the autumn of 1923 he complained more frequently of sore throats and a chronic cough, with which he sometimes spat up blood. Two doctors were consulted. Astonishingly for this date, amongst their early diagnoses was 'rheumatism'.[160] Further specialists were visited, one secretly in Florence who diagnosed cancer of the throat.[161] This was communicated only to Puccini's son 'Tonio, but not to Elvira or Puccini, who had for a long time been morbidly fearful of death. He was advised to visit Brussels to see Professor Ledoux, who had developed a new radium treatment for his condition.[162] On 5 November 1924 Puccini was admitted to hospital, taking with him the finale of *Turandot* for completion or revision. At first all was well; he even went to hear *Butterfly* in Brussels. The second stage of the treatment started on 24 November. A rubber feeding tube was passed through his nose into the stomach. Under local anaesthetic, an opening was made in the windpipe (tracheostomy) so that his airway could be maintained during the remainder of the operation, which took over three hours as radium needles were inserted into the tumour.[163] On 28 November 1924, whilst sitting in his chair, Puccini suffered a major heart attack, something to which he was already predisposed as a heavy smoker and ageing diabetic. Professor Ledoux rapidly removed the needles but to no avail. On 29 November Puccini died, probably painfully and certainly unpleasantly.[164] All this was about thirty years since Brahms's friend Theodor Billroth had first described the draconian but life-saving procedure of laryngectomy, which totally removes the larynx (voice-box) and thus the power of speech. Today it is reserved for advanced and recurrent cases, as treatment is usually based on radiotherapy. Cases caught early now can expect preservation of the larynx and an 85–90% five-year survival.

It is curious that this composer, so hugely popular with the public, stirs passions not just of sentiment and the heart but also of superciliousness. Surely he was no worse than many other men. His hobbies and indulgences are today very popular amongst the prosperous. He philandered with women, but he always came home, and in the Manfredi affair, it was Elvira who had wronged Puccini. He paid the bills and in his own way remained devoted to her, as well as remaining seared by the affair until his end. Carner observes that 'despite fine craftsmanship' *Rondine* (1917) suggested a staleness.[165] If that is so then surely it was the aftermath of the Manfredi case in 1909 and not the later throat cancer which was to blame. The famous late photograph is of a haunted man.

The remaining mystery is the failure to complete *Turandot*, the score of which was on his bedside table when he died. He is said to have left some direction as to the conductor's performance should he not live to complete the score.[166] Toscanini and Puccini's son deputed an Italian composer, Alfano, to provide a conclusion consonant with rough sketches which the master left. Alfano was ordered about by Toscanini, who at the eventual premiere laid down his baton, announcing to the audience, 'This is where the master laid down his pen', thus fulfilling Puccini's wishes.[167] The question remains whether it was his final illness (which seems the more likely) or his own persistent anguish over the Manfredi affair, with which there are obvious parallels in *Turandot*, which inhibited its conclusion. Liù, the Doria Manfredi figure in *Turandot*, selflessly kills herself, but questions remain as to the resolution of the relationship between Calaf and Turandot. Was Puccini similarly troubled with Elvira? Turandot and Elvira were not comfortable women, Turandot being much less warm, earthy or loving than most of his earlier heroines. What cannot be doubted is Puccini's legacy of uncluttered and unashamed melody, plus that persistent melancholy.

✝ SERGEI RACHMANINOV ✝
(1873–1943)

It seems that only one place is closed to me and that is my own country
– Russia

Sergei Rachmaninov, 1930

Rachmaninov's entry here is based on his dying from the spread (metastases) of a skin tumour. Like Bartók, he sits appropriately with those whose psychological health was disturbed by separation from their own country. Rachmaninov is also of medical interest because he has been said to have had Marfan's syndrome (see Britten in Chapter 8),[168] although there is scant evidence, large hands apart, that he exhibited signs of that condition. Undoubtedly he was tall, about six foot three, as well as thin, but so was Osama Bin Laden, and as yet there is no claim that he had Marfan's syndrome. My scepticism was advanced by Tony Palmer's film *The Harvest of Sorrows*, in which we see Rachmaninov's many outdoor activities, including tennis, as well as his habit of not wearing glasses away from his desk.[169] From this arose the clinical conclusion that his sight was not seriously diminished, that he lived until he was nearly seventy and that he did not have scoliosis and was unlikely to have had any of the heart complications of Marfan's syndrome. In fact some would say he was quite a striking man in a soulful way. Stravinsky described Rachmaninov as a six-and-a-half foot scowl.[170]

'"Vengeance is mine; I will repay," saith the Lord' (Romans 12). So enigmatically Rachmaninov inscribed his First Symphony, which had its premiere in March 1897 conducted by Glazunov, a much better symphonist than conductor. It is popularly believed that Glazunov had been drunk at the time. This was a fiasco, and received scathing criticism. César Cui, the least of the Mighty Handful, likened it to the Seven Plagues of Egypt.[171] Rachmaninov's somewhat melancholy disposition turned to depression and tortured self-doubt with composer's block. This was resolved by Dr Nikolai Dahl, a Muscovite neurologist and hypnotherapist.[172] The triumphant and grateful outcome was the Second Piano Concerto, dedicated to Dahl. The First Symphony is perhaps a more novel piece, not least because this virtuoso pianist was also such a fine symphonist and master of the orchestra. Anyone caught in the realisation of his tortured lack of self-confidence should listen again to the introduction to the last movement, which is so at odds with the perception of miserable Rachmaninov.

There are few more exultant and confident statements in all of classical music, although he himself wrote of lacking self-confidence as he came to dislike the First Symphony.[173] Nevertheless he said that, although the premiere had been a decisive influence on his later development, when he composed the First he had imagined there was nothing he could not do.[174] In the account he gave of this travesty to the conductor Riesemann, Rachmaninov did not incriminate Glazunov's refreshment. That arose years later from Mrs Rachmaninov.[175] He ignored the First Symphony after its premiere, and even considered destroying it.[176] The enigma is not public disfavour, or critical people such as Rimsky-Korsakov, but his own rejection of it.

By the first decade of the twentieth century Rachmaninov was successful at composition, conducting and the piano, so much so that by 1913 he was exhausted and downcast. He and his wife returned to her beloved estate, Ivanovka,[177] where he could spend time with horses and motor cars. Despite the Rachmaninovs' work for the war effort, the peasants turned them out of Ivanovka, subsequently setting fire to it in 1917. The family escaped to Europe and later set up home in both France and the USA, where they tried to re-create Ivanovka with Russian food, drink, servants and customs, even Russian doctors, and of course they conversed in their native tongue.[178] In his panorama of Russian culture, *Natasha's Dance*, Orlando Figes quotes Rachmaninov as having said in 1941: 'I am a Russian composer and the land of my birth has influenced my temperament and outlook, and music is a product of the temperament.' Elsewhere he had said, 'When I left Russia I left behind the desire to compose: losing my country I lost myself also';[179] this theme was possibly later echoed in the *Symphonic Dances* (1940), but even more by most of his greatest compositions from the time before he left Russia. This melancholy has perhaps been over-resolved into a diagnosis of clinical depression. That intermittently he became miserable throughout his life seems incontestable, but easily overstated. Surely his music was often a plangent lament, or just a yearning for a Russia which, after the first revolution of 1905, started to vanish whilst remaining memorably vivid after that of 1917. However melancholic that may be, it is an emotion quite distinct from clinical depression. The former may evoke creativity; the latter, almost by definition, physically subdues it.

Rachmaninov had told his doctor, Alexander Golitsyn, that his 1942–43 concert tour season would be his last.[180] Despite having felt fatigue and complaining of arthritis, as well as being diagnosed with pleurisy and ominously losing weight, he went ahead with a concert on 17 February 1943 in Knoxville, Tennessee. It was his last, and ended with Chopin's Funeral March. There followed a lengthy train journey back to Los Angeles.[181] By then he felt very unwell, had coughed up blood (haemoptysis) and was scared.[182] Geoffrey Norris describes his rapid death as being due to a 'rare and virulent form of cancer'.[183] This was almost certainly due to secondary deposits in the lungs (metastases) from skin cancer. These were seen on X-ray, and the diagnosis of malignant melanoma was confirmed with a biopsy.[184] Incongruously, he was laid to rest in Valhalla, New York, a thousand leagues from the Russianness of Ivanovka. So passed 'the last of the Romantics in the modern age'.[185]

✢ BÉLA BARTÓK ✢
(1881–1945)

It's not enough to be Hungarian, you must have talent too
attributed to Sir Alexander Korda

Bartók was probably stronger of mind than of physique, being a small, rather pale man. He remained fiercely proud and steeped in his native Hungary and its traditions, especially those of country folk. As a child he had an unpleasant rash, which caused him to hide during his first few years.[186] Griffiths believes it could have been the result of an inoculation for smallpox,[187] which is unlikely. In 1899 he fell ill, coughing up blood; he took months to recover,[188] the probable diagnosis being TB. In 1900, shortly before his first major public recital, he was ill again with a fever which was diagnosed as pneumonia,[189] but it may have been related to his earlier suspected TB. He convalesced successfully at Merano in the Italian Tyrol, regaining twenty-two pounds in weight.[190] Regarding the circumstantial evidence for a weak constitution, it is probably reasonable to say that his travels tracing and recording folk music from Rumania to Algeria seem more in keeping with T. E. Lawrence than with those of a frail invalid.

Bartók was an ascetic man, notwithstanding his marrying a sixteen-year-old student, Márta Ziegler, which he did privately in 1909, during an interval in her music lesson and after composing 'Portrait of a Girl' for her when she was fifteen.[191] Before marrying Márta, he had become intimate in 1907 with a violinist, Stefi Geyer, who later rejected him. It seems that his final break from Stefi, who possibly inspired his First Violin Concerto, was due at least in part to his new-found atheism, although later he joined the Unitarian Church in America. He had written to Stefi, 'I have a sad misgiving that I shall never find any consolation in life save in music.'[192] His friend and fellow composer Zoltán Kodály said that Stefi's rejection had brought him to the verge of non-existence,[193] which surely implies thoughts of suicide. Miserable in rejection, he wrote the Opus 7 First String Quartet and then fourteen bagatelles, in the thirteenth of which the so-called Stefi theme, 'Elle est morte', is quoted.[194] The *Four Dirges* and *Three Burlesques* of 1908–11 are mournful. Griffiths opines that they represent Bartók's negative side,[195] although they are perhaps tinged with irony, a quality to recur, most famously with the send-up (raspberries and all) of Shostakovich's 'Leningrad' Symphony in his own late *Concerto for*

Orchestra. We go even further into Bartók's psyche by finding that even Webern thought the Third and Fourth String Quartets 'too harsh'.[196] This frugal aridity was more likely to have derived from his musical personality than from any serious mental affliction.

In 1914, like Ravel, he was rejected for army service, being underweight.[197] During the following year he thought of emigrating, developed a creative block and again contemplated suicide. He was then apparently cheered up by a fifteen-year-old girl, Klára Gombossy.[198] Bartók's relations with teenage girls are inconsistent in his psychological make-up, which was otherwise so ascetic, although as a teacher he was said to be kind, patient and gentle. Chalmers judges that his first child-bride Márta was the mature, sunny and probably practical partner. Bartók was attracted to childlike women, becoming childlike himself with them. When he was a child his father had died, but his loving mother moved out only when Márta moved in, and possibly that seamlessness explains the incongruous persistence of the playroom. So how incongruous that the one-act pantomime *The Miraculous Mandarin* (1918–19) followed with desultory scenarios in dismal garrets, with poverty, prostitution and attempted murder. In 1922 Bartók and Márta divorced, and within months he succumbed again to youthful charms when he married another teenage student, Ditta Pásztory,[199] with whom he spent the rest of his life and whom he loved and cared for, as she did him. His mother died in late 1939, although Bartók was too upset to attend her funeral, and this seems to have cut his last real tie with Hungary. He appears to have always been a tortured and probably self-engrossed soul, saying now that he 'drowned himself in his work'.[200] By the early 1930s he was increasingly at odds with the musical establishment in Budapest. As fascism infected Europe he was fervently against the government. The cultural stupidity of the fascists is revealed by their condemnation of him, of all people, as being insufficiently nationalistic.[201]

With his physical health Bartók's story takes us to the USA. In October 1940 Béla and Ditta Bartók gave their last concert in Budapest. He played Bach and she Mozart. Then they played the Mozart Double Piano Concerto together before leaving for America.[202] Their son Péter joined his parents in 1942 and then entered the US Navy. Typically, Americans were kind and welcoming. Benny Goodman had commissioned a short rhapsody for piano, violin and clarinet in 1938 and got *Contrasts*, a longer piece.[203] But in the early 1940s Bartók completed almost nothing. He had a research job on a renewable contract at Columbia University and one later at Harvard. He even described himself as 'an ex-composer'. Periarthritis of his shoulders had been diagnosed as early as the summer of 1940, continuing in

America. For a time he could not raise his right arm. Despite its initial warmth and generosity, Bartók did not embrace America, and it started to lose interest in a man who associated almost exclusively with other Hungarians and was a rather grey figure, sometimes rude and graceless and often complaining. During a period of some success there he pronounced a fervent wish to return home to Hungary, for ever.[204]

By 1942 Bartók was tiring more, looking thin and gaunt, and had an undiagnosed fever.[205] He was depressed by world events. There were periods in excess of twenty-one days of unrelieved gloom, even despair, and cessation of composition, satisfying a textbook diagnosis of clinical depression. His Sonata for two pianos and percussion had been orchestrated; he and Ditta were the soloists at its premiere with the New York Philharmonic Orchestra under Reiner in January 1943. It was his last public performance.[206] After giving lectures at Harvard during the spring of 1943 he was clearly very unwell, and initially TB was suspected.[207] Money was short, and discreetly those two conducting giants, Serge Koussevitzky and Fritz Reiner, enabled commissions and engagements to come his way. Koussevitzky commissioned his late masterpiece, the *Concerto for Orchestra*; Bartók composed this during his first summer at Saranac Lake, in a convalescent home supported by ASCAP,* which paid for his medical treatment.[208] Whilst convalescing in the winter of 1943–44 at Asheville in North Carolina, he became energetic enough to walk in the mountains as his weight increased from eighty-seven pounds to a 'stout 7½ stone'.[209] There Bartók wrote the Sonata for solo violin for Yehudi Menuhin, which was to be his last completed work. It was well received by the public, but not by the critics.

In 1943 he was said to have polycythaemia, a pathological excess of red blood cells. In 1944 the diagnosis was at last clarified by Dr Israel Rappaport, a Hungarian. By now there were too many white cells, and that is leukaemia,[210] for which little useful treatment existed in 1944, although radiotherapy was given to his enlarged spleen.[211]

In March 1945 pneumonia was treated by the new miracle – antibiotics.[212] He worked on, completing his Third Piano Concerto five days before his death.[213] This was for Ditta to play after he had gone,[214] as financially he worried for her future. His Viola Concerto for William Primrose was also incomplete and probably still in his briefcase when he returned to New York in late August 1945 from his third and last summer retreat at Saranac Lake, where he had started composing again after a break of

* The American Society of Composers, Authors and Publishers.

one year. He rapidly deteriorated and on 22 September was admitted to the West Side Hospital, where he died on the 26 with Ditta and Péter each holding one hand.[215] Bartók had marked the second movement of the Third Concerto 'Adagio religioso'. Many years later he and Ditta were together laid to rest in Budapest, back in the country he had so ardently loved, upheld but left.

Postscript: Leukaemia Today

Much has changed since Bartók wasted away in 1945. Leukaemia in simplistic terms is cancer of the system producing white blood cells, and it arises either at the production sites in bone marrow (myeloid leukaemia) or in the lymphatic tissue, such as the spleen (lymphoblastic leukaemia). These may develop acutely or as chronic conditions. In such cases tiredness, vague ill health, sweating and fever are all well recognised. This accords well with Bartók's case history. Myeloid leukaemia shares a heritage with polycythaemia (PRV), wherewith it is the red blood cell lineage which overproduces. That is a condition with lassitude but also pruritus (itching), to which Bartók was prone. One thing against PRV with Bartók is that patients usually look plethoric, not pale and anaemic as he did. However, the key point is that PRV, Bartók's initial diagnosis, can spontaneously convert years later to myeloid leukaemia (his second diagnosis).

Today wonderful things can be done for leukaemia, although some are hugely demanding for the patients. Sadly none of this was available in 1945, so Bartók's condition was incurable. Progress came in the next decade, as we will see with Gerald Finzi.

✣ GERALD FINZI ✣
(1901–1956)

Like the sweet apple which reddens upon the topmost bough
        Dante Gabriel Rossetti, 'Beauty: A Combination from Sappho'

How different Bartók and Finzi first seem. Nevertheless, between these two approximate contemporaries there are unexpected similarities. Both felt for their native lands and country people. They seemingly made satisfactory marriages, particularly Finzi. Neither had lavish tastes. Bartók loved ethnic Hungarian furniture as Finzi did English apples, and both feared for the extinction of old ways. Their music echoes the traditions of their respective countries, as both composers went their own ways. Their musical origins were often with folk music. Finzi was very resistant to being classed as a 'pastoral composer'. Lastly, in middle age both were sick men.

Like Bartók, Finzi experienced sickness early in life. In 1913 he had been put in quarantine for a childhood infection at the school, which he hated so much that he feigned fainting fits and was taken to Switzerland.[216] This thespian device succeeded in his being taken away from school altogether. Then Finzi's acquaintance with sickness worsened. His father had half of his face removed for a cancerous growth, and three of his four siblings died.[217] He was especially moved by the death at the end of the Great War of his favourite brother, Edgar. He became and remained a conscientious objector, as well as being a serious, idealistic young man, both rural and intellectual in his outlook. In 1928 his TB of the lung was agreeably nursed back to robust health by good food and country air. The diagnosis seems to have been changed to pleurisy late in the treatment,[218] although the two are not mutually exclusive. Like Bartók, Finzi hated traffic noise, and he disliked smoke, which caused him to complain to the landlady of his cottage at Crowborough, where the chimney smoked. She wisely sent her daughter Joy to appease him. Such diplomacy resulted two years later in Gerald and Joy marrying.[219]

As the Second World War approached Finzi completed *Dies natalis* and then joined the Home Guard before being ordered in July 1941 to a desk job in London, which he loathed.[220] He was anti-authority, be it in public schools or with the forces. That said, the war was confusing for him; his origins were both Italian and Jewish. In 1943 he collapsed and was sent home for a month, his wife declaring him to be physically, mentally and spiritually drained.[221] McVeagh suspects that he was for a time clinically depressed;[222] if so, his depression was reactive and not bipolar. Weekends down in the country from London left insufficient time in which to settle down to compose, but he remained physically, as well as mentally, weary.

After the war he became more weary, lacking his usual vigour for dale, mountain or garden. The diagnosis of non-Hodgkin's lymphoma was on the basis of a lymph node biopsy and microscopic examination of his bone marrow in 1946, when he noticed a lump in his neck.[223] Non-Hodgkin's lymphoma can be slow in its development. It is a form of cancer of the lymph nodes and pathologically a neighbour of Bartók's final illness. As a family the Finzis accepted this in a quiet, business-like manner.[224] In 1950 Finzi set to music Wordsworth's 'Intimations of Immortality', with its vision of a lost past childhood. Finzi and his consultant, Professor Witts in Oxford, were pleased with his response to treatment,[225] although it is interesting that he revised *Eclogue* when he started with radiotherapy. He went on to compose the Cello Concerto, the *Grand Fantasia and Toccata* and *In terra pax*, based on a poem by Robert Bridges. This latter may have been a response to clinical improvement, although he completed it whilst undergoing radiotherapy, when the nurses had been amazed at his remaining immersed in his work, sitting on his bed and working for as long as ten hours. Whether and when he underwent radiotherapy or chemotherapy depended on how robust his blood cell counts were. Despite these health problems, life at home and composition continued normally.

In 1954 the singer John Carol Case had asked him to compose a work for baritone, *Dies natalis*. He replied enigmatically with a sweet smile, 'I'm afraid there isn't time.'[226] He was already working on the Cello Concerto, which was premiered on 19 July 1955 at the Cheltenham Festival. However, his comment may reveal an insight into his own all too frail mortality. In January 1955 he deteriorated, and Witts advised urgent removal of his spleen (splenectomy).[227] Finzi pleaded for delay; he was probably at the height of his powers and said he had much still to do. Following the surgery at the end of January, he was back working at home within a month. Quickly he returned to writing, composing and lecturing as well as having more radiotherapy. During the summer of 1956 he was well enough to enjoy the Three Choirs Festival accompanied by his friends Howard Ferguson and Ralph and Ursula Vaughan Williams.

In September 1956, Finzi took Vaughan Williams to the village at Chosen Hill, where they could see the church and hear its bells, an inspiration for *In terra pax*. There the sexton's child, whom he liked, had chickenpox and Finzi went to see him.[228] Shortly thereafter Finzi developed chest pains and a rash, which was taken at the time to be shingles.[229] It possibly was. Joy has left us a loving but businesslike account of Gerald's last two weeks. He became feverish and developed a severe headache as well as becoming confused and then apathetic. He was admitted to the Radcliffe Infirmary in Oxford, where he developed convulsions, quickly relapsing into a coma. He died of encephalitis or meningoencephalitis,[230] which is inflammation of the brain and its surrounding membranes (meninges). His wife said that so great had his sufferings become that it was a mercy his sufferings were over.[231] He was privately cremated on 2 October 1956.

He may not have contracted chickenpox as a child and so may not have acquired immunity to subsequent and similar infections from the chickenpox virus, which in adults can cause shingles and rarely the much more serious condition from which he died. Furthermore, his immunity would have been suppressed by his treatment for lymphoma. Had Finzi not taken Vaughan Williams to Chosen Hill, then on a balance of probabilities he would not have died then. It is particularly sad to contemplate a photograph of him, taken only a fortnight before he died; he looked very well, but he would always have remained vulnerable. Finzi seems to have died as he lived, as a man whose life and works expressed an intense bond with the traditional countryside of his birth and embrace. He was not a selfish man and was one who soldiered on with dignified determination. Many of his best-known and best-loved works were composed as the Sword of Damocles hovered above him.

Jules Massenet (1842–1912)

Like Rossini, Massenet was perhaps a great composer of operas, rather than a composer of great operas. According to well-researched biography,[232] until near the end of his life his issues with health were largely trivial, although he may have survived cholera during the 1866 epidemic in Paris.[233] He was prone to sore throats, bronchitis and 'rheumatism', which sometimes produced 'sick notes' enabling him to avoid functions he had no wish to attend, including Verdi's funeral.[234] After the success of *Manon* in 1884, he composed another twenty operas over the remaining twenty-eight years, as well as ballet and incidental music.

In 1910 by his own accounts his health was conspicuously failing as he visibly aged and tired. In the spring he consulted his doctor in Paris and was told he was very sick. In August of that year he went into hospital under a pseudonym. The operation was abdominal and for 'cancer'.[235] He was in hospital for two weeks, and peritonitis was said to have been averted.[236] Within two or three weeks he was eating and sleeping well. On 15 September he was well enough to give a funeral oration, although by New Year 1911 he was ill in bed once more.[237] A year later he wrote that he had 'a passing malady to be sure, but a cruel one'.[238] But he perked up and went off to Monte Carlo for the premiere of his opera *Roma*. His two final operas were given after his death; he finished *Cléopâtre* in May.[239] His last illness recorded by his friend the architect Raymond de Rigné was one of a gentle passing of a largely gentle man on 13 August 1912.[240] Nevertheless, he allegedly had to be rushed home from the hospital with Marguerite Long pretending to give him oxygen,[241] when by conventional clinical criteria he was probably already dead. He had expressly wished to die at home with his family. It had been a long illness, at the end of which the nurse stopped him trying to compose a new opera, although it was only in his declining last few months that he took to writing the written word, the last work, entitled 'Pensées posthumes', a month before he died.[242]

Exactly what he died of remains unclear. Sparse information makes abdominal cancer the broad and obvious diagnosis, beyond which we can only speculate. The recorded avoidance of peritonitis suggests that he may well have had a large bowel obstruction dealt with before it could burst to cause peritonitis. This makes carcinoma of the rectum or colon probable. His death was consistent with his life, for it was gentle, with people he loved, and just a little operatic.

Chapter 11

The Ultimate Blow:
Deafness

Silence is argument carried on by other means
Che Guevara

Introduction

THE COMPOSER AS HERO is possibly epitomised by those who
became deaf. It seems the supreme injustice. Many ask how musicians can compose when they cannot hear the result of their labours.
Beethoven showed that they can. He said, when seriously deaf, that of all
his activities composition was the easiest, and social interaction the most
difficult.[1] Martin Cooper has talked of Beethoven's 'inner life of almost
unparalleled reality and intensity, unsullied by unwelcome noise and thus
distraction, whereby the process of cerebral composition may be actually
enhanced'.[2] But one wonders. Beneath one of the Cumbrian mountains
is a memorial to a young man who, after amputation of a leg, scaled it on
crutches. Perhaps deaf composition is like that.

Fig. 7 outlines the basic anatomy and mechanism of hearing. Sound
waves enter the external meatus having been magnified by the outer ear
(pinna), which acts like a megaphone in reverse. On reaching the tympanic membrane the sound waves resonate and are transmitted across the
middle ear by three small bones (ossicles) known as malleus, incus and
stapes. The stirrup-shaped stapes is attached to a second membrane which
then transmits sound to a complex organ, the cochlea, which resembles
a baby octopus. Within this marvel of creation are tiny hairs which convert sound waves into impulses, which are electrically transmitted to the
hearing centres of the brain via the acoustic (or auditory) nerve, and so we
behold the miracle of hearing.

Deafness is either conductive, usually due to wax in the outer ear or disease in the middle ear, or sensorineural, that is, due to disease with the cochlea and/or the acoustic nerve. There are mixed patterns too. Smetana's deafness was due to syphilitic destruction of that nerve and therefore entirely sensorineural. It was typically syphilitic, with fairly sudden onset and progression to total deafness within a few months. Secondly, presby-acusis is the typical and usually inevitable cochlea sensorineural deafness of old age,[3] which affected Ralph Vaughan Williams and possibly Ethel Smyth.

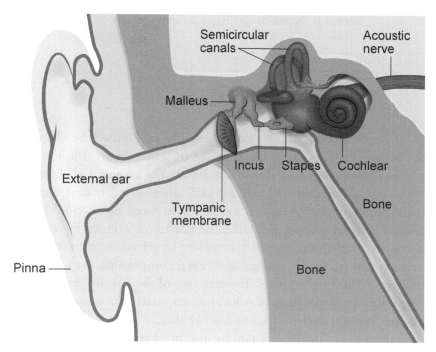

Fig. 7 Diagram of the Ear

✢ LUDWIG VAN BEETHOVEN ✢
(1770–1827)

That jealous demon, my wretched health
Ludwig van Beethoven, 1801

The greatness of Beethoven, like that of his music, was recognised during his lifetime. At his funeral the poet Grillparzer said, 'He was an artist, and who shall arise to stand beside him?'[4] His strengths were so admirable, his weaknesses so very human, that many people claim an empathy with Beethoven. Little of this may be understood without interleaving his medical history with his life history.

Firstly, sources must be declared. An early account is that by Anton Schindler, who at various times was Beethoven's assistant and secretary. He gets a mixed press and has been held responsible for destroying 264 of the approximately 400 conversation books which, by 1818, Beethoven used as a regular aid for conversation.[5] Barry Cooper disputes the destruction of 264,[6] although he describes Schindler as 'a scoundrel' who fabricated false entries in the conversation books.[7] Schindler probably had his own agenda, not least to retain favour, believing himself to be a standard-bearer for Beethoven's good reputation. Perhaps the best summary is that of Elliot Forbes, who said that Schindler himself provided the smoke that has led people to suspect a fire.[8]

Edward Larkin offered another explanation. In 1830 Schindler, with Dr Bertolini, who had been one of Beethoven's medical attendants, burned conversation books and letters because Beethoven had been notoriously outspoken in relation to politics,[9] particularly after Metternich's settlement of 1815, with which Austria became tantamount to a police state. Beethoven had spoken of the 'utter moral rottenness of the Austrian State' and advocated absolute personal freedom.[10] Meanwhile, 137 conversation books repose today in a Berlin museum. They consist of what the other people said, but not Beethoven's responses, as he still spoke, which weakens the political editorship theory.

An early biography is that by his friends Franz Wegeler and Ferdinand Ries; a recent one is that by Swafford. Beethoven's correspondence has been categorised by Emily Anderson, Kalischer and Hamburger. A classic baseline biography is that of Thayer, edited in English by Forbes. A recently published important medical account of Beethoven is that by the psychiatrist Mai, whose strength, nevertheless, is with Beethoven's history and the psychology of creativity, and less in analysing and summarising all of the enormous medical literature relating to him, admittedly no easy task. The most vital single piece of medical evidence is the autopsy report, originally in Latin, written by Professor J. Wagner in 1827.[11]

The Beginning

Sickness was a theme with variations from Beethoven's very beginning. His father, whom he despised, became an alcoholic, whereas his beloved mother died young of TB. There was a litany of infant mortality amongst Beethoven's siblings, only two seemingly disliked brothers surviving into adulthood. In 1790 Emperor Joseph died, inspiring Beethoven to compose what is possibly his first mature work, *Cantata on the Death of Emperor Joseph II*. By his late teens Beethoven was a brilliant organist and pianist. He impressed Joseph Haydn, who gave him lessons and was importunate on his behalf. Beethoven succeeded in falling out with him, as he did with most people at some stage. He could be rough, gruff, sullen and even ungrateful to his long-suffering friends, just as he could be warm, funny, kind and humane. This underlines the long-standing loyalty of old friends such as Dr Wegeler, Ries, the lawyer Stephan von Breuning, Count Waldstein and Archduke Rudolf, testifying to the essential greatness of his soul, despite the moods and tantrums. Many acknowledged his fervent goodwill and basic decency. It is also relevant that he seems to have upheld a high moral code and been something of a prude. His friend Friedrich Wähner said of him, 'Just as he withstood like a man the temptations of wine, so he seems never to have been seduced by the power of love.'[12]

Those disposed to pathologise the great have occasionally gone to town on Beethoven. Ernest Newman described him as a drunkard, a syphilitic and ruthless.[13] Even the more recent and more restrained Martin Cooper said in 1971 that Beethoven did 'indeed suffer at some time from venereal disease'.[14] For that there is no sound evidence. Larkin, who presented a good chronology of Beethoven's illnesses, quoted Rau, a banker, who remarked to Beethoven's disciple Moscheles about this 'venerated, highly acclaimed man', 'the noblest, kindest-hearted human being'.[15]

Early Intimations of Illness

From the age of seventeen Beethoven complained of abdominal symptoms including painful colic with both diarrhoea and constipation.[16] Whilst still in Bonn, the town of his birth, he received various treatments from Dr Wegeler for this. He was also said to be chesty.[17] Recounting his abdominal symptoms from adolescence, Kubba and Young suggest that Beethoven may have contracted typhoid or 'typhus' in 1796 or 1797.[18] Thayer attributed this diagnosis to Dr Aloys Weissenbach, a Salzburg surgeon.[19] Beethoven himself suggested that typhus was a possible trigger for his deafness and was unwittingly ahead of his time in accounting for all his disparate ailments with one diagnosis.[20] The terms 'typhoid' and 'typhus' were synonymous then as 'typhus' was a term generic to many gastrointestinal complaints (see Schubert in Chapter 4). Typhoid only very rarely results in deafness. Today, we never make two diagnoses where one would do. This 'typhus' story comes from his having had a sweaty fever with bowel complaints shortly before the first early intimations of deafness. Before he left Bonn for Vienna, his intestinal symptoms quickly worsened, but still he soldiered on. As Beethoven passed from the eighteenth into the early nineteenth century with the 'Pathétique' Sonata, he had already produced the First Symphony, with the Second quickly following. The first two piano concertos were followed by the third in 1803, and the six Opus 18 String Quartets already marked him as a man apart, taking novel directions into the new century. But by then other clouds were gathering. He wrote to Wegeler in June 1801 of increasing deafness over the past three years.[21]

Early Deafness

It is generally accepted that before the end of the eighteenth century Beethoven had become increasingly aware of problems with his hearing and, for several years, had been able, professionally and socially, to conceal the problem.[22] He may have deliberately used his notorious absent-minded and eccentric behaviour as a smoke screen for his own awful realisation. In the Heiligenstadt Testament of October 1802, he said his deafness had started six years previously.[23] This document has been widely suspected of being a forewarning of suicide. Barry Cooper believes it to have been the exact opposite, namely a rejection of suicide. He points to *Christus am Oelberge*, written shortly after Heiligenstadt, which deals explicitly with extreme and undeserved suffering in the belief that sufferers can take comfort from that of others.[24] In two letters of June and November 1801 to his friend and doctor Franz Wegeler, Beethoven wrote about his wretched health, saying that for the last three years his hearing had become weaker.[25] He was just as bothered by the unpleasant buzzing, humming and ringing in his ears (tinnitus) as he was by deafness.[26] In 1801 he complained that his ears 'whistled and buzzed continually, day and night'.[27]

The consequences of Beethoven's maladies extended beyond music. He had long been anxious to marry, and friends implied that he seemed to be passionately in love with one lady or another most of the time. That probably affectionate observation has been turned subsequently into spurious evidence for promiscuity and thus the inevitability of his being syphilitic,[28] as we will shortly see. Wegeler remarked that Beethoven was 'never not in love' and that 'He had always been above the frailties of the flesh.'[29] In 1801 he fell in love with a pupil, Countess Giulietta Guicciardi, who was 'not of his class'. Thayer believed that she was not indifferent to Beethoven, but that her father had objected to one who was of insufficient rank and increasingly deaf. Beethoven ended this episode by dedicating his 'Moonlight' Sonata to Giulietta.[30] A bachelor existence may have been his choice anyway.[31]

Meanwhile, various doctors recommended diverse remedies. Generally worthless, they are too numerous to describe, but perhaps Beethoven's reference to 'bumbling doctors and medical asses'[32] was justified when we consider one example. In a letter to Wegeler, quoted in full by Mai, Beethoven described how an army surgeon, Dr Vering, bandaged the bark of a poisonous tree shrub, *Daphne mezereum*, soaked in water, to his arms. As the bark dried it shrank, causing blistering. The blisters were then lanced to release the deafness! The result was painful arms and an inability to play the piano.[33]

Better advice came from Dr Johann Schmidt, who advised him to leave the dust, dirt and noise of Vienna to compose music in the countryside.[34] So we come in 1802 to the spa village of Heiligenstadt, where he rented a cottage and in the autumn wrote the Heiligenstadt Testament, in which he explained his social withdrawal because of increasing deafness, emphasising its calamity in a musician.[35] He admitted that he had contemplated suicide and then vowed against it, saying that only his art had restrained him, with a trust in God and love of his fellow men. He clearly meant to carry on, and here we see the odd combination of sadness and defiance to be heard in some of his music. Barry Cooper regards his compositions from this time to have been quite up-beat, citing the Violin Sonatas Opus

30 and the Piano Sonatas Opus 31 as well as the two sets of variations Opus 35. He immersed himself in work as a frequent antidote to misery.[36] It is also consonant with one of this book's major themes, for we encounter a composer defying enormous odds and continuing in spite of everything laid against him. The oddity is that, despite his close friendship with the lawyer Stefan von Breuning, Beethoven put the Heiligenstadt Testament away in a drawer, where it was found soon after his death. It may be that its main function was catharsis as he put events behind him. His return from Heiligenstadt became a new beginning.[37] Dramatic changes in style followed, as encountered in the 'Eroica' Symphony, despite the continuing deterioration of his hearing. Arising triumphantly once more in Vienna, early in 1803 he became composer in residence at the Theater an der Wien and premiered the Third Piano Concerto, which, along with the First and Second Symphonies and *Christus am Oelberge*, became the programme for his second benefit concert.

During the summer of 1805 Beethoven committed to paper his undying love for Josephine Deym (née Brunsvik),[38] as well as first drafts of his opera *Leonore*, initially a failure in November 1805 and later revised to become *Fidelio*. During 1806 amongst female rejections, increasing deafness and money worries, he composed the Fourth Piano Concerto, the Fourth Symphony, the Violin Concerto and the 'Razumovsky' Quartets, all resurgent pieces. As he was under great physical and mental strain, his generous patron Prince Lichnowsky took him to his castle at Grätz,[39] where a dinner party was given in October. Guests bade Beethoven to play for them. Offended, he flew into a temper, leaving Grätz that night. During his journey back to Vienna during a violent storm, Beethoven caught a chill, which traditionally is said to have worsened his deafness, a claim which Robbins Landon infers is exaggerated.[40] On his return he composed the mighty Fifth Symphony, which was probably the last he substantially heard. In 1806 Beethoven's brother, Carl, married Johanna, much to Ludwig's anxious disapproval. She was already heavily pregnant and had served a prison sentence for theft.[41] It may be that, in terms of Beethoven's mental health, family feuds and personal conflicts evoked as much anguish and mental torment as did his failing own health and hearing.[42] He was fortunate in his staunch friends, above all the emperor's youngest brother, Archduke Rudolf, who rescued the composer to some extent from the disorder into which his life had sunk. Rudolf was discreetly generous with both patronage and money.

Back in the peace and quiet of Heiligenstadt during the summer of 1807 Beethoven composed the Mass in C and probably worked on the

'Pastoral' (Sixth) Symphony, which he had started in 1803 and did not complete until 1808.[43] Throughout the first two decades of the nineteenth century other disorders of health prevailed. During 1807 a finger abscess developed, for which even amputation was considered.[44] Fortunately, lancing it was sufficient. Further abscesses affected the jaw and a foot.[45] Such repeated infections suggest reduced immunity, which might have been due to any one of several disorders. He also continued to be afflicted by chest complaints.[46]

Late Deafness

On 22 December 1808 there was the famous concert whose programme was the Fifth and Sixth Symphonies, parts of the Mass in C, the Fourth Piano Concerto and the Choral Fantasia, all in an unheated hall.[47] By now Beethoven was seriously hard of hearing but not totally deaf, and as recorded by Carl Czerny he immediately spotted an orchestral mistake during the Fantasia.[48] From the conditions into which he had relapsed Beethoven arose once again even more triumphantly, with the Fifth Piano Concerto ('Emperor') in 1809. A year later he fell in love with Therese Malfatti, by whom (or by whose family) he was rejected, despite her smartening up his often dishevelled appearance. One suspects that she was the recipient of *Für Elise*, for Elise was her nickname.[49] That year he declared: 'Had I not read somewhere that a man ought not of his own free will to take away his life so long as he could still perform a good action, I should long ago have been dead, by my own hand.'[50] He was still giving recitals, whilst increasingly withdrawing from society.

When Beethoven met Goethe at the spa of Teplitz in 1812,[51] the courtly poet and the gruff composer were possibly antipathetic to one another despite their daily walks; Goethe is said to have found him 'unruly', later describing Beethoven's Fifth Symphony to Mendelssohn as 'mad'[52] and saying that Beethoven could hear nothing. Conversely, Carl Czerny said he could sustain conversation by shouting loudly, whilst noticing that Beethoven's piano was out of tune.[53] Once more world affairs affected him as he celebrated Bonaparte's loss at the battles of Leipzig and then Vitoria in 1813. The musically controversial *Battle Symphony* was born, and he insisted upon conducting the premiere himself. Louis Spohr described his wild antics whilst conducting, intermittently losing the orchestra.[54] Spohr noticed that Beethoven could not hear pianissimo but found his way again when forte returned. Dr Karl von Bursy visited Beethoven in June

1816, attesting that conversation was very difficult but not impossible.[55] Wegeler, Ries and Andreas Wawruch all commented on the variability of Beethoven's hearing.[56] Despite everything, the composer still commented upon the pianistic skills of his few remaining pupils, and even tried to converse in Italian.

In November 1815 his brother Carl was clearly dying of consumption, and Beethoven pursued a nearly five-year bitter legal battle with his sister-in-law, Johanna, for custody of his nephew Karl, whose affection Beethoven had stifled with a heavy hand, pursuant to Karl's ultimate adoption as his ersatz son. During this period he also had difficulty with a chronic chest infection, saying he had been unwell for some time.[57] His conduct throughout did not show Beethoven as kind, gentle or humane, but just as driven, although when, temporarily, the court returned Karl to his mother, Beethoven was distraught. Not until 8 April 1820 was this judgement reversed on appeal.[58] Musically it is interesting that, for some of this three-to-four-year period, there was a reduction in composition, as personal affairs substantially cast him down. Bower suggests that during the approximate period 1815–20 Beethoven may have suffered what he had previously described as a transient psychosis,[59] similar to Ellenberger's later description of creative illness,[60] a condition precipitated by overwhelming stress with psychotic behaviour following. The patient may become obsessed by a prevailing idea for three to four years. Thereafter functional recovery is complete, which Ellenberger claimed may then be to an even higher level. In his treatise *Art and Scientific Thought* Johnson commented on the highly sophisticated and mature musical thought inherent in Beethoven's late works.[61] Systemic illness and deafness seem to have been less inhibiting to his powers of composition than this psychological disturbance provoked by family issues. However, Barry Cooper points to an 'inflammatory fever' in October 1816, which he reasonably speculates may have caused a post-viral weakness syndrome.[62]

Beethoven was greatly cheered when Broadwood sent him a new grand piano in 1818, although he had last performed publicly in May 1814, playing the 'Archduke' Trio.[63] There are nevertheless accounts of him extemporising at the piano for friends as late as 1826.[64] By 1818 he had relinquished the unequal struggle in verbal discourse, which was when conversation books appeared. In 1821 Beethoven was struck down by a severe febrile illness again, this time including jaundice;[65] this was possibly due to infective hepatitis, a harbinger of more mortal illness to come. He also spoke of a 'violent attack of rheumatism'; the two were possibly the same. In 1823 Schultz said the deafness was not as bad as he had expected and that accounts of it had been exaggerated,[66] whereas Carl Maria von Weber declared that everything had to be written down for him.[67] Sadly, neither visit is corroborated by the remaining conversation books. During 1823 Beethoven had prolonged painful inflammation of an eye, assumed to be iritis.[68] There then followed from this tormented but resilient soul the *Missa solemnis* and 'Choral' Symphony, premiered in the spring of 1824. This was when the singer Caroline Unger prompted Beethoven to face the audience's applause.[69] It was his pupil Czerny who recorded Beethoven at that time as having some residual hearing, albeit with an ear trumpet.[70] It is also interesting that the young Gerhard von Breuning suggested that Beethoven as late as 1825 could converse without recourse to the conversation books.[71]

Final Sickness

Illness persisted, probably interrupting composition, although the innovative Opus 127 String Quartet, started in 1824, was first performed in 1825. Sketches for a Tenth Symphony originate from this period and even go back to 1822.[72] By the spring of 1825 Beethoven was very ill again with his usual gastrointestinal problems, now accompanied by coughing up blood and nose bleeds.[73] We should not accept uncritically this complaint of haemoptysis as it may have been haematemesis, bleeding not from the lungs but from the stomach. It is possible to confuse the two, and haematemesis sits well with other medical details. Two string quartets, Opus 132 and Opus 130, followed and, whilst he was convalescing in Baden, his health improved. Barry Cooper refers to long, enjoyable walks in the hills and a cheerful dinner with ample champagne at this time.[74] On his sketch for the third movement of Opus 132 Beethoven wrote 'Hymn of thanks from a sick man to God on his recovery' and 'Feeling of new strength and reawakened feelings'.[75] Shortly after this, following a performance of Opus 132, he dined with Sir George Smart, who observed that 'He could still hear a little if one spoke into his left ear', as well as still being able to extemporise at the piano.[76]

In 1826 bowel problems were again accompanied by a prolonged iritis, apparently exacerbated by continuous problems with Karl, who in 1826 attempted suicide;[77] as to how seriously we may be sceptical. As Karl recuperated from his superficial gunshot wound and Ludwig from another relapse, rather strangely they went together to convalesce at Gneixendorf on the estate of Beethoven's brother Johann, now wealthy from having been a major medical supplier to Napoleon's army. It was at Gneixendorf that the legendary 'frightening the oxen' episode possibly occurred.[78] Several cows were disturbed by Beethoven's country walk, being enlivened with his eccentric behaviour including shouting, waving and muttering! Such behaviour was not unusual for the great man, even on the conductor's podium.

Beethoven stayed longer than planned and then disagreed with Johann, despite recorded signs of greater sickness having become evident. After a midnight row Beethoven, accompanied by Karl, departed for Vienna on an open cart, despite it being early December in foul weather. They had to stay overnight in a damp, dirty unheated inn.[79] Newly arrived in Vienna, Beethoven could hardly walk and was put to bed with a fever, thirst, chest pain and a hacking cough, a likely case of pneumonia.[80] With him he took the unfinished String Quintet in C, which was essentially his last composition.

Various doctors were called, some of them refusing to attend the man by whom they had previously been rudely dismissed. On 5 December 1826 Andreas Wawruch, Professor of Pathology at the Vienna General Hospital, attended, saying he was a great admirer of Beethoven. He recorded abdominal and chest pain, with difficulty breathing, gross swelling (oedema), ascites, jaundice and decreased urinary output.[81] Wawruch was joined in his attentions by Dr Malfatti, whose niece, Therese, Beethoven had courted before dismissing Malfatti himself ten years previously. On 2 January Karl left to join the army, and he never saw his uncle again.[82] Beethoven's condition then temporarily improved, probably because of several procedures undertaken by a surgeon to tap and drain huge quantities of ascitic fluid. One of the puncture wounds in the abdominal wall became and remained infected.[83] Reports vary as to the quantity of fluid drained,[84] but it was clearly in basins rather than cups. Both physicians recommended frozen punch, with ice applications to his abdomen.[85] Swafford believes that even then Beethoven may not have comprehended that his illness was terminal and describes his final completed composition, the F major String Quartet Opus 135, as full of humour, unlike some late quartets of Haydn and Mozart.[86] Nevertheless, in December 1826 Beethoven became intermittently depressed on realising finally that the end was nigh, although his spirits rose when a 42-volume set of Handel's works arrived.[87] There were episodes of gallows humour, none more so than when he announced his own death: 'Applaud friends, the comedy is over.' Shortly before he died he received the priest. On 24 March 1827 he relapsed into a coma. His last words are said to have been 'Pity, pity – too late', as he finally received some bottles of his favourite Mainz wine.[88] He died at 6p.m. on 26 March 1827 during a violent storm; the report of his raised clenched fist was possibly unsubstantiated,[89] but certainly cinematic. Clinically it is more likely that the ending, after many years of struggle, survival and triumph, passed more insidiously. Up to twenty thousand Viennese followed Beethoven's cortege.[90] To contemplate the last compositions, there is little evidence of the impending disaster and finale. Bower quotes musicologists of fame who attest to the greatness and illumination of the last works, especially the string quartets.[91] Heroic defiance was, until the end, a Beethovenian theme.

The Autopsy

The original autopsy report was lost for a time,[92] being later found in the Vienna Museum of Anatomical Pathology. The autopsy, undertaken by Dr J. Wagner, was a thorough examination for those times, apart from having no description of the bowels, gaseous distension apart. Exhumation and re-interment in 1863 and again in 1888, when Bruckner attended, have added nothing further, until a recent forensic analysis of his hair.[93] Intermittently, friends, as well as vicarious souvenir hunters, harvested locks of Beethoven's hair.[94]

The salient points were that his extremities were grossly wasted, although swollen with oedema, and there were multiple little skin bruises (petechiae).[95] His mastoid bones were large, but normal. The cap of his skull was 'of normal density', and Wagner measured its thickness as being about half the extent of the tip of his own thumb, here estimated as about 1.3cm. Frustratingly, the middle ear bones, which presumably were removed by Dr Wagner, have disappeared. The acoustic nerves were thinned, the left more than the right. The adjoining facial nerves were 'thickened', as were the accompanying arteries leading to the inner ear. The thorax (chest) was said to be normal. That implies that all was well with heart and lungs, which seems improbable. The abdominal cavity contained 'four measures' (perhaps four pints or litres) of rusty ascitic fluid. The liver was hard, nodular and reduced to half its normal size. The description was of macronodular, not micronodular, cirrhosis. This is no abstruse academic digression; it assists in refuting a Beethoven 'legend' regarding excessive alcohol intake. There was 'gravel' (small stones) in the gall bladder; 'calcareous deposits' (stones again) were also found in the kidneys, whose surrounding capsules were very thickened. The spleen was doubled in size and the pancreas, leathery in consistency, was also enlarged.

The Cause(s) of Death

The vast literature on this subject is of varied quality. Pathography can become an armchair pastime, unless the picture is obvious and/or there is sound documentation, as, by the standard of his time, there is quite often with Beethoven. The general principle of avoiding multiple diagnoses when various afflictions can be bound together in one or two disease processes seems sound.[96] Thus, from the outset, we may ask whether deafness was due to other illnesses evolving through much of Beethoven's life. Several such unifying diagnoses are now proposed. This section will conclude with reasons for rejecting or diminishing, on a balance of probabilities, alternatives given in the literature.

Cirrhosis of the Liver

The view accepted by many is that the basic cause of death was liver failure secondary to cirrhosis.[97] Schwarz has argued that whilst Beethoven had cirrhosis it was unlikely to have been the ultimate cause of death, in that such an end usually is accompanied by coma, known as hepatic encephalopathy.[98] Beethoven's ultimate cause of death was likely to have been bronchopneumonia, which probably overtook him before hepatic encephalopathy could. Pneumonia and cirrhosis are not mutually exclusive, and Beethoven had a long history of respiratory illness. He may have coughed up blood close to his end,[99] and he had complained to Dr Wawruch of breathlessness and chest pain.

A popular view has been that the most probable cause of his cirrhosis was alcoholism.[100] But this seems unlikely. It is well recorded that his favourite drinks were spring water and coffee.[101] Very late in his illness he used fortified wines and, close to death, iced punch, but on prescription, to alleviate his abdominal pain.[102] Neither is there any convincing evidence of this comfort drinking having been excessive. Such amelioration in a dying man is no basis for diagnosing alcoholism. Schindler, Wegeler and Ries said that Beethoven was temperate and that he hated drunkenness,[103] probably as a reaction to his alcoholic father, although Treitschke observed that Beethoven would ignore food and drink whilst inspired during composition.[104] Nevertheless, Beethoven wrote on 1 September 1825, 'I must also confess that the champagne got very much into my head yesterday and I had to learn again from experience that such things rather suppress than increase my efficacy'[105] – not the reflection of a typical alcoholic who cannot function without a drink first. Furthermore, the characteristic alcoholic cirrhotic liver is micronodular and not macronodular, as was clearly found with Beethoven. Mai, a recent diagnostician of Beethoven's alcohol dependence, says that Drs Malfatti, Braunhoffer and Staudenheim shared Dr Wawruch's views on Beethoven's drinking habits, which views are then left unclear.[106] However, Wawruch, like Ries, regarded Beethoven as temperate in his habits.[107] Mai claims that his poor self-care, lack of social grace and shabby appearance are typical of alcoholism,[108] and so they may be, but scruffiness can also be noted amongst staunch Methodists! Also, despite wearing shabby overcoats, Beethoven was known to be meticulous in washing his person and with his linen, not least because of his chronic diarrhoea.[109] Holz, in a letter to Otto Jahn of 1825, stated that Beethoven was 'a stout eater of food and that he drank a great deal of wine at table'. There is then the revelation that Beethoven was sometimes tipsy at jolly dinners.[110] If that is diagnostic of alcohol dependence, then what a vast number of us must be alcoholics. It is significant that he often took walks after heavy dinners.[111] How sensible, and how uncharacteristic of alcoholism. There are no accounts or features typical of the true alcoholic in terminal decline, and of course at 'jolly dinners' alcoholics typically don't bother much with the food. However, Mai tells us that his friend Bernard told Beethoven that he drank too much wine;[112] this is hardly a diagnosis of alcoholism, even if he did. On a balance of probabilities, we should discard the alcoholic label.

Macronodular cirrhosis is the characteristic pattern following viral hepatitis. It is a reasonable diagnostic suggestion with Type A, but not with Types B and C (both twentieth-century infections),[113] and with Beethoven's past history of febrile illness and jaundice. In some cases viral hepatitis can grumble on as chronic active viral hepatitis. The proposition of viral hepatitis does not explain his chronic bowel disorder, iritis, joint problems, deafness and much else, but is said to fit in with his eating oysters.[114] But a variation on this theme is more convincing, as follows.

Primary Sclerosing Cholangitis (PSC)

This is a chronic disease of uncertain aetiology suggested as a unifying diagnosis.[115] In it there is stasis in the gall bladder and its system of ducts, which convey bile to the gut to assist in digestion. If there is back-pressure in the flow of bile, that may cause jaundice and secondary cirrhosis of the liver.[116] Approximately 70% of sufferers also have inflammatory bowel disease, usually ulcerative colitis, just as 3–10% of inflammatory bowel disease sufferers proceed to liver disease.[117] And so we come full circle. It hardly matters whether PSC is a feature of ulcerative colitis or vice versa. Clearly they are intimate bedfellows, possibly having dominated Beethoven's life, as well as causing his deafness and death.

Chronic Pancreatitis

The autopsy description of the pancreas could suggest chronic pancreatitis, which, in a majority of cases, affects middle-aged alcoholic men with cirrhosis, although heavy drinking can cause chronic pancreatitis without overt cirrhosis. This would also fit with Davies's suspicions regarding diabetes.[118] Chronic pancreatitis presents with abdominal pain, often relieved by alcoholic drinks, sometimes with episodes of obstructive jaundice. The problems are that Beethoven's was an illness spread over nearly forty years, too long a survival. Furthermore, iritis, joint pains and intermittent diarrhoea or constipation, let alone deafness, would not be associated. That is quite apart from the balance of probabilities weighing against alcoholism.

Inflammatory Bowel Disease

A likely explanation for Beethoven's bowel disturbance over four decades is chronic inflammatory bowel disease,[119] such as ulcerative colitis or Crohn's disease, neither of which was recognised by doctors until after Beethoven's death. Primarily an auto-immune disease, ulcerative colitis causes many other systemic complications,[120] including arthritis, iritis and liver disease (see the section on PSC above). Once a link is made between ulcerative colitis and cirrhosis then many late features such as iritis, jaundice, oedema, 'rheumatism' and ascites are readily explained. There could be two reasons for not incriminating ulcerative colitis as a unifying cause for all of Beethoven's medical problems. Firstly, it is unclear whether or not his diarrhoea was bloody, that being a very common symptom, although absence of obvious blood should not now preclude the diagnosis. Uncertainty remains as to the degree of introspection with which composers two hundred years ago examined their own faeces. Adams found evidence of Beethoven's diarrhoea intermittently being accompanied by blood anyway;[121] Dr Wawruch spoke of 'haemorrhoidalleiden', which implies bloody piles.[122] Secondly, a unified diagnosis based upon colitis could become thwarted because of Beethoven's deafness. However, sensorineural hearing loss was described as due to auto-immunity in 1979,[123] and subsequently it has been reported as a complication of both ulcerative colitis[124] and Crohn's disease.[125] The differences between Crohn's and ulcerative colitis are beyond the scope of this book. However, Crohn's disease, unlike ulcerative colitis, is generally a painful condition and could be a better explanation for many of Beethoven's problems.

It is useful to briefly review those medical conditions which, with some foundation, have been implicated, but can be excluded on a balance of probabilities. Few of the 'standard theories' survive careful scrutiny. Not all medical reviews have made a link between a general illness with multiple systems affected on the one hand and deafness on the other.[126]

Systemic Lupus Erythematosus (SLE, aka Lupus)

A 'connective tissue disorder' was the original unifying diagnosis suggested by Larkin.[127] SLE is an auto-immune disorder in which a butterfly-shaped facial rash is pathognomonic, and it is an obvious choice because, from descriptions at the time, there are references to Beethoven's pock-marked face,[128] which are neither confirmatory nor inconsistent but could be explained by his having contracted smallpox as a child. Arthritic bone and joint afflictions prevail in SLE, and there are many references to 'rheumatism' in Mai's review. However, he was walking heartily until the end of 1826,[129] which does not support SLE. More importantly, chronic active hepatitis leading to cirrhosis is unusual in SLE and even rarer as a cause of death with it, undermining the validity of lupus as a likely diagnosis.[130]

Kidney Disease and Diabetes

Wagner's autopsy revealed thickening of the kidneys' capsule and kidney stones sufficient to persuade Schwarz that Beethoven's death could have been due to renal papillary necrosis (RPN),[131] a kidney disease with chalky deposits in the system of tiny funnels (calyces) which collect urine in the kidneys before it flows down the ureters to the bladder. That is very much a microscopic, not a naked-eye, diagnosis. It is particularly associated with long-term ingestion of non-steroidal anti-inflammatory drugs, making it a disease for our times rather than nearly two hundred years ago. Few of Beethoven's multitude of symptoms suggest RPN, least of all deafness or bowel disorder, although colitis or Crohn's disease can cause oxalate kidney stones. However, 3–17% of autopsies in cases of RPN reveal evidence of liver cirrhosis,[132] and people with liver failure may develop secondary kidney failure. Also many sufferers (17–90%) from RPN are diabetic.[133] Few of the clinical descriptions at Beethoven's time fit in with diabetes, although he was prone to diverse infections as diabetics may be, but then so are patients with auto-immune disease. RPN is interesting but, like diabetes, remains highly improbable and does not conflate with Beethoven's other afflictions and their course over four decades.

Haemochromatosis

Davies claims that Beethoven consumed considerable quantities of cheap adulterated wines, which may have caused him to develop secondary haemochromatosis.[134] This is a condition where an excess of iron is deposited in organs such as the liver in alcoholic cirrhosis. However, such iron deposition is usually mild when compared with that in true primary haemochromatosis, which is an inborn error of metabolism. So this too is an interesting speculation, but there is much more against than for the suggestion that Beethoven succumbed to a form of human 'rusting', which accounts for neither his chronic bowel problems nor his deafness. The cheap adulterated wine theory is tenuous anyway, but has led to speculation regarding plumbism (lead poisoning).[135]

Plumbism

Some of Beethoven's clinical features could be explained by this diagnosis. Lead salts were used illegally two hundred years ago to 'improve' cheap wine. Moreover, some lead-lined manufacturing or storage vessels could adulterate wine. The subject is well reviewed by Mai.[136] He diverts us into suspicions that Beethoven died of alcoholic jaundice. The straw (or hair) to cling to with this esoteric diagnosis is that Martin recently reported high levels of lead in Beethoven's hair.[137] As Mai concedes, patterns of death by poisoning rarely cover more than thirty years, and a common cause of lead in hair, especially after two hundred years, is external contamination.[138] Keynes discusses a diagnosis of plumbism made by analysing a mere eight hairs and reviews all the inherent inaccuracy, not least the poor correlation between levels of lead in blood and in hair.[139] Finally, plumbism would not account for many of Beethoven's other problems.

Sarcoidosis (aka Sarcoid)

This is a condition where a chronic inflammatory process may cause multi-system disease. It has some microscopic similarities with TB, although there is no evidence that sarcoidosis is infectious. Its inclusion in Beethoven's difficult differential diagnosis has been well argued.[140] The range of problems typical of sarcoidosis is summarised in the list below, from which its attraction to Beethoven's diagnosticians is obvious.

Incidence of Features in Sarcoidosis[141]

Liver disease: 30% of cases
Respiratory problems: 25% of cases
Joint pains/arthritis: 20% of cases
Eye problems (e.g. iritis): 8% of cases
Neurological problems: 1% of cases (including cranial nerve palsies)

Sarcoidosis is often symptomless, being diagnosed serendipitously from tests undertaken for another reason, a far cry from Beethoven's decades of painful suffering. Palferman argues alternatively that kidney stones may accompany sarcoidosis and thus explain his severe pain,[142] although the many descriptions of abdominal pain are much more redolent of bowel than kidney problems. Moreover, had Beethoven suffered multiple renal stone formation over all his adult life, it is likely that there would have been much more evidence of it at the autopsy, and that is supposing his renal function had survived decades of assault by kidney stones. Sarcoid of the bowel is rare, and when it occurs is usually painless. Neither is the autopsy description of the liver supportive of sarcoid. When cranial nerves are involved in sarcoid, which is rarely, it is usually the seventh (facial) nerve and not the eighth (acoustic) nerve which is affected. Those with sarcoid deafness also have facial weakness, which Beethoven did not. A leading advocate of sarcoidosis explains that the deafness could have been due to a pathological hardening of bone caused by an abnormally high level of calcium in the blood.[143] The incidence of abnormally raised calcium in the blood in sarcoid is only about 1%,[144] and the chances of that causing bone hardening are even less.

Syphilis

Syphilis remains an object of popular, sometimes salacious, interest. Squires was so keen on syphilis with Beethoven that he highlighted the word in block capitals.[145] Had the case been strong, such emphasis would have been unnecessary. The point may be trivial, but could demonstrate the ardent enthusiasm with which some people misdiagnose syphilis. However, with Beethoven there may still be a case to answer. The origins of the 'Beethoven's syphilis' case[146] may derive from older German papers.[147] Palferman has elegantly demolished these origins as 'Chinese whispers'.[148]

Larkin described Jacobssohn's evidence as 'worthless'.[149] The key was that in the 1879 first edition of his *Dictionary of Music and Musicians* Grove stated in a footnote that Thayer told him that he, in turn, had heard from Dr Bertolini that his senior partner, Dr Malfatti, had given Beethoven certain medicines,[150] which have been assumed to have contained mercury.[151] These prescriptions had been destroyed, allegedly to protect Beethoven's reputation and legacy, with the assumption that they were for mercury to treat syphilis. As well as a universal panacea for syphilis, so mercury was for various other conditions. Neither does Beethoven's case history suggest any of the early, let alone third-stage, features of that terrible disease. Hayden seems to imply that he would have had them had he lived longer![152] As we saw with Smetana, once syphilis starts after a long latency, deafness, if it occurs, is typically quick and then total in its development. Beethoven's deafness evolved over thirty-one years and probably was never total; this is almost incompatible with a syphilitic cause. Notwithstanding its limitations, a recent toxicological analysis of Beethoven's hair has revealed mercury to be 'undetectable' – certainly not the result one would expect had he been syphilitic.[153]

Whereas Beethoven fell in love frequently, it is mischievous to translate that into promiscuity. During what Bower regards as a psychological illness (1816–20), he claims that Beethoven's letters mention 'prostitute'.[154] The context appears to have been his allegations that his sister-in-law, Johanna, gave favours for money.[155] However, Beethoven's relations – or lack of them – with prostitutes remain uncertain. Barry Cooper believes that Beethoven's hatred was not of Johanna herself, but only of her jurisdiction over Karl.[156] He has also shown that suspicion of prostitutes arose in Beethoven's correspondence because of misinterpretation and even mistranslation in a book by Editha and Richard Sterba published in 1954.[157] Bower's views appear unsupported in his own text. In 1819 Beethoven became interested in a French book about the French pox,[158] belying the inference that he had contracted syphilis, for which there is then no firm evidence. His objective in obtaining this book (if he did) was more likely to have been his concern for Karl's future conduct in the army than his own in the past. Barry Cooper quotes Beethoven as saying that 'Sensual enjoyment without a union of souls is bestial and will always remain bestial.'[159] Larkin's assertion does not justify the claim that it was likely that Beethoven caught venereal disease, but not syphilis, something for which no sound evidence was adduced anyway.[160] Moreover if it was gonorrhoea, as Larkin suggests, then it is highly probable that, like Rossini, he would have developed and reported complications from it subsequently. Syphilitic deafness may not be rare,[161] but in the late stages it is typically associated with vertigo,[162] of which Beethoven did not complain. Donnenberg and colleagues, who are advocates of Beethoven's alleged syphilis, reported that in the 1970s 7% of patients with unattributable sensorineural hearing loss had a positive blood test for syphilis (WR or VDRL).[163] This overlooked the overwhelming random prevalence of positive tests for syphilis until the advent of penicillin,[164] and their only incremental decrease for several decades thereafter. In 1914 12–15% of all Londoners were said to be WR positive.[165] Even in the 1970s there was a residuum of people surviving latent syphilis that they had contracted before the advent of penicillin. An incidence of 7% at first seems remarkably high. However, in the absence of a control group of people who had no hearing loss but were WR positive in significantly fewer than 7% of cases, this claim is speculative.

Syphilis would not readily explain Beethoven's bowel problems or indeed much else. Hayden claims that the 'early years of hidden syphilis' may be characterised by gastrointestinal pain.[166] Recently an expert venereologist and a consultant gastroenterologist have disagreed.[167] The interior of the bowel was one of the few parts of the body not to have been ravaged by syphilis in the past. There are, however, accounts of chronic gastritis in syphilis,[168] but not lasting more than thirty-five years or causing the erratic bowel function which blighted Beethoven's life. Anyway, his problems were with his bowels, not his stomach. Although cirrhosis is sometimes found at autopsy in syphilitic subjects, only very rarely does it cause death.[169] Furthermore, ascites is rare and Beethoven had that literally by the bucketful. An argument that his moods might be explained by general paralysis of the insane (GPI) suggests a lack of familiarity with features of GPI. Beethoven was a titanic figure, far removed from the demented megalomania of GPI typified by Hugo Wolf or the transient violence perpetrated by Donizetti and Smetana (see Chapter 4). Probably the best contrary evidence would be Beethoven's late musical compositions.

Before finally dismissing syphilis we should consider an unusual form of tertiary syphilis, meningo-vascular syphilis, of which there might remain some suspicion from the autopsy report. The natural history of deafness arising from syphilis is that its onset takes some ten to twenty years to first manifest itself after the original sexual infection, although it may often be rapid in its development once it starts. That would make Beethoven between eight and eighteen when he caught the pox. Syphilis becomes even more improbable as he exhibited no features of primary or secondary syphilis before going deaf, and typically deafness in syphilis is a late complication anyway. Had syphilis been the diagnosis, he would not then have survived for four decades or more. Accordingly, the wretched evolution of untreated syphilis and then of Beethoven's long and often miserable medical history do not clinically resonate with one another. If Beethoven himself had any suspicion that he was syphilitic it is improbable that in his will he would have beseeched those responsible for his legacy to make known the cause(s) of his death. Perhaps he anticipated the advent of the 'Beethoven's syphilis' school of fiction writers.

Whipple's Disease

Whipple's disease is a very rare infectious condition that has also been suggested as a unifying diagnosis.[170] Although intestinal disturbance is usually a symptom first typically bringing a middle-aged white man to the doctor, the commonest symptoms relate to the joints. The liver, spleen, pancreas, heart and kidneys, as well as the central nervous system, can all become involved. Iritis may occur, and chest problems are common in this condition. Even commoner is skin pigmentation. So far so good, there being an apparently strong case for ascribing the diagnosis to the swarthy, chesty Beethoven. However, closer examination undermines any such confidence. The onset of Whipple's typically is in middle age – a little late for any confident diagnosis with Beethoven. The neurological picture typically would be of apathy, progressing to dementia and some-times meningitis, which does not correlate with our patient's story, despite his damaged acoustic nerves. Today it is said to be usually fatal if left untreated, upon which basis it may be excluded in Beethoven's case.

Possible Causes of Deafness Alone

This chapter so far has charted the evolution of Beethoven's deafness, of which Ealy gives a scholarly chronicle.[171] His review of correspondence puts the onset as early as 1796. Ealy could not corroborate McCabe's descrip-tion of Beethoven holding a drumstick, attached to the piano, between his teeth, to hear via sound conduction through the skull bone.[172] He does recount use of a resonance plate as reported by Gerhard von Breuning. This was placed beneath his piano and employed with an ear trumpet, one of which was almost two feet long as described by Clara Schumann's father. A vital reflection is that the correspondence after Heiligenstadt from 1802 to 1810 contains scant mention of his deafness, whereas after 1825 there is little to have us believe that any conversation could be sustained.

We now turn away from a unifying diagnosis and look at disease processes merely causing deafness, thereby accepting that one of the conditions already described would have caused all of his other problems. As long as one accepts a moderately common cause for two separate problems then such a hypothesis is tenable.* It is when two rare conditions are suggested in parallel that the balance of probabilities becomes over-stretched.

Paget's Disease

An interesting suggestion is that Paget's disease caused Beethoven's deafness,[173] on the basis of an alleged but dubious bulge in Beethoven's head described in 1927.[174] Paget's disease affects bone, some areas being weakened and adjoining areas becoming dense and thickened where bone is over-produced. Typically this affects men from middle age onwards. The commonest bones to be involved are the shin bones (tibiae), hips, spine and skull. It is known that areas of bone overgrowth can actually trap and damage nerves as they pass through narrow bony tunnels or channels. Paget's disease is a recognised cause of deafness;[175] thus the plausible theory arose that Beethoven's acoustic nerves were progressively compressed by Paget's disease of the skull. The appeal here is that we have many descriptions of the progression of Beethoven's deafness.[176] This commenced with early features of high-frequency hearing loss and complaints of loudness recruitment with tinnitus, which Hood has described as being typical of sensorineural hearing loss,[177] as we might expect with Paget's. Beethoven hated shouting and when, in 1809, Vienna was bombarded, so disagreeable was the noise to him that he retreated to the cellar with his ears muffled by pillows.[178] As long ago as 1936 deafness was said to be the commonest clinical manifestation of Paget's disease affecting the skull.[179] In a study of 116 cases of the condition,[180] surprisingly three were in the 25–29 age group, which supported Naiken's theory.[181] Naiken believed that famous sketches or caricatures of the composer reflected a typically Pagetic patient, but a cartoon is not a clinical photograph and should not be regarded as clinical evidence. The Klein bust of 1812, by which time Beethoven's deafness was well established, does not show bossing of the forehead, the characteristic of Paget's disease affecting the skull.[182] Neither

* As a rough approximation, if two conditions both have a random incidence of 1 in 500 of the population, for them to co-exist the odds become 1 in 250,000 (500 × 500). Thus, one rarer condition with an incidence of 1 in 100,000 is 2.5 times more likely as an explanation than the conjunction of the two commoner conditions.

is the autopsy description of a uniformly thickened skull vault typical of Paget's disease. Lastly, the diagnosis was refuted in Germany in 1986 on the basis of an analysis of Beethoven's remains, from which no evidence of Paget's disease was found.[183]

Otosclerosis

Despite the principle of a unifying single diagnosis, there is no absolute reason why disease processes explaining the symptom complex already described should necessarily have also been the cause for his deafness. Accordingly, let us consider a condition which would be a likely free-standing explanation for Beethoven's deafness.

The introduction to this chapter explained how three small bones transmit sound percussively. Otosclerosis is a degenerative condition in which the third bone (stapes) becomes tethered to the inner membrane, which in itself stiffens and can no longer resonate. With an inability to resonate, the conversion of sound waves into the cerebral appreciation of sound is increasingly diminished. Otosclerosis can be encountered in young adults and even children. If bilateral and left untreated, this may end in complete deafness. Today it is treated surgically by removing the stapes (stapedectomy) so that it no longer tethers the membrane, which accordingly will again resonate to some extent. Interestingly, today the commonest cause of deafness in patients with Paget's disease is otosclerosis and not trapping of the acoustic nerve, perhaps providing a final coffin nail in Naiken's theory.

Otosclerosis has been proposed as the cause of Beethoven's deafness,[184] an objection to which is that his loss was presumed to be a pure sensorineural deafness, whereas with otosclerosis there is a mixed pattern of both conductive and sensorineural loss.[185] On this basis otosclerosis has recently been declared to be 'highly unlikely' as a cause of Beethoven's deafness.[186] Surely it is impossible two hundred years later to make the distinction between pure sensorineural and mixed pattern deafness.

If we are to separate causes of deafness from the other systemic disorders, then otosclerosis coincides with the age of onset, presentation and progression, and it is common. It can also cause horrible tinnitus such as that of which Beethoven complained. An objection to otosclerosis is the good autopsy description by Dr Wagner of acoustic nerve atrophy,[187] which typically is not a feature with otosclerosis, although it does tally with sensorineural deafness.

Conclusion

Beethoven's deafness, by several accounts, was never complete.[188] The various diagnoses in Beethoven's case are summarised in the list below, and it is clear that many can be safely discarded, leaving several auto-immune disorders, of which ulcerative colitis and Crohn's disease fit the known facts. For those uncomfortable with either of those two diagnoses also explaining deafness, then otosclerosis becomes a possible addition. Not in dispute is that in those last years, with his mental and physical suffering, this great figure took classical music to places it had not previously dreamed of visiting. Surely we should deplore biography which becomes so sensational as to describe Beethoven as having 'the head of a steel-willed mental giant paradoxically poised on the decadent body of a dwarf'.[189] Perhaps the author confused Wagner's Alberich with music's most titanic figure.

Finally, it is worth considering the phenomenon whereby one sensory deprivation may evoke an exaggerated area of sensory function in a different part of the brain, which recently has been shown on brain scans.[190] Thus we may ask whether Beethoven's deafness cleared sensory pathways of extraneous noise to facilitate the intellectual and emotional conflation which is musical composition.[191] Martin Cooper suggested, a transition from the exterior to the interior,[192] whilst proposing there to be no discrepancy between Beethoven's character and his creation. This is a theory overlooking the intrusion of tinnitus. That may be what Cooper meant as 'evidence of an inner life of almost unparalleled reality and intensity'.[193] In the late string quartets, the alterations of tempo may reflect those of Beethoven's mood, although the final quartet (Opus 135) is full of humour.[194] Kerman believes that the mood of the much earlier 'La malinconia' does not seem to approach melancholy.[195] A similar account relating Schumann's mood swings to his music (see Chapter 6) is easier to make from those readily recorded vacillations, which were due to his bipolar disorder. This is quite distinct from Beethoven's quixotic temperament, which is more difficult to monitor retrospectively. An alternating pattern of sunny symphonies (Nos. 2, 4, 6, 8) and darker ones (Nos. 1, 3, 5, 7, 9) is often suggested in concert programmes, but is hard to correlate with contemporaneous accounts of his state of health or mind. However, we can compare Beethoven's heard music with that from the unheard period when he had become almost completely deaf. So perhaps the final word in our technocratic era is that tone and frequency patterns have been analysed by computer for all nine symphonies.[196] The authors found no musical structural difference between those works Beethoven heard, those he heard with sound distortion and those which he hardly heard if at all. These authors questioned the theory of auditory feedback, whereby people need to hear sounds to then use them accurately.[197] They suggest that this probably holds for ordinary mortals, but not for creative geniuses. Such theorising is more helpful than esoteric speculation about syphilis or Whipple's disease. There can be no better a scientific validation of the unflinching and brave stoicism of Ludwig van Beethoven.

Diagnoses in Beethoven's Case
(with some key references)

1   **Unifying disease processes**
    a   Probable (auto-immune disorders)[198]
        - Ulcerative colitis or Crohn's disease with liver cirrhosis[199]
    b   Improbable
        - Systemic lupus erythematosus[200]
        - Primary sclerosing cholangitis[201]
        - Whipple's disease[202]
        - Sarcoidosis[203]
        - Post-viral hepatitis, leading to cirrhosis[204]
        - Syphilis[205]
    c   Very improbable – disregard
        - Alcohol[206]
        - Renal disease[207]
        - Haemochromatosis[208]
        - Pancreatitis[209]
        - Diabetes[210]
2   **Separate causes of deafness**
    d   Very possible
        - Otosclerosis[211]
        - Auto-immune disorder[212]
    e   Improbable
        - Otitis media[213]
        - Paget's disease[214]
        - Syphilis[215]
    f   Far-fetched – disregard
        - Trauma[216]
        - Typhus[217]
        - Lead poisoning[218]
        - Mercury poisoning[219]

✛ GABRIEL FAURÉ ✛
(1845–1924)

That man's silence is wonderful to listen to
> Thomas Hardy, *Under the Greenwood Tree*, 1872

Despite speaking of his 'spleen',[220] Fauré was not a man such as Tchaikovsky who resorted to self-pity; neither was he grumpy like Debussy. Spleen is probably similar to Churchillian 'black dogs'. In common with many men who have lacked parental support he tended to befriend father figures, particularly, for most of his life, Camille Saint-Saëns. Reviewing biographies such as those of Nectoux, Orledge and Duchen reveals reasonable grounds for his 'spleen' in that, from early adult life well into middle age, he was dominated by impecunity and migraine. He depended on menial jobs as teacher and organist in order to achieve security for his wife, Marie Fremiet, and their two sons. His work often required him to spend several hours a day travelling by train.[221] Neither was his return home in the evening to Marie likely to have been cheering.[222]

Earlier on, Fauré had been a passionate and sensuous young man blessed with wit, charm and good looks. He was devastated when Marianne, daughter of the singer and socialite Pauline Viardot, broke off her engagement to him.[223] He kept her letters for the remainder of his life.[224] This was rejection just as, in many ways, he had also been rejected by his own parents. Subsequently he was serially passed over for professional recognition and advancement. After Marianne he became something of a sexual buccaneer, despite an unhappy arranged marriage in 1883 to Marie, whose father, the sculptor Emmanuel Fremiet, was Fauré's lifelong friend.[225] Marie was quiet and plain, had artistic ambitions and stayed at home of her own volition, whilst simultaneously managing to resent so doing. This combination of impecunity, a rather joyless marriage and an inability to compose because of relentless routine, would have given many of us 'spleen'. The primary source of his frustration was insufficient time to settle down to serious composition.

Despite Fauré's intermittent unhappiness, here was a man with many friends, including several mistresses. One was Emma Bardac, later to become Mme Claude Debussy, for whom he wrote *La bonne chanson* and, for her infant daughter, the *Dolly Suite*.[226] There were generous patrons who were also friends, such as the painter John Singer Sargent and the sewing machine heiress Winnaretta Singer. 'Winni' and other *fin de siècle* grand ladies admitted Fauré, with his charming manners and winning ways, to the salons of Paris, where he came to realise that he was valued for what he was. This must have been an attractive alternative to his home with Marie, who generally refused to accompany her husband to parties, trips abroad or anything else. What is striking is that their two sons, Emmanuel and Philippe, whilst remaining at home well into their twenties, remained close to Fauré until he died. They were decent young men and loyal to both parents, although Emmanuel said that his mother was 'such a reluctant wife that it was tantamount to abandoning the role'.[227] For a warm, sensual, affectionate man and always a gentle one, this must have been hard to bear. Reasons for Fauré to have been downcast come easily. Evidence that he was ever clinically seriously depressed is harder to find. Duchen comments on the apparent lack of correlation between his deafness and the nature of late compositions, especially the 'tremendous beauty' of late works such as the Piano Trio or Second Cello Sonata.[228]

During 1900 in the arena at Béziers there was an open-air premiere of the first of Fauré's two operas, *Prométhée*. Apart from Marie, who refused to attend,[229] all Fauré's women were there including a tall, beautiful musician thirty-one years his junior. It seems to have been love at first sight, and Marguerite Hasselmans remained devoted to him until he died. He remained supportive of Marie, writing to her regularly when he was away, during their entire marriage, although she seldom replied.[230] Marguerite surely gave Fauré the emotional security which he had always craved. He kept her in a Parisian flat whilst continuing to live with Marie.[231] Marguerite improved his self-confidence and ability to compose. He even retrieved the abandoned First Piano Quintet, successfully reviving it in the summer of 1903. That was when disaster struck,[232] although suspicion of deafness was first mentioned in a letter to Marie in September 1901.[233] His son Philippe recounted that Fauré heard bass notes a third higher and treble notes a third lower. The mid-range was heard normally but more faintly.[234] Sound was distorted, later fragmented and sometimes accompanied by tinnitus. There was a family history of deafness, and he was diagnosed as having otosclerosis, which was probably correct, although an English otologist (Mr Andrew Morrison) proclaimed it to be a rarer form of deafness.[235] Today he might have benefited from hearing aids, as Vaughan Williams did, but even more so by surgical removal of the stapes bone. The bitter irony was that, like Smetana, this befell him when his career had eventually taken off. He was fifty-eight.

The debate has been as to how deafness affected composition, with the suggestion that the late works became more abstract and less accessible,[236] certainly in comparison with earlier pieces that are popular today, such as the *Cantique de Jean Racine*, the *Pavane* or the Requiem. Whereas there can be a bleakness to the late String Quartet, the Piano Trio is a beautiful work. Duchen suggests that, as for Beethoven, increasing aural isolation enabled Fauré to create an exceptionally profound musical world.[237] He found speech much easier to hear than music.[238] Possibly the increased volume of late composition came as a result of this aural isolation. The alternative but prosaic reason for composition becoming more frequent was that he had more time to compose. Fauré told Marie that he seemed to compose both more quickly and easily now. Perhaps this was just because Marie was on his back less and he no longer had the train to catch. What was observed and agreed at the time is that, although he physically aged, his music retained a youthful verve.[239]

His correspondence, collected and edited by Barrie Jones, is fascinating. It is always courteous and often jaunty, but most surprising is the sheer volume of affectionate letters he sent to his remote wife. Reading through these from 1914 to his death a decade later reveals three major health issues. Each winter this heavy smoker was beset with chronic bronchitis, which was worse in the north and alleviated by trips to the French Riviera or the Alps around Annecy, where he completed the Piano Trio.[240] In 1917 he may have had pneumonia. Two years later he wrote to the singer Madeleine Grey, beseeching her to write to him on white paper, as his eyesight was fading,[241] and later he recorded, 'More and more dim – Ah! Old age.' Of his increasing deafness he seldom complained, although when he wrote to Marie in April 1919 he conceded that he could no longer hear music properly and that his hearing, like his circulation, was always worse in the morning.[242] There are clear signs from the letters of his walking becoming 'weaker' and 'feeble',[243] which is suggestive in a heavy smoker of intermittent claudication due to arteriosclerosis (hardening of the arteries). Typically with that condition patients report cramp-like calf muscle pain on walking, which is relieved only by stopping. Despite all these infirmities he continued to compose whenever he felt strong enough, and he always took work with him on his excursions and holidays away from Paris. His mantra was 'to formulate all one's desires for the best'.[244] Today, both his respiratory and probably his mobility problems and deafness would be amenable to treatment, although whether his life might thereby have been extended is uncertain.

Landormy and Herter pointed to Fauré's social withdrawal from scented drawing rooms as deafness increased being a little like Beethoven's retreats.[245] They also suggested that the Impromptus Nos. 4 and 5,

Barcarolles Nos. 7, 8 and 9 and Nocturnes Nos. 8 and 9, composed in the first few years after he went deaf, are among the loveliest things he wrote. Aaron Copland wrote just before Fauré's death of 'A Neglected Master'.[246] In Copland's judgement deafness was irrelevant to the development of composition; he could find little difference in approach between the early and late works.

Fauré last played publicly at Tours in 1921, the year Saint-Saëns died. Just before that he had accompanied Madeleine Grey in *Mirages*, which he had written for her to premiere. So good was his accompaniment that Grey had not realised that Fauré was deaf until someone told her after the performance.[247] Then Fauré's output slowed, possibly at first because of desolation with the deaths of friends and siblings, but also because his weak chest was catching up with him. By now he was a frail, exhausted old man who could work less than he wished to. He had two episodes of pneumonia in 1922, interrupting the composition of his Trio for piano, cello and clarinet (or violin).[248] In 1923 he worked intermittently between illnesses on his late String Quartet, and by then he probably realised he did not have long to live. His son later said that during his composition of the String Quartet, 'He lived in an inner joy which seemed to revive him.'[249] The work was completed in the summer of 1924, almost immediately whereafter he developed double pneumonia whilst still at Annecy.[250] On 14 October 1924 he wrote his last letter to Marie. It is reflective and concerned for her rather than himself. He said, 'Your life has been a sad one', and went on to suggest that this was because of her unfulfilled ambition, which he gently suggested was mitigated by two fine sons and their families.[251] Fauré ended, after all their difficulties, 'I kiss you from the depth of my heart.' Then four days later he bade farewell to surroundings he loved and returned to Paris. In November he summoned both his sons to his bedside. He told them that, after he had gone, his supporters would fall away. He continued, 'I did what I could – now let God be my judge.'[252] He said no more and peacefully faded away the next morning.

Here was a gentle, decent man, one of wit and charm who had spanned the enormous journey which led from Berlioz to Ravel. The sadness surely is that Fauré probably craved recognition, and when it came, especially with the great concert in his honour in June 1922, he could hardly hear anything but a distortion of sound, so perhaps, as Thomas Hardy said, silence would have been wonderful to listen to. If there is a heaven, then they surely perform Fauré's Requiem there.

Postscript

So is deafness the supreme injustice for a composer? Perhaps the small number of deaf composers reveals the incompatibility of composition with such a monstrous disability, although paradoxically Beethoven said that of all his activities composition was the one that was least impeded. Fauré commented on a greater fecundity and speed in his declining and deaf years. We saw how the totally deaf Smetana went to watch the opera. The totally blind painter is professionally finished, although interesting theories are advanced regarding Modigliani's and Monet's eyesight in old age. Curiously, Handel's blindness seems to have been more restrictive than the deafness of Beethoven or Fauré. We thus end with this book's prime conclusion, which is about triumph in adversity.

Epilogue and Coda

And to make an end is to make a beginning.
The end is where we start from.

T. S. Eliot, *Four Quartets*, 1944

After a rollercoaster ride through so much wonderful music, punctuated by personal tragedy and illness and then abbreviated by death, let us define what themes and conclusions may be drawn. Unease persists with some accounts of composers' deaths. Although uncertainty will continue regarding the exact cause of Mozart's death, that he was not poisoned is beyond all reasonable doubt, and his final illness, from either kidney or heart failure, took two and a half weeks. There have been cases, more than a hundred years ago, where analysis of contemporaneous accounts allows confident clinical conclusions, as with Beethoven or Brahms. Clearly Schubert did not die of syphilis, although he almost certainly died with it.

A recurrent theme has been the dogmatic claims made by doctors and musicologists alike. Elgar's 'last five words' may reflect more about Ernest Newman than about Elgar. Before we leave Newman, surely his overwhelming character assassination of Beethoven is appalling, defacing the memory of a titanic figure. This tendency to advance the potentially salacious, especially VD or alcohol, can render an awful disservice to the reputations of great people who deserve better, something which had concerned Beethoven himself. Newman's judgement is continued in subsequent quotation by others – and to what end? Opinions from pompous medical pin-stripes should be discarded, along with an apparent urge to publish increasingly abstruse medical opinion. Merging of the scholarly with the ludicrous was seen with various published diagnoses in the cases of Mozart and Beethoven, for both of whom over a hundred diagnoses have previously been advanced. Hopefully, future research will be presented in a manner reasoned upon a balance of probabilities. Moreover, it is a mantra of good clinical practice to never make two or more diagnoses where one would do.

We should dispose of Mozart's Tourette's syndrome and Gershwin's 'overwrought hysteria'. A recent Proms concert programme asserted that Schumann died of syphilis, with a suggestion that his hand problem had been self-inflicted;[1] both are questionable. The biographer's responsibility is to do justice to all the evidence. No musicologist should write regarding a musician's health without consulting appropriate medical experts and vice versa. That great composers are dead should not banish defences against publishing opinions which would be open to legal redress were the composers still alive. Today a person's right to sue for libel dies with that person. Surely the essence of analyses such as these must be respect for the truth and also for a person's now defenceless legacy, of which we may be custodians.

Sir George Pickering, Oxford Professor of Medicine, once said, 'The history of medicine is a monument to human folly.' Thus it may be that the strident and sometimes Soviet-style strictures of today's 'managed healthcare' will seem as foolish to our successors as blood-letting does to us today. We should not be too smug in our condemnation. Blood-letting was done because it always had been, and doctors have often been slow to embrace change or innovation. Mercury treatment for syphilis continued into the 1950s, despite penicillin. To this day challenges to new medical therapies, often made respectable only by the later passage of time, are sometimes initially opposed by established practitioners. So comment upon the quality of composers' medical care itself is a theme throughout this book. Not until we reach the late nineteenth century can a contemporary clinician regularly recognise a treatment as having been appropriate. Until then almost all treatment was at best a harmless blandishment and at worst overtly damaging. Much of it was mumbo-jumbo. The bungled surgery of Bach and Handel, the incarceration of Schumann and the extensive bleeding of many seem outrageous now. In the twentieth century the deaths of Gershwin and Ravel almost immediately after brain surgery seem unfortunate and today, like Holst's death, would today command at least a coroner's inquest. Ravel's was probably avoidable, Gershwin's operation never had much to offer him and was too late anyway. As euthanasia is currently topical, it is paradoxical that an early post-operative death spared Ravel and Gershwin further inevitable suffering. It was Schubert's gastroenteritis, treatable today, which probably spared him the later ravages of syphilis which clearly killed Donizetti, Smetana, Wolf, Delius and probably Chabrier. Interestingly, these five with Schubert were the only assured cases of composers with syphilis. Few, if any, others should be added on a balance of probabilities, despite alternative mythology.

Another chronic exaggeration now deflated is the alcoholic composer, where one looks little beyond Musorgsky, Satie and probably Glazunov, along with Field, Lambert and Arnold. There is no serious evidence for Tchaikovsky, Schubert, Mozart, Brahms, Britten or Beethoven having been alcoholic, despite alternative claims. Of more interest is that a heavy drinking tendency, as with Sibelius, may be self-controlled. Any notion of alcohol fuelling musical creativity is rejected, and this is surely why Musorgsky under-achieved. Ludwig showed from a group of hard-drinking creative types (mainly writers) that, for the majority, alcohol did more harm than good over a long time-period, despite popular notions to the contrary.[2] This led to the question: what does fuel creativity? Could madness play a part?

Ancients such as Aristotle, Plato and Socrates believed that all geniuses were at least a little mad, as in the famous Byronic epithet: 'We of the craft are all crazy.' Harold Nicolson regarded mad poets as a poetic invention.[3] Advocates of mad genius seldom comment upon the bourgeois sanity of Shakespeare, Einstein, Haydn or J. S. Bach. In 1998 Waddell, a Canadian psychiatrist, published an extensive literature review of this subject, concluding that 'Enthusiasm for associating creativity and mental illness was not upheld by the evidence.'[4] Many of the studies which she cited were unsupported by comparisons with randomly chosen control subjects. An important earlier study is Juda's, where 113 artists (in the broad sense) and 181 scientists, selected by peers for their eminence, were compared.[5] From her data there was no definite relationship between highest mental capacity and psychological ill health, although she did infer that 'artists' had a higher incidence of suicide and neurosis. Neither was there good evidence for genius being dependent upon psychotic illness. Her sub-group of twenty-seven German-speaking composers, described in her book and quoted by Slater and Meyer,[6] was no madder than the general population. Of these twenty-seven, three – Gluck, Wolf and Schumann – became psychotic or demented, wherewith composition withered. For Gluck it was dementia from successive strokes and for Wolf dementia from the advance of tertiary syphilis, which leaves only Schumann. According to my studies it is only he and Bruckner, with Gesualdo and Arnold, who clearly were mad, if only intermittently. Schumann and possibly Arnold are the only clear examples of manic-depressive bipolar psychosis in this book. Rossini and Bartók may have fallen into that modern category. Schumann's mental breakdown caused him to be incarcerated, which probably led to his cachectic death. In my preliminary review of nearly three hundred composers, apart from Schumann jumping, and Tchaikovsky and Wolf wading, non-fatally into water, only Clarke and possibly Warlock took their own lives, although Arnold certainly tried. Bruckner's intermittent madness hampered composition; obsessive anxieties over earlier symphonies compulsively led to multiple revisions rather than completion of his Ninth Symphony, but the miracle is that composition occurred at all amidst the disharmony of his mind: another case of in spite of, not because of. Serious madness or psychosis is the exception, not the rule. Like illness, it is the hurdle and not the starting pistol.

Farnworth, in his essay 'Musicality and Abnormality', claimed that great composers had drive far surpassing that of ordinary mortals without suffering any increased psychosis.[7] He concluded that psychosis had no proven connection with artistic achievement. Arnold clearly composed between, not during, psychotic episodes. Vernon judged persistent drive and hard work to be as important as high intelligence in the creative personality.[8] Post's 1994 study of creativity and psychopathology in '291 World-Famous Men',[9] fifty-two of whom were composers, reached similar conclusions. However, some of the observations were unexpected. Those classified as having no psychopathology included Bartók and Brahms and two others who died of general paralysis of the insane! Slater and Meyer concluded that most men of great achievement were normal, albeit with eccentric behaviour patterns.[10] Foucault, a French philosopher, said that 'Madness may historically have been a social diagnosis to ostracise socially deviant behaviour.'[11] Kay Jamison drew a positive correlation between creativity and cyclothymic behaviour.[12] This becomes a self-evident truth when we review many composers within these pages. Composition vacillated with distinct mood swings. We should not be surprised that people touched by genius (or 'fire'[13]) exhibit over-developed personality or mental features. Ludwig proposed that emotional lability may provide the motivation, conviction and inspiration for new creativity, implying that emotional overdevelopment, if only in the conventional view, may allow a creative person to escape the social and cultural constraints of conformity.[14]

Another approach to this question was that of Pickering, who, in *Creative Malady* suggested that Charles Darwin, Florence Nightingale and other 'invalids' advanced their creativity by hiding behind the protective screen of an assumed illness.[15] The domestic and social demands of Victorian convention were thereby avoided, allowing a creative job to continue undisturbed. Consonant with such behaviour were Tchaikovsky's shy resignation, Sibelius's forbidding gloom and the sometimes ursine manners of Brahms, Debussy, Beethoven and even Mahler, with all of whom the ferment and fervour of composition stretched the boundaries of normal behaviour.

Pickering also mentioned the effect of luck in creativity, such as Fleming's accidental discovery of penicillin.[16] Inevitably luck, bad or good, may hugely influence composition. Luck could be in the form of the spouses and partners in composers' lives. Without George Sand's loving care of Chopin at Nohant, his life might have been even shorter. The same may be said of Jelka's care of Delius. Kennedy has declared that before Elgar knew Alice, and then after her death, he composed very little great music.[17] An eminent doctor attending Rossini suggested that, without Olympe Pélissier, he could have spent many years in an asylum.[18] To such an establishment Schumann might have gone earlier, had it not been for Clara. Before leaving this topic, we may note that some of these women undoubtedly were muses, not carers. Clara Schumann was probably both, and to two men. Elgar's 'Windflower', Mahler's Almschi and Janáček's Kamila were muses, sometimes to the point of obsession.

Another question which hopefully this book answers is whether creativity is actually fuelled by illness, such as TB.[19] Recently, in a radio broadcast, a medical historian confirmed there to be no evidence that 'toxins' liberated in TB might stimulate composition.[20] No such substance has been isolated, and neither is there circumstantial evidence for one. The two most allegedly consumptive composers, Weber and Chopin, composed in spite of illness, not because of it. There were times when sickness was so overbearing as to suspend any attempt to compose. Like Weber, Chopin dreaded winter, latterly needing to have his emaciated person carried upstairs and then put to bed by a servant. There is no evidence that disease spurred him on, as Sand generously had done. In his last years Weber almost gave up composition, continuing to earn by conducting, an enterprise which probably hastened his end. Nevertheless, intimations of mortality urged some, such as Prokofiev, to commit their compositions to paper without delay. Here we must distinguish the primary conception of a composition from the mechanics of then having the music written on a score or, in Shostakovich's case, actually performed. A limitation in scholars correlating 'illness' with 'musical creativity' is that Wagner's music dramas may be placed in the same pigeonhole as Chopin's nocturnes.

I have attempted to relate the course of illness to the quantity and quality of music which composers left. There is a popular concept of composers producing their final notes from a deathbed, but it is an image appropriate in only a few cases. Borodin and Gounod were composing on the day they dropped down dead. Some ill composers continued almost regardless, wherewith Beethoven is the magnificent paragon, and it was despite, and not because of, illness. Accepting that composers' minds are different from those of average people should not surprise us. In the 2016 Paralympic Games people with major disabilities performed physical near-miracles. Their message was not to concentrate on the absence of a limb, but to focus on what the other parts can do. Perhaps the creative brain of a sick person is similar.

Tantalisingly, would composers have survived their illnesses with modern medical treatment? Over half of my cohort of seventy would. People often fantasise over the great compositions which might have resulted had Mozart, Schubert, Mendelssohn or Chopin reached sixty years or more. With the benefit of hindsight their musical output would probably have been slower, different and even disappointing. It is fascinating that several composers with a huge output, such as Mozart, Schubert or Purcell, died in their thirties. On the other hand, many of those reaching their seventies and eighties had by then slowed down or stopped composing. But we have also seen how an innate drive to compose manifests itself in other ways, as with both Delius and Ravel. The grossly disabled Delius was relieved of his musical concepts by Fenby, whilst Ravel complained pathetically of 'composing' and hearing music in his head, but of there being no means of exteriorising it from his locked-in brain disease, whilst he otherwise remained physically quite well. The strange and often irrational figure of Smetana still attempted composition whilst developing syphilitic dementia, as did Wolf.

In order to evaluate the overall question of the impact of final illness upon composition, an analysis was conducted of sixty-seven of the seventy composers (Gesualdo, Clarke and Vivaldi were excluded for lack of sufficient evidence). For the rest a prime source was the work lists in *New Grove*. The final illnesses were subdivided as follows:

- An acute ending to a long-term (chronic) illness
- Sudden, unexpected fatality
- Short-term illness
- Final decline in long-term, chronic illness
- A sudden episode probably unrelated to the chronic condition already prevailing

One group to have always intrigued historians is those who have just retired, and not because of any obvious physical or mental affliction, although in the latter case who knows? Anyway, they retired apparently of their own free will, which suggests conventional retirement in old age. Sibelius last composed in 1929, writing three pieces for violin and piano, and died peacefully twenty-eight years later. Between his wife's death in

1920 and a short time before he died in 1934, Elgar composed little of note and then, close to death, started a Third Symphony and experienced an unfulfilled wish to write an opera. Rossini emerged from decades of producing very little to compose the *Petite messe solennelle* four years before he died, possibly upon a religious impulse. His masterpiece, *William Tell*, had been premiered thirty-five years before that. Brahms and Dvořák, whilst still in apparent good health, pronounced their retirements openly, as professional people usually do. In the last few years, nevertheless, Brahms did produce some chorale preludes and had a brief affair with the clarinet before he died three years later, and Dvořák remained consumed by a wish to outdo Smetana with Czech opera, hence the fairly unsuccessful *Armida* in 1902–03, but composed nothing else. Another apparent retiree is Delius, who admittedly had been physically incapacitated for over twenty years but, as Cardus and later Elgar pointed out, he remained mentally very active. Rimsky-Korsakov and Glazunov also had periods exceeding two years when they stopped composition. Rachmaninov composed almost nothing after the *Symphonic Dances* of 1940, living for another three years.

Just as some composed until the very end, others made late autumnal farewells, of which the warmth of Verdi's *Falstaff* or Richard Strauss's *Four Last Songs* appears as a comfortable accommodation with old age. This may just suggest another hypothesis that there is perhaps a finite package of creative energy and output in each composer. Perhaps Mozart and Schubert managed a full allotment from their teens to their early thirties. Although he died at thirty-eight, Mendelssohn might have had little more original to say had he lived longer. Hans von Bülow said that Mendelssohn started as a genius, ending as a talent; musically his output declined, like his health, in the two years before his sadly premature death. Bellini composed almost nothing in his last year after completing *I puritani*, although his final illness was brief. Perhaps Sibelius, Elgar or Brahms had said all they wanted to say well before their deaths.

Many composers doubled up as soloists and/or conductors, and we have seen that today Grieg would probably have joined the jet-set of musicians as Stravinsky did. Weber was unequivocal about his late financial dedication to opera production, especially with his last masterpiece, *Oberon*. As heart disease overwhelmed Mahler, the conductor's podium was his last musical step into a rapid final illness, leaving the Tenth Symphony incomplete. There is also a small group of composers for whom, near the ends of their lives, the written word became the prime objective, of whom Nielsen, Poulenc and possibly Massenet are examples.

Triumph in adversity has been a theme throughout this book, and a list of eleven composers who were composing on the day of their death or from their deathbed emerges with Borodin, Puccini, Finzi, Holst, Gounod, Massenet, Bruckner, Prokofiev and Bartók joining Mozart and Beethoven. Then we distinguish between two lists of composers: those who, despite illness, soldiered on with little alteration in prolific composition, and those who did continue, or tried to, but with a conspicuous tailing off in both the quantity and quality of composition, this being easily attributable to ill health (see below). Twenty-five (at least) of the sixty-seven left works incomplete at death, a few of them because a sudden and unexpected illness supervened, as with Janáček, Bizet, Borodin and Mozart.

Composers who Continued as Before until Death, Despite Ill Health

    Pergolesi
    Beethoven
    Field
    Schubert
    Gounod
    Bruckner
    Musorgsky
    Massenet
    Mahler
    Puccini
    Nielsen
    Holst
    Bartók
    Prokofiev
    Finzi
    Shostakovich
    Britten

Composers whose Illnesses Caused Reduction or Cessation of Composition

    Handel
    J. S. Bach
    Gluck
    Haydn
    Mozart
    Donizetti
    Berlioz
    Schumann

Liszt
Wagner
Verdi
Smetana
Chabrier
Fauré
Wolf
Debussy
Richard Strauss
Satie
Schoenberg
Ravel
Stravinsky
Warlock
Gershwin
Copland
Arnold

As we work down the list of sixty-seven composers, we may ask with how many was a work which most of us would regard as great (whether complete or incomplete) a product of these final months. This can easily become fraught with personal preference, which I have strenuously tried to avoid. However, Table 1 is an attempt to summarise the answer. Only a quarter of our cohort (17 out of 67) conspicuously were involved with a last great composition, and eight of these works were incomplete. Surely the miracle is enshrined in the first list above, with a cohort of composers who resolved to continue as best they could until their illness finally overwhelmed them. In conclusion, my personal suspicion, that within each composer there was an innate quantity of composition, might be upheld. As a doctor, one is not surprised to encounter very varied professional responses to sickness, but illness, probably without exception, was borne bravely. Although Mahler died leaving his Tenth Symphony unfinished, there is little evidence that he was struggling with it during his final illness.

A common theme throughout much musical biography is that of inter-mittent depression (or melancholia), as opposed to psychotic depression. This was obvious with Berlioz or Bartók and others in this book, and is consistent with Jamison's views regarding cyclothymia.[21] Even those usually known for cheerfulness, such as Mozart, Nielsen or Mendelssohn, were sometimes cast down. On the other hand, many typically melancholic com-posers, such as Rachmaninov or Tchaikovsky, had passages of contentment.

Table 1 Last Great Works Composed during a Final Decline in Health

Composer	Work(s)	Continued in last few weeks	Left incomplete	Assisted or completed by a 2nd composer
Pergolesi	*Stabat mater*	✓		✓
Mozart	Requiem	✓	✓	✓
Beethoven	Opus 131 and 135 String Quartets, sketch of Tenth Symphony		✓ ✓	
Weber	*Oberon*	✓		
Schubert	String Quintet, D897 and 898 Piano Trios	✓		
Wagner	*Parsifal*			
Bruckner	Ninth Symphony	✓	✓	
Borodin	*Prince Igor*, Third Symphony	✓	✓	✓
Musorgsky	*Khovanshchina*	✓	✓	✓
Janáček	*House of the Dead*			
Mahler	10th Symphony		✓	
Puccini	*Turandot*	✓	✓	✓
R. Strauss	*Four Last Songs*			
Vaughan Williams	Ninth Symphony			
Bartók	Viola Concerto	✓		
Prokofiev	Seventh Symphony			
Finzi	*In terra pax*			
Shostakovich	Fifteenth String Quartet	✓		

Elgar's melancholia, previously described as hypochondria, should now be separated, in that he had a number of physical diseases to account for his physical and psychological symptoms, which made much of his melancholia exogenous or reactive. He was not a hypochondriac.[22] There is no sound clinical reason, despite intermittent woe and misery, to satisfy a clinical diagnosis of endogenous manic-depressive psychosis with Elgar. The musical question remains as to how reactive depression affected composers. The answer often reposes with the circumstances to which they reacted depressively. Brahms's or Mahler's recollection of events from childhood or adolescence reveal melancholy to have been reflective upon things past, and this can be followed in the music, particularly that of Mahler, who so brilliantly juxtaposed the bucolic and burlesque with tragedy, which was sometimes born of his memories. In bereavement the cause is obvious with Dvořák, Saint-Saëns and the young Verdi. With Schubert, reactions to unsuccessful love affairs, and especially the realisation that he was probably syphilitic, are ample explanation, as deafness was for Beethoven. Stalin and the KGB are surely to blame for much of Shostakovich's misery. For Tchaikovsky or Rachmaninov a tendency towards melancholy, often evident in their music, seems to have been innate, and was worsened in Rachmaninov's case, like Bartók's, by exile from his own country. Tchaikovsky was certainly tormented by sexual guilt, but even with him moods dipped and then lightened. Both musically and clinically endogenous can be separated from reactive (exogenous) depression. With the former there is apathy, inertia, mentally a blank wall: 'The world disappears. One has nothing to say', as we saw occasionally with Debussy.[23] This finally became the case with Schumann, as well as with Debussy intermittently as he contemplated 'a hole in the ground'. Reactive depression can be seen in the plangent melancholy of Rachmaninov's Second Piano Concerto, as it can in the late works of Tchaikovsky and Elgar. The music probably came as it did because of that reaction, rather than being suppressed by that blank wall. The list of compositions whose mood reflects a composer's personal experience could be endless.

What was often so admirable and reassuring is the way in which many composers shook off the misery from sometimes unbearable circumstances and ill health. So an abundant theme is the magnificent manner in which many courageously rose again to endure and to create in spite of everything. Composers generally were people of huge moral and sometimes physical courage, capable of extraordinary endurance. For the majority, their approach to adversity, sickness and musical composition was the apogee of their heroism. Debussy, Mahler and Schubert in their last few years, or Elgar and Mozart in their final weeks, were full of real personal bravery. Garcia writes that, throughout his life, Mahler turned adversity into creativity.[24] As the blind and paralysed Delius said, 'In spite of my infirmities, I manage to get something out of life'.

Perhaps the greatest act of courage may be acting in the interests of others. It was a wish to provide financial security for his family which drove Weber to work in London and not sunny Italy, knowing that the exercise might kill him, as it did. In the modern age Benjamin Britten's first concern in the management of his own illness was to immediately complete his last great role, in *Death in Venice*, for his beloved Peter Pears. Doing so delayed his heart valve surgery by months, during which the actual heart muscle stretched beyond redemption, despite great surgical skill. That delay was an act of generosity which probably shortened his life. Would Mahler have succumbed to endocarditis if he had not insisted on conducting a Busoni premiere?

After tying together some strong themes, is there a final word to say about all these composers and their awful illnesses? Their genius was innate, being driven by courage and usually sheer hard graft. They were all very vulnerable people, and different ones too. The great psychiatrist Anthony Storr wrote that the more we delve into famous people's lives, the more obvious do vagaries of character appear, not least because biographers won't let them rest in peace.[25] In a recent newspaper article, Michael White considered the scope and impact of Wagner's music dramas, comparing them with Chartres Cathedral, *War and Peace* or the ceiling of the Sistine Chapel, as amongst humankind's supreme artistic achievements.[26] Then he judged that 'great artists rarely prove to be great human beings'. Clearly he had Wagner in mind, but generally I disagree. The preceding pages repeatedly demonstrate the admirable human qualities with which many composers worked. In his treatise on world leaders dogged by ill health, the psychiatrist, neurologist and former Foreign Secretary David Owen convincingly showed that hubris became a politician's occupational disease.[27] Of our subjects for whom there is no 'composers' disease', we can replace hubris with a courageous generosity of spirit. How sad it is that many composers suffered so much, when they left a legacy with which our own lives have been infinitely enriched. We are all the custodians of their legacy.[28]

Appendix:
Accidental and/or Violent Deaths

These studies have revealed little connection between accidental or violent death and musical composition, although there are several caveats to that, and the ultimately fatal accident suffered by Jean-Baptiste Lully is often claimed to have altered or fostered the progress of orchestral conducting. Nevertheless, some surprising statistics emerge. This book covers seventy composers, albeit twenty-six of them briefly. However, an additional nine died violently or accidentally. If we add to them non-fatal injuries suffered by Mendelssohn, Puccini, Prokofiev and Ravel from traffic accidents, as well as Nielsen, then fourteen of a total group of seventy-nine suffered violent or accidental episodes (18%). These are surprisingly high figures, without an obvious explanation. Three died as a result of warfare, two are alleged to have ultimately developed sepsis secondary to boils, and two succumbed to freak accidents.

Jean-Baptiste Lully (1632–1687) famously was conducting his own *Te Deum* to give thanks for the Sun King's recovery from surgery. As he beat time, he drove his conducting staff's pointed end into his foot, which subsequently became infected.[1] Gangrene followed; he refused an amputation and died two months after the original episode.[2] The theory that, forewarned by this tragedy, conductors thereafter used a scroll, violin bow or ultimately a baton to conduct is exaggerated. By Lully's time the conducting staff was starting to decrease in popularity, although it was Weber, Berlioz, and Wagner, more than a century later, who brought the art of conducting to a picture recognisable today.[3]

Charles Valentin Alkan (1813–1888) almost by tradition died because, whilst he was seeking his Talmud from a high shelf, the bookcase fell upon him. Alternatively, matters may have been more prosaic as the concierge at his flat found him prostrate on the kitchen floor under the hat stand.[4] It has been sensibly argued that he collapsed on arriving home, grabbing the hat stand as he did so. Having been put to bed, he died there later the same day, most probably from a stroke or heart attack.[5] Otherwise, he may have fainted and collapsed whilst preparing food in the kitchen. McCallum has added mystery to Alkan's story, suggesting he was schizophrenic.[6]

César Franck (1822–1890) is generally believed to have died as a result of being hit by a horse-drawn omnibus which struck him heavily on the chest. One account had him in a cab,[7] another crossing the road.[8] Whether his death five months later was as a direct result or not seems questionable. Complications from the original injuries were more probably contributory, rather than a primary cause of death.

Ernest Chausson (1855–1899), according to Lockspeiser, died when he hit his head heavily on a wall, falling from his bicycle.[9] His biographer Scott Grover disputes this.[10]

Alexander Scriabin (1872–1915) was said by Abraham (as quoted by de La Grange) to have had an 'insane imagination' and 'incredible egomania'.[11] Bowers gives a colourful account of his various ailments culminating in his visit to London in March 1914.[12] He became unwell with an abscess on his elaborately moustached upper lip, which allegedly he had cut shaving. Like Berg, after several operations to extirpate the infection, he succumbed to septicaemia, dying in April 1915.[13] Two germs were isolated from the pus, leading to speculation whether this was a synergistic infection (that is, two bacteria aiding and abetting each other). One also wonders whether Scriabin was diabetic, which would also explain some of his earlier ailments. Nevertheless, this does seem to have been an esoteric and sad outcome from an originally very minor injury.

George Butterworth (1865–1916), an unfulfilled musical talent, posthumously won the Military Cross whilst defending 'Butterworth trench' on the Somme, where he was shot by a German sniper bullet.[14] His Commanding Officer, Brigadier Page Croft, declared him to be a brilliant musician in times of peace and an equally brilliant soldier in time of stress.[15]

Enrique Granados (1867–1916) had to return from the USA to Spain via Britain, whose passenger steamship, the *Sussex*, was sunk by a German torpedo. In trying to save his wife struggling in the water, he drowned with her.[16]

Alban Berg (1885–1935) referred to his 'miserable health', which included a tendency to develop boils.[17] In August 1935 he was attacked by a swarm of bees, becoming ill for a week.[18] From this he developed an abscess, which was treated surgically but then recurred, leading to septicaemia, from which he died on Christmas Eve.[19] Today one questions whether he was immunologically suppressed and/or diabetic. Sadly, when he died he was planning a string quartet, a new opera and a symphony. Also he had shown interest in film music – beguilingly, were these shades of Korngold?

Anton Webern (1883–1945) was resting in his daughter's garden near Salzburg when he was mysteriously shot in the abdomen by an American soldier.[20] The Second World War had ended four months earlier. The Americans then arrested his family on suspicion of black marketeering.

References

Introduction

1 O'Shea, John: *Music and Medicine: Profiles of Great Composers*, J. M. Dent and Sons Ltd, London, 1990.
2 Neumayr, Anton: *Music & Medicine*, vol. 1, *Haydn, Mozart, Beethoven, Schubert* (English trans. B. C. Clarke), Medi-Ed Press, Bloomington, IL, 1994; vol. 2, *Hummel, Weber, Mendelssohn, Schumann, Brahms, Bruckner* (English trans. B. C. Clarke), Medi-Ed Press, Bloomington, IL, 1995; vol. 3, *Chopin, Smetana, Tchaikovsky, Mahler* (English trans. D. J. Parent), Medi-Ed Press, Bloomington, IL, 1997.
3 Robbins Landon, Howard C.: *1791, Mozart's Last Year*, Thames & Hudson, London, 1989.
4 *The New Grove Dictionary of Music and Musicians* (ed. Stanley Sadie), 20 vols., Macmillan Publishers, London, 1980, and *The New Grove Dictionary of Music and Musicians,* 2nd edn (ed. Stanley Sadie and John Tyrrell), 29 vols., Macmillan Publishers, London, 2001.
5 Newman, Ernest: *The Unconscious Beethoven: An Essay in Musical Biography*, pp. 45–52, Parsons, London, 1927.
6 Stone, J.: 'Death of Mozart', *Journal of the Royal Society of Medicine* (1991) 84.179.
7 Steen, Michael: *The Lives and Times of the Great Composers*, Icon Books Ltd, London, 2010.
8 Solomon, M.: 'Franz Schubert and the Peacocks of Benvenuto Cellini', *19th Century Music* (1989) 12(3).193–206.
9 Steblin, R.: 'The Peacock's Tale: Schubert's Sexuality Reconsidered', *19th Century Music* (1993) 17(1).15–33.
10 Šostar, Z., Vodanović, M., Breitenfeld, D., et al.: 'Composers – Substance Abusers', *Alcoholism* (2009) 45.127–42.
11 Critchley, MacDonald, and Henson, R. A. (eds): *Music and the Brain: Studies in the Neurology of Music*, William Heinemann Medical Books Ltd, London, 1977.

Chapter 1

1 Burrows, John, and Wiffen, Charles (eds): *Classical Music*, Eyewitness Companions Series, Dorking Kindersley Ltd, London, 2005
2 Robbins Landon, Howard C.: *1791, Mozart's Last Year*, p. 19, Thames & Hudson, London, 1989.
3 Von Neukomm, Sigismund: *Mozarts Tod, Manuscript in the Mozarteum*, cited by Robbins Landon, *1791, Mozart's Last Year*, p.19.
4 Karhausen, L. R.: 'The Myth of Mozart's Poor Health and Weak Constitution', *Journal of Medical Biography* (1999) 7.111–17.
5 Robbins Landon, *1791, Mozart's Last Year*, p. 147.
6 Niemetschek, F.: *Leben des k.k. Kapellmeisters Wolfgang Gottlieb Mozart, nach Originalquellen beschrieben*, Herrlische Buchhandlung, Prague, 1798.

7 Mozarteum Foundation, Salzburg: *Next to Mozart: Answers to the III Most Common Questions* (ed. S. Greger-Amanshauser, C. Grosspietsch and G. Ramsauer, trans. K. Kopp), Verlag Anton Pustet, Salzburg, 2011.

8 Shaffer, Peter: 'Paying homage to Mozart', *New York Times*, 2 September 1984.

9 Simkin, Benjamin: *Medical and Musical Byways of Mozartiana*, pp. 165–6, Fithian Press, Santa Barbara, CA, 2001.

Simkin, B.: 'Mozart's Scatological Disorder', *British Medical Journal* (1992) 305.1563–7.

Davies, P. J.: 'Mozart's Scatological Disorder', *British Medical Journal* (1993) 306.521–2.

Karhausen, L. R.: 'Mozart's Scatological Disorder', *British Medical Journal* (1993) 306.522.

Keynes, Milo: 'The Personality and Illnesses of Wolfgang Amadeus Mozart', *Journal of Medical Biography* (1994) 2.217–32.

Eibl, J. H., and Senn, W.: *Mozarts Bäsle-Briefe*, Bärenreiter-Verlag, Karl Vötterle GmbH & Co., K.G., Kassel, 1978.

10 Anderson, Emily: *The Letters of Mozart and his Family*, 3rd edn, p. 89, Macmillan Press, London, 1985.

11 Mozarteum Foundation, *III Most Common Questions*, p. 23.

12 Davies, P. J.: 'Mozart's Manic-Depressive Tendencies – 1', *Musical Times* (1987) 128.123–6.

13 Ibid.

14 Mozarteum Foundation, *III Most Common Questions*, p. 53.

15 O'Shea, John: *Music and Medicine*, 'W. A. Mozart', p. 26, J. M. Dent & Sons Ltd, London, 1990.

16 Ibid., p. 25.

17 Mozarteum Foundation, *III Most Common Questions*, p. 60.

18 O'Shea, *Music and Medicine*, p. 30.

19 Fluker, J. L.: 'Mozart: His Health and Death', *The Practitioner* (1972): 209.841–5.

Turner, W. J.: *Mozart: The Man and his Works*, p. 361, Victor Gollancz Ltd, London, 1938.

20 Karhausen, 'The Myth of Mozart's Poor Health and Weak Constitution', pp. 111–17.

21 Anderson, Emily (ed.): *The Letters of Mozart and his Family*, 3rd edn, pp. 228–30, 232, Macmillan Press, London, 1985.

22 Karhausen, 'The Myth of Mozart's Poor Health and Weak Constitution', pp. 111–17.

Keynes, 'The Personality and Illnesses of Wolfgang Amadeus Mozart', pp. 217–32.

Fluker, 'Mozart: His Health and Death', pp. 841–5.

Davies, P. J: 'Mozart's Illnesses and Death – 1, The Illnesses 1756–1790', *Musical Times* (1984) 125.437–42.

Jenkins, J. S.: 'The Medical History and Death of Mozart', *Journal of the Royal College of Physicians of London* (1991) 25.351–3.

Carp, L.: 'Mozart: His Tragic Life and Controversial Death', *Bulletin of the New York Academy of Medicine* (1970) 46.267–79.

Davies, P. J.: 'Mozart's Illnesses and Death', *Journal of the Royal Society of Medicine* (1983): 76.776–85.

23 Karhausen, 'The Myth of Mozart's Poor Health and Weak Constitution', pp. 111–17.

24 Halliwell, Ruth: *The Mozart Family*, pp. 99–101, Clarendon Press, Oxford, 1998.

25 Davies, 'Mozart's Illnesses and Death' (1983), pp. 776–85.

26 Jenkins, 'The Medical History and Death of Mozart', pp. 351–3.

     Anderson, *Letters of Mozart*, pp. 234, 237–47.

27 Keynes, 'The Personality and Illnesses of Wolfgang Amadeus Mozart', p. 217.

28 Karhausen, 'The Myth of Mozart's Poor Health and Weak Constitution', p. 115.

29 Puech, P. F., Puech, B., and Tichy, G.: 'Identification of the Cranium of W. A. Mozart', *Forensic Science International* (1989) 41.101–10.
     Puech, B., Puech, P. F., Tichy, G., et al.: 'Craniofacial Dysmorphism in Mozart's Skull', *Journal of Forensic Sciences* (1989) 34.487–90.

30 Fluker, 'Mozart: His Health and Death', p. 843.

31 Carp, 'Mozart: His Tragic Life and Controversial Death', p. 269.

32 Davies, 'Mozart's Illnesses and Death' (1983), p. 779.

33 Keynes, 'The Personality and Illnesses of Wolfgang Amadeus Mozart', pp. 217–18.

34 Carp, 'Mozart: His Tragic Life and Controversial Death', p. 269.

35 Mozarteum Foundation, *111 Most Common Questions*, p. 95.

36 Robbins Landon, Howard C.: *The Mozart Compendium: A Guide to Mozart's Life and Music*, pp. 113–20, Thames & Hudson, London, 1990.

37 Davies, 'Mozart's Illnesses and Death – 1, The Illnesses 1756–1790', p. 439.

38 Mozarteum Foundation, *111 Most Common Questions*, p. 156.

39 Puech, B., Puech, P. F., Dhellemes, P., et al.: 'Did Mozart Have a Chronic Extra-Dural Haematoma?', *Injury* (1989): 20.327–30.
     Mozarteum Foundation, *111 Most Common Questions*, p. 158.

40 Keynes, 'The Personality and Illnesses of Wolfgang Amadeus Mozart', p. 230.

41 Puech, Puech, Dhellemes et al., 'Did Mozart Have a Chronic Extra-Dural Haematoma?', p. 327.

42 Mozarteum Foundation, *111 Most Common Questions*, p. 158.

43 Puech, Puech and Tichy, 'Identification of the Cranium of W. A. Mozart', pp. 101–10.
     Puech, Puech, Tichy et al, 'Craniofacial Dysmorphism in Mozart's Skull', pp. 487–90.
     Puech, Puech, Dhellemes et al., 'Did Mozart Have a Chronic Extra-Dural Haematoma?', pp. 327–30.
     Puech, P. F.: 'Apartenne proprio a Mozart il cranio espoto a Salisburgo', *La stampa*, 21 October 1987.

44 O'Shea, *Music and Medicine*, p. 28.

45 Puech, Puech, Tichy et al., 'Craniofacial Dysmorphism in Mozart's Skull', p. 487.

46 Puech, Puech and Tichy, 'Identification of the Cranium of W. A. Mozart', p. 101.

47 Puech, Puech, Dhellemes et al., 'Did Mozart Have a Chronic Extra-Dural Haematoma?', pp. 327–30.

48 Ibid., p. 329.

49 Greger-Amanshauser, S.: personal communication (2012).

50 Ibid.

51 Paton, A., Pahor, A. L., and Graham, G. R.: 'Looking for Mozart's Ears', *British Medical Journal* (1986) 293,1622–4.

52 Davies, P. J.: 'Mozart's Left Ear, Nephropathy and Death', *Medical Journal of Australia* (1987) 147.581–5 (p. 581).

53 Gerber, P. H.: 'Mozarts Ohr', *Deutsch Medizinische Wochenschrift* (1898) 24.351–2.

54 Davies, 'Mozart's Left Ear, Nephropathy and Death', p. 582.
     O'Shea, *Music and Medicine*, p. 28.

55 Hilson, D.: 'Malformation of Ears as a Sign of Malformation of Genito-Urinary Tract', *British Medical Journal* (October 1957), 2 (5048), pp. 785–9.
     Vincent, R. W., Ryan, R. F., and Longenecker, C. G.: 'Malformation of Ear Associated with Urogenital Abnormalities', *Plastic and Reconstructive Surgery* (1961) 28.214–20.

56 Davies, 'Mozart's Left Ear, Nephropathy and Death', p. 583.

57 Karhausen, L. R.: 'Mozart Ear and Mozart Death', *British Medical Journal*(1987) 294.511–12.
    Karhausen, L. R.: 'Contra-Davies: Mozart's Terminal Illness', *Journal of the Royal Society of Medicine* (1991) 84.734–6.

58 Karhausen, 'Mozart Ear and Mozart Death', pp. 511–12.
    Karhausen, 'Contra-Davies: Mozart's Terminal Illness', p. 734.

59 Wasserman, E., Sagel, I., and Bingol, N.: 'Renal Disease, Polycystic Adult Type' in *Birth Defects Compendium* (ed. D. Bergsma), pp. 925–6, Macmillan, London, 1979.

60 Fog, R., and Regeur, L.: 'Did W. A. Mozart Suffer from Tourette's Syndrome?', p. 214, Proceedings of World Congress of Psychiatry, Vienna, 1985.

61 Swerdlow, N. R.: 'Current Controversies and the Battlefield Landscape', *Current Neurology and Neuroscience Reports* (2005) 5.329–31.
    Ashoori, A., and Jankovic, J.: 'Mozart's Movements and Behaviour, a Case of Tourette's Syndrome', *Journal of Neurology, Neurosurgery, and Psychiatry* (2007) 78.1171–5.

62 Kammer, T.: 'Mozart in the Neurological Department – Who Had the Tic?' *Neurology and Neurosciences* (2007) 22.184–92.

63 Leckman, G. F., Bloch, M. H., King, R. A. et al: 'Phenomenology of Tics and Natural History of Tic Disorders' in *Tourette's Syndrome* (eds J. T. Walkup, J. W. Mink, and P. J. Hollenbeck), *Advances in Neurology* (2006) 99.1–16.

64 Swerdlow, 'Current Controversies and the Battlefield Landscape', p. 330.
    Lombroso, P. J., and Scahill, L., 'Tourette Syndrome and Obsessive-Compulsive Disorder', *Brain and Development* (2008) 30.231–7.

65 Swerdlow, 'Current Controversies and the Battlefield Landscape', p. 330.
    Lombroso and Scahill, 'Tourette Syndrome and Obsessive-Compulsive Disorder', pp. 231, 233.

66 Davies, 'Mozart's Illnesses and Death', p.777.

67 Simkin, *Medical and Musical Byways*, pp. 165–6.

68 Ibid., p. 213.

69 Simkin, 'Mozart's Scatological Disorder', p. 1563.
    Ashoori and Jankovic, 'Mozart's Movements and Behaviour, a Case of Tourette's Syndrome', p. 1172.

70 Eibl and Senn, *Mozarts Bäsle-Briefe*.

71 Simkin, *Medical and Musical Byways*, pp. 170–1.

72 Eibl and Senn, *Mozarts Bäsle-Briefe*.

73 Anderson, *Letters of Mozart*, p. 60.

74 Simkin, *Medical and Musical Byways*, p. 170.

75 Anderson, *Letters of Mozart*, p. 60.

76 Rosselli, John: *The Life of Mozart*, p. 12, Cambridge University Press, 1998.

77 Mozarteum Foundation, *111 Most Common Questions*, p. 39.

78 Sacks, O.: 'Tourette's Syndrome and Creativity: Exploiting the Ticcy Witticisms and Witty Ticcicisms', *British Medical Journal* (1992) 305.1515–16.

79 Swerdlow, 'Current Controversies and the Battlefield Landscape', p. 330.

80 Winternitz, E.: 'Gnagflow Trazom: An Essay on Mozart's Script, Pastimes and Nonsense Letters', *Journal of the American Musicological Society* (1958) 11.200–16.

81 Karhausen, L. R.: 'Did Mozart Have Tourette's Syndrome?' *Perspectives in Biology and Medicine* (1995) 39.152–5.
    Karhausen, L. R.: 'Weeding Mozart's Medical History', *Journal of the Royal Society of Medicine* (1998) 91.546–50.

82 Pichler, Karoline: *Memoirs* (1843–44) in Deutsch, *Biography*, pp. 556–7, quoted by Mozarteum Foundation, *III Most Common Questions*, p. 99.

83 Sacks, 'Tourette's Syndrome and Creativity: Exploiting the Ticcy Witticisms and Witty Ticcicisms', p. 1515.

84 Simkin, *Medical and Musical Byways*, p. 30.

85 Karhausen, 'Did Mozart Have Tourette's Syndrome?'

86 Kammer, 'Mozart in the Neurological Department – Who Had the Tic?', p. 184.

87 Sacks, 'Tourette's Syndrome and Creativity: Exploiting the Ticcy Witticisms and Witty Ticcicisms', pp. 1515–16.

88 Köppen, L.: *Mozarts Tod*, Köppen Verlag, Cologne, 2005.

89 Stafford, William: *The Mozart Myths: A Critical Reassessment*, p. 53, Stanford University Press, Stanford, 1991.

90 Franzen, C.: 'Syphilis in Composers and Musicians, Mozart Beethoven, Paganini, Schubert, Schumann, Smetana', *European Journal of Clinical Microbiology & Infectious Diseases* (2008) 27.1151–7.

91 Fluker, 'Mozart: His Health and Death', p. 844.

92 Davies, 'Mozart's Left Ear, Nephropathy and Death', p. 584.

93 Bär, Carl: *Mozart: Krankheit, Tod, Begräbnis*, Schriftenreihe der Internationalen Stiftung Mozarteum Salzburg, Bärenreiter, Kassel, 1966.
    Davies, P. J.: 'Mozart's Illnesses and Death – 2. The Last Year and the Fatal Illness', *Musical Times* (1984) 125.554–61.

94 Hirschmann, J. V.: 'What Killed Mozart?' *Archives of Internal Medicine* (2001) 161.1381–9.

95 Robbins Landon, *1791, Mozart's Last Year*, p. 226.

96 Carp, 'Mozart: His Tragic Life and Controversial Death', p. 277.

97 Robbins Landon, *1791, Mozart's Last Year*, p. 175.

98 Ibid., p. 174.

99 Kerner, D,: 'Mozarts Tod bei Alexander Puschkin', *Deutsches Medizinisches Journal* (1969) 26.743–7.

100 Stafford, *Mozart Myths*, p. 53.

101 Davies, 'Mozart's Left Ear, Nephropathy and Death', p. 584.

102 Glover, Jane: *Mozart's Women: His Family, his Friends, his Music*, p. 178, Pan Books, London, 2006.
     Mozarteum Foundation, *III Most Common Questions*, p. 149.

103 Davies, 'Mozart's Manic-Depressive Tendencies – 1', pp. 123–6.

104 Jenkins, 'The Medical History and Death of Mozart', p. 351.
     Jenkins, J.S: 'Mozart's Last Months and Controversial Death', *Journal of Medical Biography*(1994) 2.185–6.

105 Anderson, *Letters of Mozart*, p. 234.

106 Robbins Landon, *1791, Mozart's Last Year*, p. 99.

107 Guillery, E. N.: 'Did Mozart Die of Kidney Disease? A Review from the Bicentennial of his Death', *Journal of the American. Society ofNephrology* (1992) 2.1671–6.

108 Anderson, *Letters of Mozart*, pp. 242–3.

109 Novello, Mary and Vincent: *A Mozart Pilgrimage, Being the Travel Diaries of Vincent and Mary Novello in the Year 1829* (transcribed and compiled by Nerina Medici di Marignano, ed. Rosemary Hughes, London, 1955), quoted by Robbins Landon, *1791, Mozart's Last Year*, p. 155.

110 Robbins Landon, *1791, Mozart's Last Year*, p. 173.

111 Ibid., p. 173.

112 Novello, *A Mozart Pilgrimage*, quoted by Robbins Landon, *1791, Mozart's Last Year*, p. 155.

113 Sakula, A.: 'Was Amadeus Mozart Poisoned?', *History of Medicine* (January–February 1980) 6–9.

114 Davies, 'Mozart's Illnesses and Death – 1, The Illnesses, p. 439.

115 Keynes, 'The Personality and Illnesses of Wolfgang Amadeus Mozart'.
Fluker, 'Mozart: His Health and Death'.
Jenkins, 'The Medical History and Death of Mozart'.
Yu, A. S. L., and Brenner, B. M.: 'Diagnosing Mozart's Mortal Illness: An Exercise in Cranio-Nephrology', *Journal of the American. Society of Nephrology* (1992) 2.1666–70.
Treves, R.: 'Mozart's Death', *Annals of the Rheumatic Diseases* (1991) 50.963–4.
Stone, J.: 'Death of Mozart', *Journal of the Royal Society of Medicine* (1991) 84.179.
Wheater, M.: 'Mozart's Last Illness – a Medical Diagnosis', *Journal of the Royal Society of Medicine*(1990) 83.586–9.
Zegers, R. H. C., Weighl, A., and Steptoe, A.: 'The Death of W. A. Mozart: An Epidemiological Perspective', *Annals of Internal Medicine* (2009) 151.274–8.

116 Davies, 'Mozart's Illnesses and Death – 2. The Last Year and the Fatal Illness', p. 555.

117 Jenkins, 'The Medical History and Death of Mozart', p. 352.

118 Davies, 'Mozart's Left Ear, Nephropathy and Death', p. 583.

119 Robbins Landon, *1791, Mozart's Last Year*, p. 158.

120 Davies, 'Mozart's Left Ear, Nephropathy and Death', p. 583.

121 Glover, *Mozart's Women*, p. 178.

122 Robbins Landon, *1791, Mozart's Last Year*, pp. 151–2.

123 Mozarteum Foundation, *111 Most Common Questions*, p. 149.

124 Robbins Landon, *1791, Mozart's Last Year*, p. 149.

125 Guillery, 'Did Mozart Die of Kidney Disease? A Review from the Bicentennial of his Death', p. 1673.

126 Robbins Landon, *1791, Mozart's Last Year*, p. 178.

127 Karhausen, 'Mozart's Terminal Illness: Unravelling the Clinical Evidence', *Journal of Medical Biography* (2001) 9.34–48.

128 Treves, 'Mozart's Death', p. 963.

129 Karhausen, 'Mozart's Terminal Illness: Unravelling the Clinical Evidence', p. 35.
Keynes, 'The Personality and Illnesses of Wolfgang Amadeus Mozart', p. 222.

130 Robbins Landon, *1791, Mozart's Last Year*, pp. 165–6.

131 Karhausen, 'Mozart's Terminal Illness: Unravelling the Clinical Evidence', p. 35.

132 Robbins Landon, *1791, Mozart's Last Year*, p. 147.

133 Mozarteum Foundation, *111 Most Common Questions*, p. 156.

134 Ibid., p. 153.

135 Breitenfeld, D., Mikula, I., Breitenfeld, T., et al.: 'Wolfgang Amadeus Mozart (1756–1791): Pathography, Sociopsychosomatic Factors that Precipitated Mozart's Final Illness', *Alcoholism* (1992) 28.107–10.

136 Karhausen, 'Contra-Davies: Mozart's Terminal Illness', p. 735.

137 Ibid., pp. 734–6.
Davies, P. J.: 'Mozart's Death: A Rebuttal of Karhausen, Further Evidence for Schönlein-Henoch Purpura', *Journal of the Royal Society of Medicine*(1991) 84.737–40.

138 Greger-Amanshauser, personal communication (2012).

139 Bär, *Mozart: Krankheit – Tod – Begräbnis*.

140 Davies, 'Mozart's Illnesses and Death' (1983), pp. 776–85.

141 Sakula, 'Was Mozart Poisoned?', pp. 6–9.

142 Davies, 'Mozart's Illnesses and Death' (1983), pp. 783–4.
     Davies, 'Mozart's Left Ear, Nephropathy and Death', p. 585.
143 Keynes, 'The Personality and Illnesses of Wolfgang Amadeus Mozart', p. 223.
144 Karhausen, 'Contra-Davies: Mozart's Terminal Illness', p. 735.
145 Davies, 'Mozart's Left Ear, Nephropathy and Death', p. 584.
     Davies, 'Mozart's Illnesses and Death', pp. 780, 784.
146 Davies, 'Mozart's Illnesses and Death' (1983), pp. 781–2.
147 Zegers, Weighl and Steptoe, 'The Death of W. A. Mozart: An Epidemiological Perspective', p. 275.
148 Karhausen, 'Contra-Davies: Mozart's Terminal Illness', p. 734.
149 *Greither, A.,* 'Die Todeskrankheit Mozarts'. *Deutsch Medizinische Wochenschrift (1967) 92.723–5.*
150 Karhausen, 'Contra-Davies: Mozart's Terminal Illness', p. 734.
151 Davies, 'Mozart's Illnesses and Death' (1983), pp. 776–85.
152 Robbins Landon, *1791, Mozart's Last Year*, pp. 179–80.
153 Davies, 'Mozart's Left Ear, Nephropathy and Death', p. 584.
154 Karhausen, 'Mozart's Terminal Illness: Unravelling the Clinical Evidence', p. 43.
155 Karhausen, 'Contra-Davies: Mozart's Terminal Illness', p. 735.
     Jahn, Otto: *Life of Mozart* (trans. P. D. Townsend), vol. 3, p. 354, Novello Ewer & Co., London, 1882.
156 Davies, 'Mozart's Death: A Rebuttal of Karhausen', p. 737.
157 Ibid., p. 737.
158 Eybler, J.: ,Selbstbiographie', *Allgemeine musikalische Zeitung*, Leipzig, 24 May 1826.
159 Wheater, 'Mozart's Last Illness – A Medical Diagnosis', p. 587.
     Davies, 'Mozart's Illnesses and Death' (1983), p. 781.
160 Davies, 'Mozart's Illnesses and Death – 2. The Last Year and the Fatal Illness', p. 557.
161 Robbins Landon, *1791, Mozart's Last Year*, p. 180.
162 Davies, 'Mozart's Manic-Depressive Tendencies – 1', pp. 123–6.
     Davies, 'Mozart's Manic-Depressive Tendencies – 2', pp. 191–6.
163 Davies, 'Mozart's Manic-Depressive Tendencies – 2', pp. 195–6.
164 Anderson, *Letters of Mozart*, pp. 242–7.
165 Steptoe, A., Reivich, K., and Seligman, M. E. P.: 'Composing Mozart's Personality', *The Psychologist* (February 1993) 69–71.
166 Davies, 'Mozart's Illnesses and Death – 2', p. 554.
167 Reichsmann, F.: 'Life Experiences and Creativity of Great Composers: A Psychosomaticist's View', *Psychosomatic Medicine* (1981) 43.291–3.
168 Davies, 'Mozart's Left Ear, Nephropathy and Death', p. 585.
169 Karhausen, 'Contra-Davies: Mozart's Terminal Illness', p. 734.
170 Treves, 'Mozart's Death', p. 963.
171 Bywaters, E. G. L., Isdale, I., and Kempton, J. J.: 'Schönlein-Henoch Purpura: Evidence for a Group A β Haemolytic Streptococcal Aetiology', *Quarterly Journal of Medicine* (1957) 26.161–75.
     Nielsen, H. E.: 'Epidemiology of Schönlein-Henoch Purpura', *Acta Paediatrica Scandinavica* (1988) 77.125–31.
172 Farley, T. A.:., Gillespie, S., Rasoulpour, M., et al.: 'Epidemiology of a Cluster of Henoch-Schönlein Purpura', *American Journal of Diseases of Children* (1989) 143.798–803.
173 Robbins Landon, *1791, Mozart's Last Year*, pp. 174–5.
174 Hirschmann, 'What Killed Mozart?', pp. 1384–5.

175 Greger-Amanshauser, personal communication (2012).

176 Hirschmann, 'What Killed Mozart?', pp. 1387–8.

177 Greger-Amanshauser, personal communication (2012).

178 Galatopoulos, Stelios: *Bellini: Life, Times, Music*, p. 339, Sanctuary Publishing Ltd, London, 2002.

179 Rosselli, John: *The Life of Bellini*, Musical Lives, p. 3, Cambridge University Press, Cambridge, UK, 1996.

180 Steen, Michael: *The Lives and Times of the Great Composers*, 'Bellini', p. 284, Icon Books Ltd, London, 2010.

181 Rossini, G.: 'I puritani', *La revue et gazette musicale*, 19 April 1835.

182 Galatopoulos, *Bellini: Life, Times, Music*, p. 350.

183 Orrey, Leslie: *Bellini*, The Master Musicians Series, p. 56, J. M. Dent & Sons Ltd, London, 1969.

184 Rosselli, *The Life of Bellini*, p. 127.

185 Orrey, *Bellini*, pp. 157–60.

186 Rosselli, *Life of Bellini*, p. 147.

187 Galatopoulos, *Bellini: Life, Times, Music*, pp. 391–2.

188 Ibid., pp. 391–2.

189 Ibid., p. 392.

190 Ibid., p. 392.

191 Ibid., pp. 393–4.

192 Ibid., p. 394.

193 Ibid., pp. 393–4 and p. 433 note 14.

194 Ibid., p. 395.

195 Ibid., pp. 396–7.

196 Bodley-Scott, R., and de Sabata, V., both quoted by Galatopoulos, *Bellini: Life, Times, Music*, p. 433, note 17.

197 Ibid.

198 Wilks, S.: 'Morbid Appearances in the Intestines of Miss Banks', *Medical Times Gazette* (1859) 2.264–5.

199 Curtiss, Mina: *Bizet and his World*, p. 411, Alfred A. Knopf, New York, 1958.

200 Ibid.

201 Gallet, L.: *Notes d'un librettiste* (Paris, 1891), quoted by W. Dean, *Georges Bizet: His Life and Work*, The Master Musicians Series, p. 123, J. M. Dent & Sons Ltd, London, 1965.

202 Curtiss, *Bizet and his World*, p. 416.

203 Dean, *Georges Bizet*, p. 123.

204 Curtiss, *Bizet and his World*, p. 417.

205 Ibid.

206 Ibid., p. 418.

207 Dean, *Georges Bizet*, p. 126.

208 Ibid., p. 127.

209 Curtiss, *Bizet and his World*, pp. 419–20.

210 Ibid., p. 416.

211 Gelma, E,: 'Quelques souvenirs sur Georges Bizet', *L'Alsace française*, 10 December 1938.
    Gelma, E.: ‚La mort du musicien Georges Bizet', *Cahiers de psychiatrie* (Strasbourg 1948).

212 Dean, *Georges Bizet*, p. 127.

213 Hucke, H., and Monson, D. E.: 'Pergolesi, Giovanni Battista' in *New Grove Dictionary of Music and Musicians*, 2nd edn (ed. Stanley Sadie and John Tyrrell), vol. 19, p. 391, Macmillan Publishers, London, 2001.

214 Ibid., p. 390.

215 Ibid., p. 391.

216 King, Robert: *Henry Purcell*, pp. 238–50, Thames & Hudson, London, 1994.

217 Ibid.

218 Ibid., pp. 225–7.

219 Zimmerman, Franklin B.: *Henry Purcell 1659–1695: His Life and Times*, 2nd edn, p. 255, University of Pennsylvania Press, Philadelphia, 1983.

220 Holman, Peter: *Henry Purcell*, p. 22, Oxford University Press, Oxford, 1994.

221 King, *Henry Purcell*, p. 226.

222 Westrup, Jack A.: *Purcell*, The Master Musicians Series, rev. edn, p. 84, J. M. Dent & Sons Ltd, London, 1980.

223 King, *Henry Purcell*, p. 227.

224 Brown, Clive: *A Portrait of Mendelssohn*, p. 493, Yale University Press, New Haven, 2003.

Chapter 2

1 Neumayr, Anton: *Music & Medicine* (English trans. B. C. Clarke), vol. 1, *Haydn, Mozart, Beethoven, Schubert*, 'Joseph Haydn', pp. 76–7, Medi-Ed Press, Bloomington, IL, 1994.

2 Young, Percy: *Haydn*, Masters of Music, p. 40, Ernest Benn Ltd, London, 1969.

3 Jones, David W.: *The Life of Haydn*, Musical Lives, p. 94, Cambridge University Press, Cambridge, UK, 2009.

4 Ibid., p. 196.

5 Neumayr, *Music & Medicine*, vol. 1, 'Joseph Haydn', p. 30.

6 Jones, *Life of Haydn*, pp. 212–25.

7 Neumayr, *Music & Medicine*, vol. 1, 'Joseph Haydn', p. 62.

8 Ibid., pp. 55–6.

9 Ibid., pp. 55–6.

10 Ibid., pp. 65–6.

11 Ibid., p. 68.

12 Ibid., p. 72.

13 Ibid., p. 73.

14 Jones, *Life of Haydn*, p. 225.

15 Steen, Michael: *The Lives and Times of the Great Composers*, 'Haydn', p. 132, Icon Books, London, 2010.
   Geiringer K. and I. Haydn: *A Creative Life in Music*, p. 189, Geo. Allen and Unwin, London, 1982.

16 Larsen, Jens P.: 'Haydn, Joseph' in *The New Grove Dictionary of Music and Musicians* (ed. Stanley Sadie), vol. 8, pp. 349–50, Macmillan Publishers, London, 1980.

17 Neumayr, *Music & Medicine*, vol. 1, 'Joseph Haydn', pp. 86–92.

18 Steen, *The Lives and Times of the Great Composers*, 'Saint-Saëns', p. 617.

19 Rees, Brian: *Camille Saint-Saëns*, pp. 221–2, Chatto and Windus, London, 1999.

20 Ibid., p. 241.

21 Harding, James: *Saint-Saëns and his Circle*, Chapman and Hall, London, 1965.

22 Rees, *Camille Saint-Saëns*, pp. 189–93.

Rees, Brian: personal communication (2013).

23 Rees, *Camille Saint-Saëns*, p.191.

24 Steen, *The Lives and Times of the Great Composers*, 'Saint-Saëns', pp. 622–4.
Rees, *Camille Saint-Saëns*, pp. 252, 254, 280–1, 371, 391.

25 Harding, *Saint-Saëns and his Circle*.
Watson, Lyle, *Camille Saint- Saëns: His Life and Art*, Kegan Paul, London, 1923.
Hervey, Arthur, *Saint-Saëns*, John Lane, London, 1921.

26 Rees, *Camille Saint-Saëns*, p. 280.

27 Ibid., p. 252.

28 Ibid., Chapter 9, 'Collapse and Recovery', pp. 280–98.

29 Ibid., p. 369.

30 Ibid., pp. 432–6.

31 Ibid., p. 433.

32 Cooper, Martin: *French Music: From the Death of Berlioz to the Death of Fauré*, p. 201, Oxford University Press, Oxford, 1951.

33 Rees, *Camille Saint-Saëns*, p. 441.

34 Kennedy, Michael: *Portrait of Elgar*, p. 286, Clarendon Paperback, 3rd edn, Oxford University Press, Oxford, 1993.

35 Ibid., p. 282.

36 Ibid., p. 129.

37 Ibid., p. 305.

38 Ibid., p. 305.

39 Ibid., p. 290.

40 Kennedy, Michael: *The Life of Elgar*, Musical Lives, pp. 40–7, Cambridge University Press, Cambridge, UK, 2004.
Kennedy, *Portrait of Elgar*, pp. 51–2.

41 Harcup, J.: 'Edward Elgar – a Medical Enigma?' *Elgar Society Journal* (2012) 17.16–31.

42 Harcup, J., and Noble, J.: 'Edward Elgar, Moaner or Loner?', *Journal of Medical Biography* (2016) 24.135–8.

43 Harcup, 'Edward Elgar – a Medical Enigma?', p. 16.

44 Ibid., pp. 26–7.

45 Ibid., p. 28.

46 Ibid., p. 27.

47 Ibid., p. 28.

48 Kennedy, M.: personal communications (2012, 2013 and 2014).

49 Ibid.

50 Ibid.

51 Northrop Moore, Jerrold: *Edward Elgar: A Creative Life*, p. 773, Oxford University Press, Oxford, 1984.

52 Harcup, 'Edward Elgar – a Medical Enigma?', p. 28.

53 De-la-Noy, Michael: *Elgar the Man*, pp. 211–12, Allen Lane, Penguin Books Ltd, 1983.

54 Harcup, 'Edward Elgar – a Medical Enigma?', pp. 22, 29.

55 Ibid., pp. 19–22.
Harcup and Noble, 'Edward Elgar, Moaner or Loner?', pp. 135–8.

56 Harcup, 'Edward Elgar – a Medical Enigma?', p. 21.

57 Ibid., p. 21.

58 Kennedy, *The Life of Elgar*, p. 173.

59 De-la-Noy, *Elgar the Man*, p. 199.

60 Reed, William H.: *Elgar As I Knew Him*, p. 179, Victor Gollancz Ltd, London, 1936.

61 Kennedy, *Portrait of Elgar*, p. 329.

62 Kennedy, *The Life of Elgar*, pp. 185–6.

63 Northrop Moore, *Edward Elgar*, pp. 815–18.
Evening Standard, 23 February 1934.

64 Harcup, 'Edward Elgar – a Medical Enigma?', p. 31.

65 Kennedy, personal communications (2012, 2013 and 2014).

66 Harcup, 'Edward Elgar – a Medical Enigma?', p. 31.

67 Ibid., p. 29.

68 Ibid., p. 30.

69 Ibid., pp. 30–1.

70 Kennedy, *Portrait of Elgar*, p. 329.

71 Ibid., p. 328.
Kennedy, *The Life of Elgar*, p. 197.

72 Kennedy, *Portrait of Elgar*, p. 327.

73 Harcup, 'Edward Elgar – a Medical Enigma?', p. 23.

74 Newman, Ernest: Letter to Gerald Abraham published in *The Sunday Times*, 6 November 1955, and quoted again in *The Listener*, 23 July 1959.

75 Kennedy, *Portrait of Elgar*, p. 330.
De-la-Noy, *Elgar the Man*, pp. 231–2.

76 De-la-Noy, *Elgar the Man*, pp. 231–2.

77 Kennedy, personal communications (2012, 2013 and 2014).

78 Goss, Glenda Dawn: *Sibelius: A Composer's Life and the Awakening of Finland*, pp. 73, 101, University of Chicago Press, Chicago, 2009.

79 Layton, Robert: *Sibelius*, The Master Musicians Series, 4th edn, p. 54, J. M. Dent & Sons Ltd, London, 1992.

80 Nupen, Christopher: *Jean Sibelius (The Early Years, Maturity and Silence)*, Allegro Films, 2006.

81 Ekman, Karl: *Jean Sibelius: His Life and Personality* (trans. Edward Birse), Chapter 7, 'In the Outer World', pp. 63–73, Alan Wilmer Ltd, London, 1936.

82 Goss, *Sibelius*, pp. 101–4.

83 Steen, *The Lives and Times of the Great Composers*, 'Sibelius', p. 741.

84 Goss, *Sibelius*, p. 417.

85 Ibid., p. 344.

86 Ekman, *Jean Sibelius*, p. 161.

87 Ibid., 179.

88 Ibid., p. 179.

89 Ibid., p. 179.

90 Goss, *Sibelius*, p. 405.

91 Ekman, *Jean Sibelius*, pp. 232–5.

92 Goss, *Sibelius*, pp. 232–5.

93 Ibid., p. 417.

94 Barnett, Andrew: *Sibelius*, p. 327, Yale University Press, New Haven and London, 2007.

95 Ekman, *Jean Sibelius*, p. 243.

96 Levas, Santeri: *Sibelius: A Personal Portrait*, p. 73, J. M. Dent & Sons Ltd, London, 1972.

97 Ibid., p. 124.

98 Goss, *Sibelius*, p. 345.

99 Layton, *Sibelius*, p. 62.

100 Levas, *Sibelius*, p. 127.
Layton, *Sibelius*, p. 62.
101 Schonberg, Harold C.: *The Lives of the Great Composers*, 3rd edn, 'Sibelius', pp. 452–5, Abacus, London, 1998.
102 Barnett, *Sibelius*, p. 327.
103 Layton, *Sibelius*, p. 58.
104 Ibid., p. 58.
105 Ibid., p. 58.
106 Ibid., pp. 58–9.
107 Ibid., p. 57.
108 Ibid., Appendix B, pp. 209–25.
109 Goss, *Sibelius*, pp. 437–8.
110 Ibid., pp. 437–8.
111 Goss, *Sibelius*, p. 424.
112 Barnett, *Sibelius,* p. 349.
113 Redlich, Hans, F.: *Claudio Monteverdi: Life and Works* (trans. K. Dale), p. 16, Oxford University Press, Oxford, 1952.
114 Redlich, *Claudio Monteverdi*, pp. 16–17.
Schonberg, *The Lives of the Great Composers*, 'Monteverdi', p. 10.
115 Redlich, *Claudio Monteverdi*, p. 15.
116 Ibid., p. 18.
117 Ibid., p. 19.
118 Schrade, Leo: *Monteverdi: Creator of Modern Music*, p. 267, Victor Gollancz, London 1979.
Redlich, *Claudio Monteverdi*, pp. 23–5.
119 Redlich, *Claudio Monteverdi*, p. 28.
120 Ibid., pp. 33–4.
121 Schonberg, *The Lives of the Great Composers*, p. 16.
122 Redlich, *Claudio Monteverdi*, p. 37.
123 Schrade, *Monteverdi*, pp. 344 and 349.
124 Fabbri, Paolo: *Monteverdi* (trans. Tim Carter), p. 266, Cambridge University Press, Cambridge, UK, 1994.
125 Phillips-Matz, Mary Jane: *Verdi: A Biography*, p. 718, Oxford University Press, Oxford and New York, 1993.
126 Ibid., p. 718.
127 Rosselli, John: *The Life of Verdi*, Musical Lives, p. 184, Cambridge University Press, Cambridge, UK, 2000.
128 Budden, Julian: *Verdi*, The Master Musicians, p. 138, Oxford University Press, Oxford, 2008.
129 Ibid., p. 142.
130 Walker, Frank: *The Man Verdi*, p. 508, J. M. Dent & Sons Ltd, London, 1962.
131 Phillips-Matz, *Verdi*, p. 760.
132 Ibid., p. 760.
133 Ibid., p. 751.
134 Rosselli, *The Life of Verdi*, p. 186.
135 Budden, *Verdi*, p. 146.
136 Rosselli, *The Life of Verdi*, p. 186.
Budden, *Verdi*, p. 146.
137 Philips-Matz, *Verdi*, p. 764.

138 Jacob, Heinrich E.: *Johann Strauss: A Century of Light Music* (trans. Marguerite Wolff), p. 286, Hutchinson & Co. Ltd, London, 1940.

139 Crittenden, Camille: *Johann Strauss and Vienna: Operetta and the Politics of Popular Culture*, p. 22, Cambridge University Press, Cambridge, UK, 2006 (first publ. 2000).

140 Kemp, Peter: 'Johann (Baptist) Strauss (ii)' in *The New Grove Dictionary of Music and Musicians*, 2nd edn (ed. Stanley Sadie and John Tyrrell), vol. 24, p. 480, Macmillan Publishers, London, 2001.

141 Jacob, *Johann Strauss*, p. 305.

142 Ibid., p. 306.

143 Ibid., p. 307.

144 Ibid., pp. 307–8.

145 Hollander, Hans: *Leoš Janáček* (trans. Paul Hamburger), p. 42, John Calder, London, 1963.

146 Lock, Stephen: 'Janáček's Illnesses' in John Tyrrell, *Janáček: Years of a Life*, vol. 1, *(1854–1914): The Lonely Blackbird*, Chapter 64, pp. 245–7, Faber & Faber, London, 2006.

147 Steen, *The Lives and Times of the Great Composers*, 'Janáček', p. 718.

148 Tyrrell, John: 'Janáček, Leoš' in *The New Grove Dictionary of Music and Musicians*, 2nd edn (ed. Stanley Sadie and John Tyrrell), vol. 12, p. 774.

149 Hollander, *Leoš Janáček*, p. 127.

150 Ibid., p. 85.

151 Zemanová, Mirka: *Janáček: A Composer's Life*, pp. 252–3, John Murray, London, 2002.

152 Kennedy, Michael: *Richard Strauss*, The Master Musicians Series, p. 115, J. M. Dent & Sons Ltd, London, 1988.

153 Ibid., p. 114.

154 Youmans, Charles: *The Cambridge Companion to Richard Strauss*, p. 239, Cambridge University Press, Cambridge, UK, 2010.

155 Kennedy, *Richard Strauss*, p. 117.

156 Ibid., p. 117.

157 Gilliam, Bryan: *The Life of Richard Strauss*, Musical Lives, p. 181, Cambridge University Press, Cambridge, UK, 1999.

158 Kennedy, *Richard Strauss*, p. 117.

159 Kennedy, Michael, *Richard Strauss, Man, Musician and Enigma*, p. 400, Cambridge University Press, Cambridge, UK, 1999.

160 Gilliam, *The Life of Richard Strauss*, p. 182.

161 Ibid., p. 181.

162 Ibid., p. 182.

163 Ibid., p. 182.

164 Kennedy, M.: personal communications (2013).

165 Kennedy, Michael: *The Works of Ralph Vaughan Williams*, p. 369, Oxford University Press, Oxford, 1964.

166 Ibid., p. 373.

167 Vaughan Williams, Ursula: *A Biography of Ralph Vaughan Williams*, p. 399, Oxford University Press, Oxford, 1964.

168 Day, James: *Vaughan Williams*, The Master Musicians Series, p. 71, J. M. Dent & Sons Ltd, London, 1972.

169 Day, James: *Vaughan Williams*, The Master Musicians, 3rd edn, p. 97, Oxford University Press, Oxford, 1998.

Chapter 3

1　London, S. J.: 'Beethoven: Case Report of a Titan's Last Crisis', *Archives of Internal Medicine* (1964) 113.442–8.
2　O'Shea, J. G.: '"Two minutes with Venus, two years with mercury" – Mercury as an Anti-Syphilitic Chemotherapeutic Agent', *Journal of the Royal Society of Medicine* (1990) 83.392–5.
3　Gardiner, John Eliot: *Music in the Castle of Heaven*, Allen Lane, London, 2013.
4　Taylor, John: *The History of the Travels and Adventures of the Chevalier Taylor, Opthalmiater*, vol. 1, p. 25, London, 1761.
5　Jones, Henry: *The Life and Extraordinary History of the Chevalier John Taylor, (by his Son, John Taylor)*, vol. 1, p. 196, London, 1761.
6　Keates, Jonathan: *Handel: The Man and his Music*, p. 355, Pimlico, London, 2009.
7　Taylor, *History of the Travels and Adventures of the Chevalier Taylor*, p. 25.
8　Baer, K. A.: 'Johann Sebastian Bach (1685–1750) in Medical History', *Bulletin of the Medical Library Association* (1951) 39.206–11.
9　Boyd, Malcolm: *Bach*, p. 190, Oxford University Press, Oxford, 2000.
10　Forkel, Johann Nikolaus: *Über Johann Sebastian Bachs Leben, Kunst und Kunstwerke*, Hoffmeister and Kuhnel, Leipzig, 1802.
　　Ober, W. B.: 'Bach, Handel and "Chevalier" John Taylor M.D., Opthalmiater', *New York State Journal of Medicine* (1969) 69.1797–1807.
　　Williams, Peter: *The Life of Bach*, p. 191, Cambridge University Press, Cambridge, UK, 2004.
11　Boyd, *Bach*, p. 190.
12　Wolff, Christoph: *Johann Sebastian Bach: The Learned Musician*, p. 442, Oxford University Press, Oxford, 2001.
13　Williams, *The Life of Bach*, p. 190.
14　Ibid., p. 139.
15　Wolff, *Johann Sebastian Bach*, p. 444.
16　Boyd, *Bach*, p. 189.
17　Williams, *The Life of Bach*, p. 188. Wolff, *Johann Sebastian Bach*, p. 447.
18　Williams, *The Life of Bach*, p. 188–9.
　　Wolff, *Johann Sebastian Bach*, p. 447.
19　Ober, 'Bach, Handel and "Chevalier" John Taylor M.D., Opthalmiater', p. 1799.
20　Baer, 'Johann Sebastian Bach (1685–1750) in Medical History', pp. 207–8.
21　Boyd, *Bach*, p. 190.
22　Ober, 'Bach, Handel and "Chevalier" John Taylor M.D., Opthalmiater', p. 1799.
　　Baer, 'Johann Sebastian Bach (1685–1750) in Medical History', pp. 207–8
23　Boyd, *Bach*, p. 190.
　　Baer, 'Johann Sebastian Bach (1685–1750) in Medical History', p. 207.
24　Wolff, *Johann Sebastian Bach*, pp. 449–50.
25　Baer, 'Johann Sebastian Bach (1685–1750) in Medical History', p. 207.
26　Wolff, *Johann Sebastian Bach*, pp. 449–50.
27　Boyd, *Bach*, p. 190.
28　Ibid.
29　Wolff, *Johann Sebastian Bach*, p. 449.
30　Ibid.
31　Baer, 'Johann Sebastian Bach (1685–1750) in Medical History', p. 207.
32　Mizler, L. C.: obituary of J. S. Bach, *Musikalische Bibliothek* (Leipzig, 1752) 3.

33 Wolff, *Johann Sebastian Bach*, p. 443.
34 Williams, *The Life of Bach*, p. 191.
35 Kranemann, Detlef: 'Johann Sebastian Bachs Krankheit und Todesursache, Versuch einer Deutung', *Bach-Jahrbuch* (1990) 53–64.
36 Terry, Charles S.: *Bach: A Biography*, p. 264, London, 1925.
37 Burrows, Donald: *Handel*, The Master Musicians, p. 374, Oxford University Press, Oxford, 1996.
     Keynes, M.: 'Handel and his Illnesses'. *Musical Times* (1982) 123.613.
38 Keates, *Handel*, p. 308.
39 Young, Percy M.: *Handel*, The Master Musicians Series, p. 65, J. M. Dent & Sons Ltd, London, 1979.
40 Mainwaring, John: *Memoirs of the Life of the Late George Frederic Handel*, Dodsley, London, 1760.
41 Young, *Handel*, pp. 85–6.
42 Frosch, W. A.: 'The Case of George Frederic Handel', *New England Journal of Medicine* (1989), 321.765–9.
43 Keates, *Handel*, p. 236.
44 Burrows, *Handel*, p. 195.
45 Keates, *Handel*, p. 236.
46 Burrows, *Handel*, p. 272.
47 Ibid., p. 272.
48 Ibid., p. 286.
49 Keates, *Handel*, pp. 236, 291.
     Frosch, 'The Case of George Frederic Handel', p. 767.
50 Slater, E. and Meyer, A.: 'Contributions to a Pathography of the Musicians: 2. Organic and Psychotic Disorders', *Confinia Psychiatrica* (1960) 3.129–45 (p. 139).
51 Keynes, M.: 'Handel's Illnesses', *Lancet* 1980, 2 (8208–9), pp. 1354–5.
     Frosch, 'The Case of George Frideric Handel', p. 767.
52 Ober, 'Bach, Handel and "Chevalier" John Taylor M.D., Opthalmiater', p. 1800.
53 O'Shea, John: *Music and Medicine: Medical Profiles of Great Composers*, 'George Frederick Handel', p. 17, J. M. Dent & Sons Ltd, London, 1990.
54 Burrows, *Handel*, p. 338.
55 Young, *Handel*, p. 85.
56 Ibid., pp. 85–6.
57 Burrows, *Handel*, p. 405.
58 O'Shea, *Music and Medicine*, p. 18.
59 Ober, 'Bach, Handel and "Chevalier" John Taylor M.D., Opthalmiater', p. 1802.
60 Ibid., pp. 1800–1.
61 Hunter, D.: 'Handel's Illnesses, the Narrative Tradition of Heroic Strength and the Oratorio Turn', *Eighteenth Century Music* (2006) 3.253–67.
62 Young, *Handel*, p. 67.
63 Frosch, 'The Case of George Frideric Handel', p. 767.
64 Hunter, 'Handel's Illnesses', p. 261.
65 Ibid., p. 767.
66 Burrows, *Handel*, pp. 332–3, 363, 365, 370.
67 Keates, *Handel*, pp. 343, 354.
68 Ibid., pp. 355–6.
69 Keates, *Handel*, p. 356.
     Keynes, 'Handel and his Illnesses', p. 614.

70 Keates, *Handel*, pp. 356–7.

71 Holst, Imogen: *Gustav Holst: A Biography*, p. 12, Oxford University Press, London, 1958.

72 Ibid., p. 14.

73 Ibid., p. 14.

74 Ibid., p. 17.

75 Palmer, Tony: *In the Bleak Mid-Winter*, Tony Palmer Films, TPDVD173, 2011.

76 Holst, *Gustav Holst*, pp. 32–3.

77 Ibid., p. 49.

78 Ibid., pp. 85–6.

79 Ibid., pp. 85–6.

80 Ibid., p. 103.

81 Head, Raymond: personal communication (2013).

82 Holst Archive, Britten-Pears Foundation, Aldeburgh, reviewed by this author November 2013.

83 Holst, *Gustav Holst*, pp. 114–15.

84 Ibid., p. 104.

85 Ibid., pp. 127–8.

86 Ibid., p. 141.

87 Ibid., p. 141.

88 Short, Michael: *Gustav Holst: The Man and his Music*, pp. 199–200, Circaidy Gregory Press, Hastings, 2014.

89 Holst, *Gustav Holst*, p. 163.

90 Ibid., p. 165–6.

91 Short, *Gustav Holst*, p. 209.

92 Holst, *Gustav Holst*, p. 168.

93 Ibid., p. 168.

94 Gustav Holst, death certificate 28May 1934, Holst Archive, Aldeburgh.

95 Boult, Sir Adrian: letter of condolence, 1934, Holst Archive, Aldeburgh.

96 Holst Archive, Britten-Pears Foundation, Aldeburgh, reviewed by this author November 2013.

97 Hingtgen, C. M.: 'The Painful Perils of a Pair of Pianists: The Chronic Pain of Clara Schumann and Sergei Rachmaninov', *Seminars in Neurology* (1999) 19 (Suppl. 1).29–34.

98 Bliss, Sir Arthur: letter of condolence, 1934, Holst Archive, Aldeburgh.

99 Carp, L.: 'George Gershwin – Illustrious American Composer: His Fatal Glioblastoma', *American Journal of Surgical Pathology* (1979) 3.473–8.
Silverstein, A.: 'The Brain Tumour of George Gershwin and the Legs of Cole Porter', *Seminars in Neurology* (1999) 19 (Suppl. 1).3–9.
Ljunggren, B.: 'The Case of George Gershwin', *Neurosurgery* (1982) 10.733–6.

100 Greenberg, Rodney: *George Gershwin*, p. 210, Phaidon Press, London, 1998.

101 Silverstein, 'The Brain Tumour of George Gershwin', p. 4.

102 Ewen, David: *A Journey to Greatness: The Life and Music of George Gershwin*, p. 136, W. H. Allen, London, 1956.

103 Ljunggren, 'The Case of George Gershwin', p. 735.

104 Silverstein, 'The Brain Tumour of George Gershwin', p. 4.

105 Ljunggren, 'The Case of George Gershwin', p. 734.

106 Armitage, Merle: *George Gershwin, Man and Legend*, p. 82, Books for Library Press, Freeport, NY, 1958.

Silverstein, 'The Brain Tumour of George Gershwin', p. 4.

107 Silverstein, 'The Brain Tumour of George Gershwin', p. 5.

108 Carp, 'George Gershwin – Illustrious American Composer: His Fatal Glioblastoma', p. 475.

109 Peyser, Joan: *The Memory of All That*, pp. 261–2, Simon & Schuster, New York, 1993.

110 Greenberg, *George Gershwin*, pp. 210–12.

111 Silverstein, 'The Brain Tumour of George Gershwin', p. 4.

112 Greenberg, *George Gershwin*, p. 212.

113 Evans, R. W.: 'Complications of Lumbar Puncture', *Neurologic Clinics* (1998) 16.83–103.

114 Greenberg, *George Gershwin*, p. 212.

115 Carp, 'George Gershwin – Illustrious American Composer: His Fatal Glioblastoma', p. 475.

116 Greenberg, *George Gershwin*, p. 213.

117 Silverstein, 'The Brain Tumour of George Gershwin', p. 5.

118 Ibid., p. 5.

119 Carp, 'George Gershwin – Illustrious American Composer: His Fatal Glioblastoma', p. 475.

120 Ibid., p. 475.
Silverstein, 'The Brain Tumour of George Gershwin', p. 5.

121 Carp, 'George Gershwin – Illustrious American Composer: His Fatal Glioblastoma', p. 475.
Silverstein, 'The Brain Tumour of George Gershwin', p. 5.

122 Silverstein, 'The Brain Tumour of George Gershwin', p. 5.

123 Carp, 'George Gershwin – Illustrious American Composer: His Fatal Glioblastoma', pp. 475–6.
Silverstein, 'The Brain Tumour of George Gershwin', p. 6.
Ljunggren, 'The Case of George Gershwin', p. 735.

124 Greenberg, *George Gershwin*, p. 209.

125 Fabricant, N. D.: 'George Gershwin's Fatal Headache', *Eye, Ear, Nose and Throat Monthly* (1958) 37.332–4.

126 Nichols, Roger: *Ravel*, Yale University Press, New Haven and London, 2011.

127 Ibid., p. 182.

128 Ibid., p. 394.

129 Baeck, E.: 'Was Maurice Ravel's Illness a Cortico-Basal Degeneration?', *Clinical Neurology and Neurosurgery* (1996) 98.57–61 (p. 58).

130 Baeck, E.: 'The Longstanding Medical Fascination with "le cas Ravel"' in *Ravel Studies* (ed. Deborah Mawer), pp. 187–208, Cambridge University Press, Cambridge, UK, 2010.

131 O'Shea, *Music and Medicine*, 'Maurice Ravel', p. 203.

132 Nichols, *Ravel*, p. 195.

133 Henson, R. A.: 'Maurice Ravel's Illness: A Tragedy of Lost Creativity', *British Medical Journal* (1988) 296.1585–8.

134 Ibid., p. 1586.

135 Baeck, 'Was Maurice Ravel's Illness a Cortico-Basal Degeneration?', p. 57.
Baeck, 'The Longstanding Medical Fascination', pp. 188–9.

136 Henson, 'Maurice Ravel's Illness: A Tragedy of Lost Creativity', p. 1587.

137 Orenstein, Arbie: *Ravel – Man and Musician*, p. 103, Dover Publications, New York, 1991.

138 Kerner, D.: 'Ravels Tod', *Münchener Medizinische Wochenschrift* (1975), 117 591–6.

139 Nichols, *Ravel*, p. 301.

140 Baeck, E.: 'The Terminal Illness and Last Compositions of Maurice Ravel', *Neurology and Neuroscience* (2005) 19.137.

141 Howat, Roy: personal communication (2013).

142 Cybulska, E. M.: 'Bolero Unravelled: A Case of Musical Perseveration', *Psychiatric Bulletin* (1997) 21.576–7.

143 Nichols, *Ravel*, p. 302.

144 Ibid., pp. 305–6.

145 Ibid., pp. 322–3.

146 Henson, 'Maurice Ravel's Illness: A Tragedy of Lost Creativity', p. 1586.

147 Nichols, *Ravel*, p. 331.

148 Ibid., p. 331.

149 Ibid., p. 332.

150 Otte, A., De Bondt, P., Van de Wiele, C., et al.: 'The Exceptional Brain of Maurice Ravel', *Medical Science Monitor* (2003) 9.RA 154–9.
Otte, A., Juengling, F. D. and Nizsche, E. U.: 'Rethinking Mild Head Injury', *Journal of Vascular Investigation* (1998) 4.45–6.

151 Otte, De Bondt, Van de Wiele et al., 'The Exceptional Brain of Maurice Ravel', p. 157.
Otte, Juengling and Nizsche, 'Rethinking Mild Head Injury', pp. 45–6.

152 Henson, 'Maurice Ravel's Illness: A Tragedy of Lost Creativity', p. 1586.
Otte, Juengling and Nizsche, 'Rethinking Mild Head Injury', pp. 45–6.

153 Nichols, *Ravel*, p. 331.

154 Ibid., p. 131.

155 Ibid., p. 334.

156 Ibid., p. 337.

157 Ibid., p. 338.

158 Alajouanine, T.: 'Aphasia and Artistic Realisation', *Brain* (1948) 71.229–41.

159 Ibid.

160 Nichols, *Ravel*, p. 331.

161 Alajouanine, 'Aphasia and Artistic Realisation', pp. 232–4.

162 Howat, personal communication (2013).

163 Henson, 'Maurice Ravel's Illness: A Tragedy of Lost Creativity', p. 1587.

164 Dalessio, D. J.: 'Maurice Ravel and Alzheimer's Disease', *Journal of the American Medical Association* (1984) 252.3412–13.

165 Baeck, 'The Terminal Illness and Last Compositions of Maurice Ravel', p. 136.

166 Baeck, 'Was Maurice Ravel's Illness a Cortico-Basal Degeneration?'.
Baeck, 'The Longstanding Medical Fascination'.
Baeck, E.: 'Maurice Ravel and Right Hemisphere Activity', *European Journal of Neurology* (2002) 9.321.
Baeck, 'The Terminal Illness and Last Compositions of Maurice Ravel'.

167 Baeck, 'Was Maurice Ravel's Illness a Cortico-Basal Degeneration?', p. 60.

168 Ibid., p. 61.

169 Amaducci, L., Grassi, E., and Boller, E.: 'Maurice Ravel and Right Hemisphere Musical Creativity: Influence of Disease on his Last Musical Works', *European Journal of Neurology* (2002) 9.75–82.

170 Alonso, R. J., and Pascuzzi, R. M.: 'Ravel's Neurological Illness', *Seminars in Neurology* (1991) 19 (Suppl. 1).53–7.

171 Baeck, 'The Terminal Illness and Last Compositions of Maurice Ravel', p. 132.

172 Cybulska, 'Bolero Unravelled: A Case of Musical Perseveration', p. 577.

173 Baeck, 'Maurice Ravel and Right Hemisphere Activity', p. 321.

174 Amaducci, Grassi and Boller, 'Maurice Ravel and Right Hemisphere Musical Creativity: Influence of Disease on his Last Musical Works', pp. 75–82.
Marins, E. M.: 'Maurice Ravel and Right Hemisphere Activity', *European Journal of Neurology* (2002) 9.320–21.

175 Baeck, 'The Terminal Illness and Last Compositions of Maurice Ravel', p. 137.
Baeck, 'The Longstanding Medical Fascination', p. 205.

176 Baeck, 'Maurice Ravel and Right Hemisphere Activity', p. 321.

177 Joseph, Charles, M.: *Stravinksy Inside Out*, p. 261, Yale University Press, New Haven, 2001.

178 Craft, Robert: 'The Nostalgic Kingdom of Maurice Ravel' in *Current Convictions*, pp. 187–91, Secker and Warburg, London, 1978.

179 Howat, personal communication (2013).

180 Nichols, *Ravel*, p. 343.

181 Baeck, 'Was Maurice Ravel's Illness a Cortico-Basal Degeneration?', p. 58.

182 Henson, 'Maurice Ravel's Illness: A Tragedy of Lost Creativity', p. 1587.
O'Shea, *Music and Medicine*, p. 207.

183 Nichols, *Ravel*, p. 332.

184 Baeck, 'Was Maurice Ravel's Illness a Cortico-Basal Degeneration?', p. 59.
Henson, 'Maurice Ravel's Illness: A Tragedy of Lost Creativity', p. 1587.

185 Long, Marguerite: *Au piano avec Maurice Ravel*, p. 168, Juillard, Paris, 1971.

186 Henson, 'Maurice Ravel's Illness: A Tragedy of Lost Creativity', p. 1587.

187 Ibid., p. 1587.
Baeck, 'Was Maurice Ravel's Illness a Cortico-Basal Degeneration?', p. 59.

188 Tondreau, R.: 'Egas Moniz (1874–1955)', *Radiographics* (1985) 5.996–7.

189 Dandy, W. E.: 'Roentgenography of the Brain after the Injection of Air into the Spinal Canal', *Annals of Surgery* (1919) 70.397–403.

190 Gibbs, F. A., Davis, H., and Lennox, W. G.: 'The EEG in Epilepsy and in Conditions of Impaired Consciousness', *Archives of Neurology and Psychiatry* (1935) 34.1133–48.

191 Baeck, 'The Longstanding Medical Fascination', pp. 196–7.

192 Baeck, 'The Longstanding Medical Fascination', p. 200.
Henson, 'Maurice Ravel's Illness: A Tragedy of Lost Creativity', p. 1587.

193 Baeck, 'The Longstanding Medical Fascination', p. 197.

194 Nichols, *Ravel*, p. 344.

195 Ibid.

196 Seeley, W. W., Matthews, B. R., Crawford R. K., et al.: 'Unravelling Bolero, Progressive Aphasia, Transmodal Creativity and Right Posterior Neocortex', *Brain* (2008) 131.39–49.

197 Miller, B., Ponton, M., et al.: 'Enhanced Artistic Creativity with Temporal Lobe Degeneration', *Lancet* (1996) 348.1744–5.

198 Harrison, P.: 'The Effects of Deafness on Musical Composition', *Journal of the Royal Society of Medicine* (1988) 81.598–601.

199 Nichols, *Ravel*, pp. 350–1.

200 Grey, Madeleine: *Mémoires d'une chanteuse française* (ed. Gérard Zwang), p. 119, note 132, L'Harmattan, Paris, 2008.

201 Amaducci, Grassi and Boller, 'Maurice Ravel and Right Hemisphere Musical Creativity', p. 77.

202 Dalessio, 'Maurice Ravel and Alzheimer's Disease', p. 3413.
203 Noble, J.: 'Malady Makers', *BBC Music Magazine*, August 2014
   Nichols, R.: 'Ravel', *BBC Music Magazine*, September 2014.
   Noble, J.: 'Ravel Response (to Roger Nichols)', *BBC Music Magazine*, October 2014.
204 Cavallera, G. M., Guidici, S., and Tommassi, L.: 'Shadows and Darkness in the Brain of a Genius: Aspects of Neuropsychological Literature about the Final Illness of Maurice Ravel (1875–1937)', *Medical Science Monitor* (2012) 18.1–8.
205 Warren, J. D., and Rohrer, J. D.: 'Ravel's Last Illness: A Unifying Hypothesis', *Brain* (2008) 132.114.
206 Kanat, A., Kayaci, S., Yazar, U., and Yilmaz, A.: 'What Makes Ravel's Deadly Craniotomy Interesting? Concerns of One of the Famous Craniotomies in History', *Acta Neurochirurgica* (2010) 152.737–42.
207 Cavallera, Guidici and Tommassi, 'Shadows and Darkness in the Brain of a Genius'.

Chapter 4

1 Wassermann, A. von, Neisser, A., and Bruch, C.: 'Eine serodiagnostische Reaktion bei Syphilis', *Deutsche Medizinische Wochenschrift* (1906) 32.745–6.
2 Franzen, C.: 'Syphilis in composers and musicians – Mozart, Beethoven, Paganini, Schubert, Schumann, Smetana', *European Journal of Clinical Microbiology and Infectious Diseases* (2008) 27.1151–7.
   Rothschild, B. M.: 'History of Syphilis', *Clinical Infectious Diseases* (2005) 40.1454–63.
3 Waivers, L. E.: 'Did Columbus Discover More than America?', *North Carolina Medical Journal* (1989) 50.687–90.
4 Rothschild, 'History of Syphilis'.
5 Gjestland, T.: 'An Epidemiological Investigation of the Natural Course of the Syphilitic Infection, Based upon a Re-Study of the Boeck-Bruusgard Material', *Acta Derm-Venerologica* (Stockholm) (1955) 35 Suppl. 34.
6 Romandi, F.: 'Re-Examining Syphilis: An Update on Epidemiology, Clinical Manifestation and Management', *Annals of Pharmacotherapy* (2008) 42.226–36.
7 O'Shea, J. G.: '"Two minutes with Venus, two years with mercury" – Mercury as an Anti-Syphilitic Chemotherapeutic Agent', *Journal of the Royal Society of Medicine* (1990) 83.392–5.
8 Ibid.
9 Gjestland, 'An Epidemiological Investigation of the Natural Course of the Syphilitic Infection, Based upon a Re-Study of the Boeck-Bruusgard Material'.
10 Allberger, F.: 'Julius Wagner-Jauregg (1857–1940)', *Journal of Neurology, Neurosurgery and Psychiatry* (1997) 62.221.
11 Hayden, Deborah, *Pox: Genius, Madness and the Mysteries of Syphilis*, p. 54, Basic Books Group, New York, 2003.
12 Ibid., p. 42.
13 Newbould, Brian: *Schubert: The Music and the Man*, p. 388, Victor Gollancz, London, 1999.
14 Ibid., p. 183.
15 Osborne, Charles: *Schubert and his Vienna*, pp. 94–5, Weidenfeld and Nicolson, London, 1985.
16 Newbould, Brian: *Schubert and the Symphony: A New Perspective*, p. 184, Toccata Press, London, 1992.

17 Newbould, *Schubert: The Music and the Man*, pp. 424–43.
18 Ibid., p. 183.
19 Ibid., p. 179.
   Deutsch, Otto E.: *Schubert: Memoirs by his Friends* (transl. Rosamond Ley and John Nowell), p. 266, A&C Black, London, 1959.
20 Rold, R. L.: 'Schubert and Syphilis', *Journal of Medical Biography* (1995) 3.232–5.
   Sams, Eric: 'Schubert's Illness Re-Examined', *Musical Times* (1980) 121).15–22.
21 McKay, Elizabeth Norman: *Franz Schubert: A Biography*, p. 194, Clarendon Press, Oxford, 1997.
22 Sams, 'Schubert's Illness Re-Examined', pp. 15–22.
23 McKay, *Franz Schubert*, p. 159.
24 Rold, 'Schubert and Syphilis', p. 233.
   Solomon, M.: 'Franz Schubert and the Peacocks of Benvenuto Cellini', *19th Century Music* (1989) 12(3).193–206.
25 Solomon, 'Franz Schubert and the Peacocks of Benvenuto Cellini', pp. 202–3.
26 Ibid., p. 202.
27 Sams, 'Schubert's Illness Re-Examined', p. 18.
28 Steblin, R.: 'The Peacock's Tale: Schubert's Sexuality Reconsidered', *19th Century Music* (Summer 1993) 17.15–33.
29 McKay, *Franz Schubert*, pp. 125, 155–6.
30 Sams, 'Schubert's Illness Re-Examined', p. 15.
31 Newbould, *Schubert: The Music and the Man*, p. 211.
32 O'Shea, John: Music *and Medicine: Medical Profiles of Great Composers*, 'Schubert', p. 110, J. M. Dent & Sons Ltd, London, 1990.
33 Reed, John: *Schubert: The Final Years*, p. 214, Faber & Faber, London, 1972.
34 Sams, 'Schubert's Illness Re-Examined', p. 16.
35 Ibid., pp. 16–17.
36 Ibid., p. 17.
37 McKay, *Franz Schubert*, pp. 289–90.
38 Sams, 'Schubert's Illness Re-Examined', p. 21.
39 Rold, 'Schubert and Syphilis', p. 233.
40 McKay, *Franz Schubert*, pp. 311, 317.
41 Reed, *Schubert: The Final Years*, p. 215.
42 McKay, *Franz Schubert*, p. 320.
43 Reed, John: *Schubert*, The Master Musicians, p. 166, Oxford University Press, 1997.
44 Newbould, *Schubert: The Music and the Man*, pp. 128–31.
45 Reed, *Schubert* (1997), p. 166.
46 Sams, 'Schubert's Illness Re-Examined', p. 22.
47 Sams, 'Schubert's Illness Re-Examined', p. 21.
48 Rold, 'Schubert and Syphilis', p. 234.
   McKay, *Franz Schubert*, pp. 321–5.
49 Newbould, *Schubert: The Music and the Man*, p. 274.
50 McKay, *Franz Schubert*, p. 324.
51 Ibid., p. 325.
52 Ibid., pp. 324–5.
53 Walker, F.: 'Schubert's Last Illness', *Monthly Musical Record* (1947) 27.232.
54 McKay, *Franz Schubert*, p. 329.
55 Newbould, *Schubert: The Music and the Man*, p. 276.
56 McKay, *Franz Schubert*, p. 324.

57 Kurth, R.: lecture given at University of Kansas, March 1989, quoted by Newbould in *Schubert: The Music and the Man*, p. 276.
Bevan, P. G.: lecture given at University of Hull, April 1995, quoted by Newbould in *Schubert: The Music and the Man*, p. 276.
58 Sams, 'Schubert's Illness Re-Examined', p. 21.
McKay, *Franz Schubert*, pp. 329–30.
59 McKay, *Franz Schubert*, pp.327–8.
60 Ibid., pp. 328–30.
61 Sams, 'Schubert's Illness Re-Examined', p. 21.
62 Rold, 'Schubert and Syphilis', p. 234.
63 Bevan, lecture given at University of Hull, April 1995, quoted by Newbould in *Schubert: The Music and the Man*, p. 276.
64 Sams, 'Schubert's Illness Re-Examined', p. 21.
65 Clapham, John: *Smetana*, The Master Musicians Series, pp. 23–30, J. M. Dent and Sons Ltd, London, 1972.
66 Feldmann, H.: 'The Otological Aspects of Bedrich Smetana's Disease' (trans. E. Levin), *Music Review* (1971) 32.233–47.
67 Clapham, *Smetana*, p. 27.
68 Ibid., p. 29.
69 Ibid., p. 38.
70 Feldmann, 'The Otological Aspects of Bedrich Smetana's Disease', pp. 233–47.
71 Clapham, *Smetana*, p. 42.
Feldmann, 'The Otological Aspects of Bedrich Smetana's Disease', p. 234.
72 Clapham, *Smetana*, p. 42.
73 Ibid., p. 42.
74 Ibid., p. 43.
75 Feldmann, 'The Otological Aspects of Bedrich Smetana's Disease', pp. 235–6.
76 Clapham, *Smetana*, p. 44.
77 Feldmann, 'The Otological Aspects of Bedrich Smetana's Disease', p. 239.
78 Katz, D.: 'Smetana's First String Quartet: Voice of Madness or Triumph of Spirit?', *Musical Quarterly* (1997) 81.516–36.
79 Large, Brian: *Smetana*, p. 322–3, Duckworth, London, 1970.
80 Clapham, *Smetana*, p. 46.
81 Ibid., pp. 51, 47.
82 Ibid., p. 49.
83 Ibid., p. 50.
84 Large, *Smetana*, p. 370.
85 Clapham, *Smetana*, p. 51.
86 Ibid., p. 53.
87 Large, *Smetana*, pp. 370–2.
88 Ibid., pp. 372–3.
89 Katz, 'Smetana's First String Quartet: Voice of Madness or Triumph of Spirit?', p. 519.
90 Ibid., p. 518.
91 Clapham, *Smetana*, pp. 47, 54.
Large, *Smetana*, pp. 382–4.
92 Large, *Smetana*, p. 381.
93 Clapham, *Smetana*, pp. 55–6.
94 Clapham, *Smetana*, p. 56.

      Large, *Smetana*, pp. 390–3.

 95 Large, *Smetana*, p. 393.

 96 Levin, Ernst: 'Smetana's Post Mortem', Appx. E, in John Clapham, *Smetana*, pp. 150–2.

 97 'Bedřich Smetana', Wikipedia, accessed October 2016.

 98 Ramba, Jiří: *Famous Czech Skulls*, pp. 157–9, Galen, Prague, 2nd edn, 2009.

 99 Fenby, Eric: *Delius As I Knew Him*, p. 253, Faber & Faber Ltd, London, 1981.

100 Lee-Browne, Martin, and Guinery, Paul: *Delius and his Music*, p. 64, Boydell Press, Woodbridge, 2014.

      Wainapel, S.F.: 'Frederick Delius: Medical Assessment', *New York State Journal of Medicine* (1980) 80.1886–7.

      Jefferson, Alan: *Delius*, The Master Musicians Series, p. 33, J. M. Dent and Sons Ltd, London, 1972.

101 Lee-Browne and Guinery, *Delius and his Music*, pp. 259.

102 Wainapel, 'Frederick Delius', pp. 1886–7.

103 Lee-Browne and Guinery, *Delius and his Music*, p. 292.

104 Fenby, Eric: *Delius*, The Great Composers Series, p. 73, Faber & Faber, London, 1971.

105 Jefferson, *Delius*, p. 77.

106 Ibid., p. 80.

107 Ibid., pp. 82–3.

108 Payne, A., and Anderson, R.: 'Delius, Frederick', Grove Online, accessed 20 April 2010.

109 Fenby, *Delius As I Knew Him*, p. 9.

      Fenby, *Delius*, p. 77.

110 Foss, H.: 'The Instrumental Music of Frederick Delius', *Tempo* (1952–53) 26.30–7.

111 Jefferson, *Delius*, p. 84.

112 Russell, Ken: *Delius: Song of Summer*, BBC TV (1968), available on DVD, Archive Television, BBC Worldwide Ltd, 2001.

113 Ibid.

114 Warlock, Peter: *Delius* (rev. Hugo Foss), p. 183, The Bodley Head, London, 1952.

115 Cardus, Neville: *A Composer's Eleven*, p. 215, Jonathan Cape, London, 1958.

116 Redwood, Christopher (ed.): *A Delius Companion*, p. 93, John Calder, London, 1976.

117 Ibid., p. 93.

118 Elgar, Sir Edward: My Visit to Delius, *Daily Telegraph*, 1 July 1933.

119 Fenby, *Delius As I Knew Him*, p. 40.

120 Jefferson, *Delius*, p. 91.

121 Carley, Lionel: *Delius: A Life in Letters (1909–1934)*, pp. 446–7, Scholar Press, Aldershot, 1988.

122 Jefferson, *Delius*, p. 91.

123 Kennedy, Michael: personal communication (July 2014).

124 Walker, Frank: *Hugo Wolf*, p. 77, J. M. Dent & Sons Ltd, London, 1951.

125 Ibid., p. 77.

126 Sams, Eric, and Youens, Susan: 'Wolf, Hugo' in *The New Grove Dictionary of Music and Musicians*, 2nd edn (ed. Stanley Sadie and John Tyrrell), vol. 27, p. 465, Macmillan Publishers, London, 2001.

127 Newman, Ernest: *Hugo Wolf*, p. 62. Dover Publications, New York, 1966.

128 Walker, *Hugo Wolf*, pp. 191–2, 268, 279.

129 Sams and Youens, 'Wolf, Hugo', p. 470.

130 Ibid., p. 470.

131 Walker, *Hugo Wolf*, p. 303.

132 Ibid., p. 410.

133 Newman, *Hugo Wolf*, p. 144.

134 Walker, *Hugo Wolf*, p. 415.

135 Ibid., p. 420.

136 Ibid., p. 420.

137 Ibid., p. 424.

138 Ibid., p. 425.

139 Ibid., p. 432 and ibid. p. 438.

140 Ibid., p. 439.

141 Sams and Youens, 'Wolf, Hugo', p. 472.

142 Walker, *Hugo Wolf*, p. 442.

143 Ibid., p. 447.

144 Sams and Youens, 'Wolf, Hugo', p. 488.

145 Steen, Michael: *The Lives and Times of the Great Composers*, 'Donizetti', p. 293, Icon Books Ltd, London, 2010.

146 Weinstock, Herbert: *Donizetti and the World of Opera in Italy, Paris and Vienna in the First Half of the 19th Century*, p. 106, Methuen & Co., London, 1964.
Ashbrook, William: *Donizetti and his Operas*, pp. 550–2, Cambridge University Press, Cambridge, UK, 1982.

147 Smart, Mary Ann, and Budden, Julian: 'Donizetti, (Domenico) Gaetano' in *The New Grove Dictionary of Music and Musicians*, 2nd edn, vol. 7, p. 477.

148 Weinstock, *Donizetti and the World of Opera*, pp. 116, 126.

149 Ibid., p. 116.

150 Ibid., p. 116.

151 Ibid., p. 227.

152 Ibid., p. 227.

153 Ashbrook W. and Budden, Julian: 'Donizetti, (Domenico) Gaetano' in *The New Grove Dictionary of Music and Musicians*, 1980, vol. 5, p. 556.

154 Ashbrook, *Donizetti and his Operas*, pp. 184–90.

155 Ibid., p. 192.

156 Steen, *The Lives and Times of the Great Composers*, 'Donizetti', p. 300.

157 Weinstock, *Donizetti and the World of Opera*, pp. 234, 237.

158 Steen, *The Lives and Times of the Great Composers*, 'Donizetti', pp. 301.

159 Weinstock, *Donizetti and the World of Opera*, pp. 267–8.

160 Steen, *The Lives and Times of the Great Composers*, 'Donizetti', p. 301.

161 Ashbrook, *Donizetti and his Operas*, pp. 202, 671.

162 Donizetti Society website, accessed October 2016.

163 Ashbrook, *Donizetti and his Operas*, pp. 190–1.
Smart and Budden, 'Donizetti', p. 477.

164 Engel, Louis: *From Mozart to Mario: Reminiscences of Half a Century*, vol. 2, p. 70, Richard Bentley and Son, London, 1886.

165 Delage, R.: 'Ravel and Chabrier', *Musical Quarterly* (1975) 61.4.

166 Poulenc, Francis: *Emmanuel Chabrier*, p. 8, La Palatine, Paris, 1961.

167 Huebner, Steven: 'Chabrier, (Alexis-)Emmanuel' in *The New Grove Dictionary of Music and Musicians*, 2nd edn, vol. 5, p. 404.

168 Ibid., p. 405.

169 Ibid. p. 405.

170 Howat, Roy: personal communication (May 2015).

171 Hayden, *Pox*, pp. 71–88, 97–111.

Chapter 5

1 Šostar, Z., Vodanović, M., Breitenfeld, D., et al.: 'Composers – Substance Abusers', *Alcoholism* (2009) 45.127–42.

2 Kessel, Neil, and Walton, Henry: *Alcoholism*, pp. 15–22, Penguin Books, Harmondsworth, 1965.

3 World Health Organization: *Problems Related to Alcohol Consumption*, WHO Technical Report Series, No. 650, Geneva, World Health Organization, 1980.

4 Kessel and Walton, *Alcoholism*, pp. 16–27.

5 Leontaridi, R.: *Alcohol Misuse: How Much Does it Cost?*, Cabinet Office Strategy Unit, London, September 2003.

6 Kessel and Walton, *Alcoholism*, p. 60.

7 Tait, Ian: personal communication (2012).

8 Kessel and Walton, *Alcoholism*, p. 16.

9 Smith, Barry: *Peter Warlock: The Life of Philip Heseltine*, p. 277, Oxford University Press, 1994.

10 Macdonald, Hugh: 'Skryabin, Alexander (Nikolayevich)' in *The New Grove Dictionary of Music and Musicians* (ed. Stanley Sadie), vol. 17, p. 371, Macmillan Publishers, London, 1980.

11 Meredith, Anthony, and Harris, Paul: *Malcolm Arnold: Rogue Genius*, pp. 74–5, Thames/Elkin, London, 2004.

12 Ibid., p. 110.

13 Ibid., pp. 112, 179.

14 Ibid., p. 182.

15 Ibid., p. 217.

16 Ibid., 232–5.

17 Cole, Hugo: *Malcolm Arnold: Introduction to his Music*, p. 6, Faber Music, London, 1989.

18 Meredith and Harris, *Malcolm Arnold*, pp. 335–7.

19 Ibid., p. 362–3.

20 Ibid., p. 391.

21 Ibid., p. 396–8.

22 Ibid., p. 454.

23 Ibid., p. 400.

24 Ibid., p. 511.

25 Lambert, Constant: in *Music Ho!*, 'Erik Satie and his Musique d'Ameublement', pp. 115–26, Hogarth Press, London, 1985.

26 Crichton, Ronald: 'Lambert, (Leonard) Constant' in *The New Grove Dictionary of Music and Musicians*, vol. 10, p. 395.

27 Shead, Richard: *Constant Lambert*, Simon Publications, p. 118, London, 1973.

28 Crichton, 'Lambert, (Leonard) Constant', p. 396.

29 Shead, *Constant Lambert*, p. 173.

30 Ibid., p. 172.

31 Ibid., p. 160.

32 Temperley, Nicholas: 'Field, John' in *The New Grove Dictionary of Music and Musicians*, vol. 6, p. 535.

33 Piggott, Patrick: *The Life and Music of John Field, 1782–1837: Creator of the Nocturne*, pp. 22–4, University of California Press, Berkeley and Los Angeles,1973.
   Temperley, 'Field, John', p. 535.

34 Piggott, *The Life and Music of John Field*, pp. 65, 71.
   Temperley, 'Field, John', p. 535.

35 Piggott, *The Life and Music of John Field*, p. 65.

36 Temperley, 'Field, John', p. 535.

37 Ibid.

38 Piggott, *The Life and Music of John Field*, p. 97.

39 Ibid., pp. 96–7.

40 Ibid., p. 97.

41 Temperley, 'Field, John', p. 535.

42 Piggott, *The Life and Music of John Field*, p. 97.

43 Ibid., pp. 98–9.

44 Orledge, Robert: *Satie the Composer*, Music in the Twentieth Century, p. xix, Cambridge University Press, Cambridge, UK, 1990.

45 Orledge, Robert: 'Satie, Erik' in *The New Grove Dictionary of Music and Musicians*, 2nd edn (ed. Stanley Sadie and John Tyrrell), vol. 22, p. 313, Macmillan Publishers, London, 2001.

46 Ibid., p. 313.

47 Ibid., p. 314.

48 Orledge, Robert: *Satie the Composer*, p. 65.

49 Ibid., pp. 19–20.

50 Ibid., p. 19.

51 Gillmor, Alan: *Erik Satie*, p. 113, Macmillan Press Ltd, London, 1988.

52 Ibid., p. 97.

53 Orledge, *Satie the Composer*, p. 39.

54 Kessel and Walton, *Alcoholism*, pp. 57–64.

55 Lambert, *Music Ho!*, pp. 115–26.

56 Calvocoressi, M. D.: *Mussorgsky*, The Master Musicians Series (completed and revised by Gerald Abraham), p. 7, J. M. Dent & Sons Ltd, London, 1974.
   Emerson, Caryl: *The Life of Musorgsky*, p. 25, Cambridge University Press, Cambridge, UK, 1999.

57 Brown, David: *Musorgsky: His Life and Works*, The Master Musicians, p. 5, Oxford University Press, 2010.

58 Emerson, *The Life of Musorgsky*, p. 21.

59 Calvocoressi, *Mussorgsky*, pp. 9–10.

60 Seroff, Victor: *Modest Moussorgsky*, p. 34–5, Funk & Wagnalls, New York, 1968.

61 Ibid., pp. 37–8.

62 Ibid., p. 45.

63 Emerson, *The Life of Musorgsky*, p. 32.

64 Seroff, *Modest Moussorgsky*, pp. 33–4, 36.

65 Brown, *Musorgsky*, p. 357.

66 Seroff, *Modest Moussorgsky*, pp. 102–3.

67 Ibid., pp. 103–4.

68 Ibid., pp. 52–4.

69 Calvocoressi, *Mussorgsky*, p. 18.

70 Seroff, *Modest Moussorgsky*, pp. 63–5.

71 Calvocoressi, *Mussorgsky*, p. 28.

72 Emerson, *The Life of Musorgsky*, p. 78.
    Calvocoressi, *Mussorgsky*, p. 33.
73 Calvocoressi, *Mussorgsky*, p. 32.
74 Brown, *Musorgsky*, pp. 74–5, 116.
75 Ibid., p. 130.
76 Seroff, *Modest Moussorgsky*, pp. 124–6.
77 Ibid., p. 126.
78 Emerson, *The Life of Musorgsky*, p. 122–3.
79 Brown, *Musorgsky*, pp. 249–50.
80 Seroff, *Modest Moussorgsky*, p. 154–5.
81 Brown, *Musorgsky*, p. 297.
82 Seroff, *Modest Moussorgsky*, p. 158.
83 Ibid., p. 158.
84 Ibid., pp. 162–3.
85 Ibid., p. 162.
86 Brown, *Musorgsky*, p. 339.
87 Seroff, *Modest Moussorgsky*, p. 164.
88 Ibid., p. 165.
89 Calvocoressi, *Mussorgsky*, pp. 59–60.
90 Ibid.
91 Brown, *Musorgsky*, pp. 356–7.
    Seroff, *Modest Moussorgsky*, pp. 173–5.
92 Emerson, *The Life of Musorgsky*, p. 153.
93 Seroff, *Modest Moussorgsky*, pp. 174–5.
94 Ibid., p. 174.
95 Ibid., p. 175.
96 Calvocoressi, *Mussorgsky*, p. 60.
97 Emerson, *The Life of Musorgsky*, p. 95.
98 Schonberg, Harold: *The Lives of the Great Composers*, 'Russian Nationalism and the Mighty Five', p. 406, Abacus, London, 2010.
99 Schwarz, Boris: 'Glazunov, Alexander Konstantinovich' in *The New Grove Dictionary of Music and Musicians*, vol. 7, p. 428.
100 Seroff, *Modest Moussorgsky*, p. 176.
101 Schwarz, 'Glazunov, Alexander Konstantinovich', p. 428.
102 Norris, Geoffrey: *Rachmaninoff*, The Dent Master Musicians, 2nd edn, pp. 22–3, J. M. Dent & Sons Ltd, London, 1993.
103 Ibid., p. 23.
    Venturim, Daniel J.: *Alexander Glazunov. His Life and Works*, p. 20, Aero Printing, Delphos, Ohio, 1992.
104 Norris, *Rachmaninoff*, p. 23.
105 Schwarz, 'Glazunov, Alexander Konstantinovich', p. 428.
106 Fay, Laurel E.: *Shostakovich: A Life*, p. 21, Oxford University Press, Oxford, 2000.
107 Ibid., p. 292, note 13.
    Volkov, Solomon: *Testimony: The Memoirs of Dmitri Shostakovich* (trans. Antonina W. Bouis), p. 35, Hamish Hamilton, London, 1979.
108 Volkov, *Testimony*, p. 35.
109 Ibid., p. 36.
110 Schwarz, 'Glazunov, Alexander Konstantinovich', p. 429.
    Venturim, *Alexander Glazunov*, pp. 36–7.

111 Volkov, *Testimony*, p. 127.
112 Frolova-Walker, Marina: Personal Communication, November, 2017.
113 Schwarz, 'Glazunov, Alexander Konstantinovich', pp. 428–9.
114 Fay, *Shostakovich*, p. 292, note 13.
115 Fay, Laurel E.: 'Shostakovich vs Volkov: Whose Testimony?' *Russian View* (October 1980) 484–93.
116 Schwarz, 'Glazunov, Alexander Konstantinovich', pp. 428–9.
117 Venturim, *Alexander Glazunov*, p. 47.

Chapter 6

1 Juda, A.: 'The Relationship between Highest Mental Capacity and Psychic Abnormalities', *American Journal of Psychiatry* (1949) 106.296–307.
Ludwig, A. M.: 'Reflections on Creativity and Madness', *American Journal of Psychotherapy* (1989) 153.4–14.
Frosch, W. A..: 'Madness and Music', *Comprehensive Psychiatry* (1987) 28.315–22.
2 Ludwig, 'Reflections on Creativity and Madness', pp. 4–5.
3 Ostwald, Peter F.: *Schumann: Music and Madness*, p. 274, Victor Gollancz Ltd, London, 1985.
Jensen, Eric Frederick: *Schumann*, The Master Musicians, p. 279, Oxford University Press, Oxford, 2001.
4 Musgrave, Michael: *The Life of Schumann*, Musical Lives, p. 166, Cambridge University Press, Cambridge, UK, 2011.
5 Rietschel, E. T., Rietschel, M., and Beutler, B.: 'How the Mighty have Fallen: Fatal Infectious Diseases of Divine Composers', *Infectious Disease Clinics of North America* (2004) 18.311–339 (pp. 314–16).
Franken, F. H.: *Die Krankheiten grosser Komponisten*, vol. 4, 'Robert Schumann', Florian Noetzel Verlag GmbH, Wilhelmshaven, 1997.
6 Ostwald, *Schumann: Music and Madness*, p. xiii.
7 Musgrave, *The Life of Schumann*, p. 175.
Rietschel, 'How the Mighty have Fallen', p. 315.
8 Abraham, Gerald: 'Schumann, Robert (Alexander)' in *The New Grove Dictionary of Music and Musicians* (ed. Stanley Sadie), p. 831, Macmillan Publishers, London, 1980.
9 Musgrave, *The Life of Schumann*, p. 20.
Ostwald, P. F.: 'Robert Schumann and his Doctors', *American Journal of Social Psychiatry* (1983) 3.5–15 (p. 6).
10 Ostwald, 'Robert Schumann and his Doctors', p. 6.
11 Sams, E.: 'Schumann's Hand Injury', *Musical Times* (1971) 112.1156–9.
12 Jensen, *Schumann*, pp. 22–3.
13 Sams, 'Schumann's Hand Injury', pp. 1156–9.
Ostwald, *Schumann: Music and Madness*, p. 82.
14 Henson, R. A., and Urich, H.: 'Schumann's Hand Injury', *British Medical Journal* (1978) 1.900–3.
15 Jensen, *Schumann*, p. 69.
16 Ibid., p. 69.
17 Henson and Urich, 'Schumann's Hand Injury', pp. 900–3.
18 Jensen, *Schumann*, p. 70.
19 Ibid., p. 70.

20 Sams, 'Schumann's Hand Injury', p. 1156.

21 Ibid., p. 1156.

22 Henson and Urich, 'Schumann's Hand Injury', p. 901.

23 Eismann, G.: *Robert Schumann 1827–1838* (ed. G. Eismann), vol. 1, p.74, VEB Deutscher Verlag für Musik, Leipzig, 1971 (originally published 1957).

24 Ostwald, *Schumann: Music and Madness*, p. 75.

25 Worthen, John: *Robert Schumann, Life and Death of a Musician*, pp. 72–3, Yale University Press, London, 2010.

26 Slater, E., and Meyer, A.: 'Contributions to a Pathography of the Musicians: 1. Robert Schumann', Confinia Psychiatrica (1959) 2.65–94.
   Slater, Eliot: 'Schumann's Illness' in *Robert Schumann: The Man and his Music* (ed. Alan Walker), pp. 406–14, Barrie and Jenkins Ltd, London, 1972.

27 Henson and Urich, 'Schumann's Hand Injury', p. 901.
   Ostwald, *Schumann: Music and Madness*, p. 90.

28 Henson and Urich, 'Schumann's Hand Injury', p. 901.

29 Ibid., p. 901.

30 Ibid., p. 901.
   Ostwald, *Schumann: Music and Madness*, pp. 89–90.

31 Ostwald, *Schumann: Music and Madness*, pp. 177–8.

32 Carerj, L.: 'Le Mano Invalida di Robert Schumann', *Nuova rivista musicale italiana* (1979) 13.609–19.

33 Henson and Urich, 'Schumann's Hand Injury', p. 901.

34 Stanley, J. K.: 'Radial Tunnel Syndrome', *Journal of Hand Therapy* (2006) 19.180–4.

35 Charness, M. E.: 'Upper Extremity Disorders of Musicians' in *Occupational Disorders of the Upper Extremity* (ed. L. H. Millender, D. S. Louis and B. P. Simmonds), pp. 117–51, Churchill Livingstone, New York, 1992.

36 Henson and Urich, 'Schumann's Hand Injury', p. 902.

37 Ibid., p. 902.

38 Barton, N. J., Hooper, G., Noble, J., and Steel, W. M.: 'Occupational Causes of Disorders in the Upper Limb', *British Medical Journal* (1992) 304.309–11.

39 Henson and Urich, 'Schumann's Hand Injury', p. 901.

40 Pickering, George: *Creative Malady: Illness in the Lives of Charles Darwin, Florence Nightingale, Mary Baker Eddy, Sigmund Freud, Marcel Proust, Elizabeth Barrett Browning*, George Allen and Unwin Ltd, London, 1972.

41 Lederman, R. J.: 'Robert Schumann', *Seminars in Neurology* (1999) 19 (Suppl. 1).17–24 (p. 19).

42 Musgrave, *The Life of Schumann*, p. 58.

43 Ostwald, *Schumann: Music and Madness*, p. 97.

44 Ibid., pp. 151–6.

45 Ibid., p. 175.

46 Ibid., pp. 173–5.

47 Ibid., p. 186.

48 Ostwald, *Schumann: Music and Madness*, p. 194.

49 Ostwald, 'Robert Schumann and his Doctors', p. 11.
   Lederman, 'Robert Schumann', p. 20.

50 Lederman, 'Robert Schumann', p. 20.

51 Slater and Meyer, 'Contributions to a Pathography of the Musicians: 1. Robert Schumann', p. 76.

52 Musgrave, *The Life of Schumann*, p. 127.

53 Ostwald, *Schumann: Music and Madness*, p. 204.

54 Ibid., p. 219.

55 Ibid., p. 238.

56 Ibid., pp. 253–4.

57 Ibid., pp. 240–1.

58 Musgrave, *The Life of Schumann*, pp. 159–60.

59 Ibid., pp. 159–60.
  Jensen, *Schumann*, pp. 270–1.

60 Jensen, *Schumann*, pp. 270–1.

61 Ostwald, *Schumann: Music and Madness*, p. 257.

62 Ibid., pp. 255–6.

63 Jensen, *Schumann*, p. 264.

64 Ostwald, *Schumann: Music and Madness*, p. 271.

65 Ibid., p. 272.

66 Musgrave, *The Life of Schumann*, p. 165.

67 Ibid., p. 165.

68 Ibid., p. 166.

69 Ibid., p. 166–7.

70 Jensen, *Schumann*, p. 314.

71 Slater and Meyer, 'Contributions to a Pathography of the Musicians: 1. Robert Schumann', p. 77.

72 Musgrave, *The Life of Schumann*, p. 167.
  Jensen, *Schumann*, p. 317.

73 Musgrave, *The Life of Schumann*, p. 167.

74 Jensen, *Schumann*, p. 317.

75 Ostwald, *Schumann: Music and Madness*, p. 285.

76 Jensen, *Schumann*, p. 317.
  Ostwald, *Schumann: Music and Madness*, p. 290.

77 Ostwald, *Schumann: Music and Madness*, pp. 288–9.

78 Jensen, *Schumann*, pp. 321–3.

79 Sams, 'Schumann's Hand Injury', p. 1158.

80 Jensen, *Schumann*, pp. 321–3.

81 Musgrave, *The Life of Schumann*, p. 170.

82 Ostwald, *Schumann: Music and Madness*, p. 286.

83 Jensen, *Schumann*, p. 326.

84 Ostwald, *Schumann: Music and Madness*, p. 279.

85 Lederman, 'Robert Schumann', p. 20.
  Ostwald, *Schumann: Music and Madness*, p. 279.

86 Ostwald, 'Robert Schumann and his Doctors', p. 12.
  Musgrave, *The Life of Schumann*, pp. 278 and 291–2.

87 Jensen, *Schumann*, p. 331.

88 Ibid.

89 Ostwald, *Schumann: Music and Madness*, p. 278.

90 Jensen, *Schumann*, p. 333.

91 Ostwald, *Schumann: Music and Madness*, p. 292.

92 Ibid., p. 292.

93 Ibid., p. 293.

94 Ibid., pp. 295–8.

95 Jänisch, W., and Nauhaus, G.: 'Autopsy Report of the Corpse of the Composer

Robert Schumann: Publication and Interpretation of a Rediscovered Document',
Zentralblatt Fur Allgemeine Pathologie und Pathologische Anatomie (1986) 132.129–36.

96 Ostwald, *Schumann: Music and Madness*, pp. 204 and 298.

97 Ibid., p. 75.

98 Ostwald, P. F.: 'Florestan, Eusebius, Clara, and Schumann's Right Hand', *19th Century Music* (1980) 4.17–31 (p. 18).
Jensen, *Schumann*, p. 329.

99 Ostwald, 'Robert Schumann and his Doctors', p. 11.
Ostwald, *Schumann: Music and Madness*, pp. 193–4.

100 O'Shea, John: *Music and Medicine: Profiles of Great Composers*, 'Robert Schumann', p. 136, J. M. Dent & Sons Ltd, London, 1990.

101 Worthen, John: *Robert Schumann: Life and Death of a Musician*, p. 368.

102 Ostwald, *Schumann: Music and Madness*, pp. 299–300.

103 Worthen, *Robert Schumann*, p. 374.

104 Ibid., pp. 366–8.

105 Jensen, *Schumann*, p. 329.

106 Slater and Meyer, 'Contributions to a Pathography of the Musicians: 1. Robert Schumann', pp. 92–3.

107 Ostwald, *Schumann: Music and Madness*, pp. 291–3.

108 Ibid., p. 292.

109 Sams, 'Schumann's Hand Injury', pp. 1156–9.
Ostwald, *Schumann: Music and Madness*, p. 75.

110 Sams, E., 'Schumann's Hand Injury: Some Further Evidence'. *Musical Times* (1972) 113.456.

111 Henson and Urich, 'Schumann's Hand Injury', p. 902.

112 Sams, 'Schumann's Hand Injury: Some Further Evidence', p. 456.

113 Ibid., p. 456.

114 Sams, 'Schumann's Hand Injury', p. 1156.

115 Ibid., p. 1157.

116 Ostwald, *Schumann: Music and Madness*, p. 272.

117 Ibid., p. 277.

118 Ibid., p. 305.

119 Slater and Meyer, 'Contributions to a Pathography of the Musicians: 1. Robert Schumann', p. 91.

120 Jensen, *Schumann*, pp. 308–9.

121 Grühle, H.: 'Brief über Robert Schumanns Krankheit an P. J. Möbius', *Zentralblatt für Nervenheilkunde* (1906) 29.805–10.
Ostwald, *Schumann: Music and Madness*, pp. 300–1.

122 Jensen, *Schumann*, p. 330.

123 Adorno, Theodor W.: *Mahler: A Musical Physiognomy*, p. 66, University of Chicago Press, Chicago, 1996.

124 Floros, Constantin: *Anton Bruckner: The Man and the Work* (English trans. Ernest Bernhardt-Kabisch), 2nd rev. edn, p. 99, Peter Lang GmbH, Frankfurt am Main, 2015.

125 Watson, Derek: *Bruckner*, The Master Musicians, 2nd edn, pp. 40–1, Oxford University Press, Oxford, 1997.

126 Redlich, Hans F.: *Bruckner and Mahler*, The Master Musicians Series, pp. 7–8, J. M. Dent & Sons Ltd, London, 1963.

127 Ibid., p. 7.

128 Ibid., p. 8.

129 Floros, *Anton Bruckner*, p. 16.

130 Watson, *Bruckner*, p. 14.

131 Floros, *Anton Bruckner*, pp. 22–4.
     Watson, *Bruckner*, pp. 15, 18, 19, 48–9.

132 Watson, *Bruckner*, p. 39.

133 Floros, *Anton Bruckner*, p. 20.

134 Ibid., p. 20.

135 Neumayr, Anton: *Music & Medicine*, vol. 2, *Hummel, Weber, Mendelssohn, Schumann, Brahms, Bruckner* (trans. B. C. Clarke), 'Bruckner', p. 507, Medi-Ed Press, Bloomington, Illinois, 1995.

136 Horton, Julian: *Bruckner's Symphonies: Analysis Reception and Cultural Politics*, pp. 247, 256–7, Cambridge University Press, Cambridge, UK, 2004.

137 Redlich, *Bruckner and Mahler*, pp. 28–9.

138 Floros, *Anton Bruckner*, p. 18.
     Neumayr, *Music & Medicine*, vol. 2, 'Bruckner', p. 507.

139 Neumayr, *Music & Medicine*, vol. 2, 'Bruckner', p. 508.

140 Ibid., pp. 508–9.

141 Ibid., p. 510.

142 Ibid., pp. 510–12.

143 Watson, *Bruckner*, p. 25.

144 Ibid., pp. 25–6.

145 Ibid., p. 48.

146 Neumayr, *Music & Medicine*, vol. 2, 'Bruckner', pp. 522–3.

147 Ibid., p. 517.

148 Ibid., p. 521.

149 Ibid., p. 523.

150 Watson, *Bruckner*, pp. 38–9.

151 Ibid., p. 39.

152 Cooke, Deryck: 'The Bruckner Problem Simplified', *Musical Times* (January–May 1969) 110, 59–62.

153 Watson, *Bruckner*, p. 48.

154 Neumayr, *Music & Medicine*, vol. 2, 'Bruckner', pp. 530–2.

155 Ibid., pp. 532–3.

156 Ibid., pp. 532–3.

157 Ibid., pp. 532–6.

158 Ibid., p. 527.

159 Ibid., pp. 538–40.

160 Ibid., pp. 543–4.

161 Ibid., pp. 541–3.

162 Ibid., p. 540.

163 Ibid., p. 548.

164 Ibid., p. 551.

165 Floros, *Anton Bruckner*, p. 157.

166 Neumayr, *Music & Medicine*, vol. 2, 'Bruckner', p. 551.

167 Cooke, 'The Bruckner Problem Simplified'.

168 Poznansky, Alexander: *Tchaikovsky: The Quest for the Inner Man*, p. 608, Lime Tree, London, 1993.

169 Poznansky, Alexander: *Tchaikovsky's Last Days: A Documentary Study*, p. 134, Clarendon Press, Oxford, 1996.

170 Neumayr, Anton: *Music & Medicine*, vol. 3, *Chopin, Smetana, Tchaikovsky, Mahler* (English trans. D. J. Parent), 'Tchaikovsky', p. 216, Medi-Ed Press, Bloomington, Illinois, 1997.

171 Ibid., p. 217.

172 Ibid., p. 217.

173 Ibid., p. 220.

174 Garden, Edward: *Tchaikovsky*, The Master Musicians Series, p. 20, J. M. Dent & Sons Ltd, London, 1973.

175 Ibid., p. 20.

176 Neumayr, *Music & Medicine*, vol. 3, 'Tchaikovsky', pp. 231–2.

177 Holden, Anthony, *Tchaikovsky*, pp. 356–7, Bantam Press, London, 1995
Wiley, Roland J., *Tchaikovsky*, p. 446, The Master Musicians, Oxford University Press, 2009.

178 Holden, Anthony: *Tchaikovsky*, pp. 61, 316.

179 Poznansky, *Tchaikovsky's Last Days*, p. 11.

180 Neumayr, *Music & Medicine*, vol. 3, Tchaikovsky', p. 236.

181 Poznansky, *Tchaikovsky's Last Days*, p. 9.

182 Ibid., pp. 1–5.

183 Ibid., pp. 4–5.

184 Poznansky, A.: 'Tchaikovsky: The Man Behind the Myth', *Musical Times* (1992) 13.175–82.

185 Holden, *Tchaikovsky*, p. 313.
Brown, David: *Tchaikovsky: A Biographical and Critical Study*, vol. 4, *The Final Years 1885–93*, p. 474, Victor Gollancz, London, 1991.

186 Garden, *Tchaikovsky*, p. 72.

187 Poznansky, 'Tchaikovsky: The Man Behind the Myth', p. 179.
Garden, *Tchaikovsky*, pp. 74–5.

188 Garden, *Tchaikovsky*, p. 73.

189 Poznansky, *Tchaikovsky's Last Days*, pp. 15–16.

190 Holden, *Tchaikovsky*, p. 132.

191 Poznansky, *Tchaikovsky's Last Days*, p. 16.

192 Garden, *Tchaikovsky*, p. 77.
Poznansky, 'Tchaikovsky: The Man Behind the Myth', pp. 180–1.

193 Holden, *Tchaikovsky*, p. 149.

194 Garden, *Tchaikovsky*, pp. 77–8.

195 Ibid., p. 78.

196 Ibid., p. 78.

197 Ibid., p. 78.

198 Ibid., pp. 77–8.

199 Holden, *Tchaikovsky*, pp. 172, 176.

200 Ibid., p. 174.

201 Brown, David: *Tchaikovsky: A Biographical and Critical Study*, vol. 3, *The Years of Wandering 1878–85*, p. 119, Victor Gollancz, London, 1986.

202 Garden, *Tchaikovsky*, p. 100.

203 Poznansky, *Tchaikovsky: The Quest for the Inner Man*, p. 192.

204 Ibid., p. 202.

205 Ibid., p. 202.

206 Garden, Edward, and Gotteri, Nigel: *'To My Best Friend': Correspondence between Tchaikovsky and Nadezhda von Meck* (trans. Galina von Meck), Clarendon Press, Oxford, 1993.

207 Poznansky, *Tchaikovsky's Last Days*, p. 20.

208 Ibid., p. 20.

209 Poznansky, *Tchaikovsky: The Quest for the Inner Man*, p. 489.

210 Brown, *Tchaikovsky: A Biographical and Critical Study*, vol. 4, p. 190.

211 Orlova, Alexandra: *Tchaikovsky: A Self-Portrait*, pp. 373–6, Oxford University Press, Oxford, 1990.

212 Garden, *Tchaikovsky*, pp. 131–2.

213 Brown, David: *Tchaikovsky: The Man and his Music*, p. 393, Faber & Faber Ltd, London, 2006.

214 Poznansky, *Tchaikovsky: The Quest for the Inner Man*, p. 556.

215 Brown, *Tchaikovsky: A Biographical and Critical Study*, vol. 4, p. 466.

216 Poznansky, *Tchaikovsky's Last Days*, pp. 26–7.

217 Poznansky, *Tchaikovsky: The Quest for the Inner Man*, p. 52.
Poznansky, *Tchaikovsky's Last Days*, p. 75.

218 Poznansky, *Tchaikovsky's Last Days*, pp. 26–7, 44.

219 Henschel, Sir George: *Musings and Memories of a Musician*, p. 365, Macmillan and Co. Ltd, London, 1918.

220 Brown, *Tchaikovsky: A Biographical and Critical Study*, vol. 4, p. 475.

221 Poznansky, *Tchaikovsky's Last Days*, p. 171.

222 Ibid., p. 44.

223 Holden, *Tchaikovsky*, p. 360.

224 Poznansky, *Tchaikovsky: The Quest for the Inner Man*, p. 583.

225 Encyclopedia of Brogkauz and Efron, St Petersburg, vol. 37A (1903), pp. 507–15, quoted by Holden, *Tchaikovsky*, p. 472, note 12.

226 Holden, *Tchaikovsky*, pp 359–60.

227 Poznansky, *Tchaikovsky: The Quest for the Inner Man*, p. 596.

228 Brown, *Tchaikovsky: A Biographical and Critical Study*, vol. 4, p. 481.

229 Poznansky, *Tchaikovsky's Last Days*, pp. 27–8.

230 Ibid., p. 28.

231 Ibid., p. 28.

232 Ibid., p. 28.

233 Ibid., pp. 67, 171.

234 Poznansky, *Tchaikovsky: The Quest for the Inner Man*, p. 579.

235 Poznansky, *Tchaikovsky's Last Days*, p. 71.

236 Ibid., pp. 73–5.

237 Ibid., p. 81.

238 Ibid., p. 83.

239 Ibid., p. 86.

240 Ibid., pp. 121–41.

241 Poznansky, *Tchaikovsky: The Quest for the Inner Man*, p. 592.

242 Poznansky, 'Tchaikovsky's Suicide: Myth or Reality', *19th Century Music* (1988) 11/3, pp. 199–220.

243 Poznansky, *Tchaikovsky's Last Days*, pp. 130, 137, 139–40.

244 Ibid., pp. 173–80.

245 Poznansky, 'Tchaikovsky's Suicide: Myth or Reality', p. 208.

246 Poznansky, *Tchaikovsky's Last Days*, p. 177.

247 Brown, *Tchaikovsky: A Biographical and Critical Study*, vol. 4, p. 482.

248 Brown, David: 'Tchaikovsky' in *The New Grove Dictionary of Music and Musicians*, vol. 18, p. 628.

249 Brown, *Tchaikovsky: A Biographical and Critical Study*, vol. 4, p. 485.

250 Brown, *Tchaikovsky: The Man and his Music*, p. 435.

251 Brown, *Tchaikovsky: A Biographical and Critical Study*, vol. 4, pp. 482–5.

252 Ibid., pp. 478, 483–4.
Holden, *Tchaikovsky*, p. 376.

253 Orlova, *Tchaikovsky*, pp. 411–14.

254 Wiley, *Tchaikovsky*, p. 444.

255 Holden, *Tchaikovsky*, p. 373.

256 Holden, *Tchaikovsky*, p. 373.
Poznansky, *Tchaikovsky: The Quest for the Inner Man*, p. 605.

257 Holden, *Tchaikovsky*, p. 374.

258 Berberova, N., Brown, M., and Karlinsky, S.: 'Tchaikovsky's Suicide Reconsidered: A Rebuttal', *High Fidelity* (1981) 31, pp. 49–51.

259 Woodside, M., 'Comment & Chronicle', *19th Century Music* (1990) 13.273–4.

260 Holden, *Tchaikovsky*, p. 374.

261 Poznansky, *Tchaikovsky's Last Days*, pp. 71–6.
Brown, *Tchaikovsky: A Biographical and Critical Study*, vol. 4, p. 479.

262 Poznansky, *Tchaikovsky's Last Days*, pp. 76–7.

263 Brown, *Tchaikovsky: A Biographical and Critical Study*, vol. 4, pp. 479–80.
Poznansky, *Tchaikovsky's Last Days*, p. 81.

264 Stuttaford, Thomas: 'How Did the Great Composer Die?', *The Times*, 4 November 1993.

265 Sweeting, Adam: 'How Did Tchaikovsky Die?', *Daily Telegraph*, 15 January 2007.

266 Poznansky, *Tchaikovsky's Last Days*, pp. 216–17.

267 Ibid., p. 214.

268 Mari, F., Polletini, A., Lippi, D., and Bertol, E.: 'The Mysterious Death of Francesco I de'Medici and Bianca Capello', *British Medical Journal* (2006) 331.1299–1301.

269 Kingston, R. L., Hall, S., and Sioris, L.: 'Clinical Observations and Medical Outcome in 149 Cases of Arsenate Ant Killer Ingestion', *Clinical Toxicology* (1993) 31.581–91.

270 Poznansky, 'Tchaikovsky's Suicide: Myth or Reality', p. 207.

271 Poznansky, *Tchaikovsky's Last Days*, p. 218.

272 Holden, *Tchaikovsky*, p. 398.

273 Hindemarsh, J. T.: 'Caveats in Hair Analysis in Chronic Arsenic Poisoning', *Clinical Biochemistry* (2002) 35.1–11.

274 Holden, *Tchaikovsky*, p. 379.

275 Brown, 'Tchaikovsky', p 626.

276 Brown, *Tchaikovsky: The Man and his Music*, p. 435.

277 Wiley, *Tchaikovsky*, p. 443.

278 Poznansky, *Tchaikovsky's Last Days*, p. 11.

279 Holden, *Tchaikovsky*, p. 394.

280 Ibid., p. 337.

281 Ibid., p. 339.

282 Ibid., p. 350.

283 Poznansky, *Tchaikovsky's Last Days*, p. 89.

284 Ibid., pp. 76–8.

285 Brown, David: *Tchaikovsky Remembered*, pp. 210–11, Faber & Faber, London, 1993.

Poznansky, *Tchaikovsky's Last Days*, p. 81.

286 Brown, *Tchaikovsky Remembered*, p. 212.

287 Poznansky, *Tchaikovsky: The Quest for the Inner Man*, p. 573.

288 Brown, *Tchaikovsky: A Biographical and Critical Study*, vol. 4, p. 481.

289 Ibid., p. 481.

290 Poznansky, *Tchaikovsky: The Quest for the Inner Man*, p. 602.

291 Zajaczkowski, Henry: 'The Quest for the Inner Man' (Book Review), *Musical Times* (1992) 133.574.

292 Stuttaford, 'How Did the Great Composer Die?'.

293 Neumayr, *Music & Medicine*, vol. 3, Tchaikovsky', p. 240.

294 Poznansky, *Tchaikovsky: The Quest for the Inner Man*, p. 590.

295 Poznansky, *Tchaikovsky's Last Days*, pp. 170–71.

296 Ober, W. B.: 'Carlo Gesualdo, Prince of Venosa: Murder, Madrigals and Masochism', *Bulletin of the New York Academy of Medicine* (1973) 7 634–45 (p. 635).

297 Ibid., pp. 635–6.

298 Ibid., pp. 635–6.

299 Gray, Cecil, and Heseltine, Philip: *Carlo Gesualdo*, p. 74, Kegan Paul, Trench, Trubner & Co. Ltd, London, 1926.

300 Ober, 'Carlo Gesualdo', p. 637.

301 Ibid., pp. 639–40.

302 Ibid., p. 638.

303 Watkins, Glenn: *Gesualdo: The Man and the Music,* 2nd edn, p. 83, Clarendon Press, Oxford, 1991.

304 Ober, 'Carlo Gesualdo', pp. 644–5.

305 Gray and Heseltine, *Carlo Gesualdo: Musician & Murderer*, pp. 126–8.

306 Ober, 'Carlo Gesualdo', pp. 644–5.

307 Watkins, *Gesualdo: The Man and the Music*, p. 82.

308 Carstairs, Morris, in Stengel, Erwin: *Suicide and Attempted Suicide*, p. 8, Pelican, Penguin Books Ltd, Harmondsworth, 1964.

309 Warlock, Peter: *Delius*, The Bodley Head, London, 1923 (rev. 1952 by Hugo Foss).

310 Shaw, Watkins: 'Clarke, Jeremiah (i)' in *The New Grove Dictionary of Music and Musicians*, vol. 4, pp. 446–8.

311 Smith, Barry: *Peter Warlock: The Life of Philip Heseltine*, p. 277, Oxford University Press, Oxford, 1994.

312 Gray, Cecil: *Peter Warlock: A Memoir of Philip Heseltine*, pp. 218–19, Jonathan Cape, London, 1934.

313 Ibid., p. 215.

314 Collins, Brian: *Peter Warlock: The Composer*, pp. 55, 80, Scholar Press, Aldershot, 1996.

315 Smith, *Peter Warlock*, pp. 279–80.

316 Ibid., pp. 282–3.

317 Gray, *Peter Warlock*, pp. 290–5.

318 Ibid.

319 Smith, *Peter Warlock*, pp. 281–2.

320 Ibid., p. 281.

321 Sewell, Brian: 'Why I will Never Love my Father', *Daily Mail*, 14 November 2011.

322 Brooks, Richard: 'Sewell's Father was Sex Sadist Composer', *Sunday Times*, 13 November 2011.

323 Shaw, 'Clarke, Jeremiah (i)', pp. 446–8.

324 'Famous Suicides by Firearms in UK', Wikipedia, accessed December 2014.

325 Copley, Ian. A.: *The Music of Peter Warlock*, p. 23, Dennis Dobson, London, 1979.

326 Jamison, Kay R.: *Touched by Fire: Manic-Depressive Illness and the Artistic Temperament*, p. 40, Simon and Schuster, New York, 1993.

327 Harcup, J., 'Edward Elgar – a Medical Enigma?', *Elgar Society Journal* (2012) 17.20.

Chapter 7

1 Figes, Orlando: *The Whisperers*, Allen Lane, New York and London, 2007.

2 Fay, Laurel: *Shostakovich: A Life*, pp. 14–15, Oxford University Press, Oxford, 2000.

3 Ibid., p. 21.

4 Ibid., p. 37.

5 Ibid., p. 84.

6 Wilson, Elizabeth: *Shostakovich: A Life Remembered*, pp. 128–9, Faber & Faber, London, 2006.

7 McBurney, Gerard: 'Whose Shostakovich?' in *A Shostakovich Casebook* (ed. M. Hamrick-Brown), p. 287, Indiana University Press, Bloomington, 2002.

8 Wilson, *Shostakovich*, pp. 143–4.

9 Lesser, Wendy: *Music for Silenced Voices: Shostakovich and his Fifteen Quartets*, Yale University Press, New Haven and London, 2011.

10 Fay, *Shostakovich*, p. 102.

11 Wilson, *Shostakovich*, p. 152.

12 Fay, *Shostakovich*, p. 121.

13 Lesser, *Music for Silenced Voices*, p. 36.

14 Ibid., p. 38.

15 Ibid., p. 46.

16 Wilson, *Shostakovich*, p. 203.
Fay, *Shostakovich*, p. 205.

17 Norris, Christopher: 'Shostakovich: Politics and Musical Language' in *Shostakovich: The Man and his Music* (ed. C. Norris), p. 171, Lawrence and Wishart, London, 1982.

18 Taruskin, Richard: *On Russian Music*, p. 304, University of California Press, 2009.
Wilson, *Shostakovich*, pp. 211–12.

19 Nabokov, Nicolas: *Old Friends and New Music*, p. 205, Hamish Hamilton, London, 1951.

20 Fay, *Shostakovich*, pp. 211–12.

21 Ibid., p. 185

22 Ibid., p. 198.

23 Ibid., p. 217.

24 Lesser, *Music for Silenced Voices*, pp. 159–60.

25 Ibid., pp. 147–9.

26 Fay, *Shostakovich*, p. 210.

27 Wilson, *Shostakovich*, p. 440.

28 Pascuzzi, R. M.: 'Shostakovich and Amyotrophic Lateral Sclerosis', *Seminars in Neurology* (1999) 19(1).63–6.

29 Fay, *Shostakovich*, pp. 210, 215.

30 Ibid., p. 222.

31 Ibid., pp. 228–9.

32 Ibid., p. 227.

33 Lesser, *Music for Silenced Voices*, pp. 207–8.

34 Fay, *Shostakovich*, p. 249.

35 Lesser, *Music for Silenced Voices*, p. 208.
36 Fay, *Shostakovich*, p. 252.
37 Lesser, *Music for Silenced Voices*, pp. 210–11.
38 Ibid.
   Fay, *Shostakovich*, p. 255.
39 Fay, *Shostakovich*, p. 264.
40 Pascuzzi, 'Shostakovich and Amyotrophic Lateral Sclerosis', p. 64.
41 Turner, M. R., Parton, M. J., Shaw, C. E., et al.: 'Prolonged Survival in Motor Neurone Disease: A Descriptive Study of the King's Database', 1990–2002', *Journal of Neurology, Neurosurgery, and Psychiatry* (2003) 74.995–7.
42 Pascuzzi, 'Shostakovich and Amyotrophic Lateral Sclerosis', pp. 65–6.
43 Fay, *Shostakovich*, p. 259.
44 Lesser, *Music for Silenced Voices*, pp. 233–4.
45 Fay, *Shostakovich*, pp. 264–5.
46 Ibid., p. 267.
47 Ibid., p. 271.
48 Lesser, *Music for Silenced Voices*, pp. 246–7.
49 Ibid.
50 Fay, *Shostakovich*, pp. 273–4.
51 Ibid., p. 278.
52 Ibid., p. 269.
53 Fay, *Shostakovich*, p. 278.
54 Stradling, R.: 'Shostakovich and the Soviet System 1925–75' in *Shostakovich: The Man and his Music* (ed. C. Norris), p. 190.
55 Fay, *Shostakovich*, p. 276.
56 Vishnevskaya, Galina: *Galina: A Russian Story*, p. 490, Sceptre, London, 1986.
57 Lesser, *Music for Silenced Voices*, pp. 266–7.
58 Ibid., p. 261.
59 Lesser, *Music for Silenced Voices*, pp. 270–1.
60 Fay, *Shostakovich*, p. 285.
61 Ibid.
62 Volkov, Solomon (ed.): *Testimony: The Memoirs of Dmitri Shostakovich* (trans. Antonina W. Bouis), Hamish Hamilton, London, 1979.
63 Jaffé, Daniel: *Sergei Prokofiev*, p. 212, Phaidon, London, 2007.
64 Gutman, David: *Prokofiev*, The Illustrated Lives of the Great Composers, p.133, Omnibus Press, London, 1990.
65 Jaffé, *Sergei Prokofiev*, p. 32.
66 Ibid., p. 53.
67 Ibid., p. 57.
68 Ibid., pp. 66–7.
69 Jaffé, *Sergei Prokofiev*, p. 71.
   Nice, David: *Prokofiev, From Russia to the West 1891–1935*, p. 158, Yale University Press, New Haven and London, 2003.
70 Morrison, Simon: *The Love and Wars of Lina Prokofiev*, p. 99, Harvill Secker, London, 2013.
71 Robinson, Harlow: *Sergei Prokofiev*, pp. 313–19, Robert Hale, London, 1987.
   Seroff, Victor: *Sergei Prokofiev: A Soviet Tragedy*, pp. 163–4, Leslie Frewin, London, 1969.
   Nice, *Prokofiev*, pp. 331, 336.

72 Robinson, *Sergei Prokofiev*, pp. 313–19.
73 Seroff, *Sergei Prokofiev*, pp. 163–4.
74 Hingtgen, C. M.: 'The Tragedy of Sergei Prokofiev', *Seminars in Neurology* (1999) 19(1).59–61.
75 Jaffé, *Sergei Prokofiev*, p. 128.
76 Ibid., p. 151.
77 Ibid., pp. 159–60.
78 Gutman, *Prokofiev*, p. 159.
79 Morrison, *The Love and Wars of Lina Prokofiev*, p. 206.
80 Ibid., pp. 196–8.
81 Jaffé, *Sergei Prokofiev*, pp. 169.
     Gutman, *Prokofiev*, p. 162.
82 Jaffé, *Sergei Prokofiev*, pp. 164–5.
83 Morrison, *The Love and Wars of Lina Prokofiev*, p. 245.
84 Ibid., p. 244.
85 Gutman, *Prokofiev*, p. 169.
86 Ibid,, p. 178.
87 Hingtgen, 'The Tragedy of Sergei Prokofiev', p. 60.
88 Redepenning, Dorothea: 'Prokofiev, Sergey' in *The New Grove Dictionary of Music and Musicians*, 2nd edn (ed. Stanley Sadie and John Tyrrell), vol. 20, p. 417, Macmillan Publishers, London, 2001.
89 Gutman, *Prokofiev*, p. 178.
90 Jaffé, *Sergei Prokofiev*, p. 180.
91 Ibid., p. 187.
92 Hingtgen, 'The Tragedy of Sergei Prokofiev', p. 60.
93 Jaffé, *Sergei Prokofiev*, p. 184.
94 Gutman, *Prokofiev*, p. 184.
95 Hingtgen, 'The Tragedy of Sergei Prokofiev', p. 60.
96 Gutman, *Prokofiev*, p. 193.
97 Ibid., p. 191.
98 Jaffé, *Sergei Prokofiev*, p. 196.
99 Gutman, *Prokofiev*, p. 202
100 Jaffé, *Sergei Prokofiev*, p. 204.
101 Ibid., p. 211.
102 Gutman, *Prokofiev*, p. 202.
103 Jaffé, *Sergei Prokofiev*, pp. 211–12.
104 Hingtgen, 'The Tragedy of Sergei Prokofiev', p. 60.
     Jaffé, *Sergei Prokofiev*, p. 212.
105 Hingtgen, 'The Tragedy of Sergei Prokofiev', p. 60.
106 Ibid., p. 60.
107 Gutman, *Prokofiev*, p. 181.
108 Holoman, D. Kern: *Berlioz*, p. 592, Faber & Faber, London, 1989.
109 Macdonald, Hugh: *Berlioz*, The Master Musicians, p. 24, Oxford University Press, Oxford, 2000.
110 Bloom, Peter: *The Life of Berlioz*, Musical Lives, p. 166, Cambridge University Press, Cambridge, UK, 1998.
111 Cairns, David: *Berlioz*, vol. 1, *The Making of an Artist 1803–32*, p. 463, Sphere Books Ltd, London, 1989.
112 Holoman, *Berlioz*, p. 195.

113 Cairns, *Berlioz*, vol. 1, pp. 386–7.
114 Ibid., p. 208.
115 Holoman, *Berlioz*, p. 11.
116 Bloom, *The Life of Berlioz*, p. 15.
117 Cairns, *Berlioz*, vol. 1, p. 116.
118 Holoman, *Berlioz*, pp. 44–6.
119 Cairns, *Berlioz*, vol. 1, p. 297.
120 Bloom, *The Life of Berlioz*, p. 35.
121 Ibid., pp. 39, 57–8.
    Holoman, *Berlioz*, pp. 115.
122 Holoman, *Berlioz*, pp. 115–16.
123 Bloom, *The Life of Berlioz*, p. 58.
124 Cairns, *Berlioz*, vol. 1, pp. 339–40.
125 Bloom, *The Life of Berlioz*, p. 62.
126 Ibid., p. 63.
127 Holoman, *Berlioz*, pp. 150–1.
128 Bloom, *The Life of Berlioz*, p. 65.
129 Holoman, *Berlioz*, p. 150.
130 Ibid., pp. 202, 348–54.
131 Bloom, *The Life of Berlioz*, p. 91.
132 Holoman, *Berlioz*, p. 195.
133 Ibid., pp. 196–7.
134 Bloom, *The Life of Berlioz*, pp. 132–3.
135 Ibid., p. 107.
136 Holoman, *Berlioz*, p. 283.
137 Ibid., p. 301.
138 Ibid., pp. 311–12.
139 Ibid., p. 464.
140 Ibid., p. 407.
141 Ibid., p. 566.
142 Bloom, *The Life of Berlioz*, p. 170.
143 Holoman, *Berlioz*, p. 503.
144 Ibid., p. 572.
145 Ibid., p. 495.
146 Baker, Theodore: 'Pauline Viardot to Julius Rietz, Letters of Friendship', *Musical Quarterly* (1916) 2.42–5.
147 Bloom, *The Life of Berlioz*, p. 156.
148 Ibid., p. 157.
149 Holoman, *Berlioz*, p. 585.
150 Macdonald, *Berlioz*, pp. 65–6.
151 Ibid., p. 66.
152 Ibid., pp. 66–7.
153 Elliot, J. H.: *Berlioz*, The Master Musicians Series, p. 105, J. M. Dent & Sons Ltd, London, 1967.
154 Holoman, *Berlioz*, p. 587.
155 Elliot, *Berlioz*, pp. 106–7.
156 Holoman, *Berlioz*, pp. 589–92.
157 Ibid., p. 589.
158 Ibid., p. 590.

159 Ibid., p. 591.

160 Ibid., p. 592.

161 Elliot, *Berlioz*, p. 107.

162 Holoman, *Berlioz*, p. 407.

163 Burney, Charles: *An Eighteenth Century Musical Tour in Central Europe and the Netherlands* (ed. Percy A. Scholes), Dr. Burney's Musical Tours, 2, p. 93, Oxford University Press, London, 1959.

164 Ibid., p. 90.

165 Croll, Gerhard, and Dean, Winton: 'Gluck, Christoph Willibald' in *The New Grove Dictionary of Music and Musicians* (ed. Stanley Sadie), vol. 7, p. 457, Macmillan Publishers, London, 1980.

166 Ibid., pp. 457–60.

167 Howard, Patricia: *Gluck: An Eighteenth Century Portrait*, pp. 180–1, Clarendon Press, Oxford, 1995.
Croll and Dean, 'Gluck, Christoph Willibald', p. 465.

168 Croll and Dean, 'Gluck, Christoph Willibald', p. 466.
Howard, *Gluck*, pp. 204–6.

169 Croll and Dean, 'Gluck, Christoph Willibald', p. 466.
Howard, *Gluck*, pp. 223–4.

170 Howard, *Gluck*, pp. 223, 230.
Slater, E. and Meyer, A.: 'Contributions to a Pathography of the Musicians: 2. Organic and Psychotic Disorders', *Confinia Psychiatrica* (1960) 3.129–45 (p. 130).

171 Cooper, Martin: *Gluck*, p. 266, Chatto & Windus, London, 1935.

172 Croll and Dean, 'Gluck, Christoph Willibald', p. 466.

173 Cooper, *Gluck*, pp. 266–7.

174 Ibid., p. 267.

175 Langham-Smith, R: 'The Ooze of the Erotic Priest', programme notes for *Faust*, Royal Opera House, Covent Garden, London, 2012.

176 Harding, James: *Gounod*, pp. 162–5, Stein & Day, New York, 1973.

177 Ibid., pp. 172–3.

178 Cooper, Martin: 'Gounod, Charles-François' in *The New Grove Dictionary of Music and Musicians*, vol. 7, pp. 583–4.

179 Harding, *Gounod*, p. 182.

180 Ibid., p. 169.

181 Ibid., p. 185.

182 Huebner, Steven: 'Gounod, Charles-François' in *The New Grove Dictionary of Music and Musicians*, 2nd edn, vol. 10, p. 223.

183 Harding, *Gounod*, p. 221.

184 Ibid., pp. 222–3.

185 Ibid., p. 224.

186 Brown, Clive: *A Portrait of Mendelssohn*, p. 3, Yale University Press, New Haven, 2003.

187 Ibid., pp. 3–9.
Radcliffe, Philip: *Mendelssohn*, 3rd edn, The Master Musicians Series, p. 4, J. M. Dent & Sons Ltd, London, 1990.

188 Brown, *A Portrait of Mendelssohn*, p. 409.

189 Ibid., p. 488.

190 Mercer-Taylor, Peter, *The Life of Mendelssohn*, Musical Lives, p. 54, Cambridge University Press, Cambridge, UK, 2000.

191 Neumayr, Anton: *Music & Medicine*, vol. 2, *Hummel, Weber, Mendelssohn, Schumann, Brahms, Bruckner* (English trans. B. C. Clarke), 'Felix Mendelssohn', pp. 163–5, Medi-Ed Press, Bloomington, IL, 1995.

192 Radcliffe, *Mendelssohn*, pp. 31–4.

193 Neumayr, *Music & Medicine*, vol. 2, 'Mendelssohn', pp. 183–5.

194 Ibid., p. 184.

195 Ibid., pp. 184–5.
   Cherington, M., Smith, R., and Nielsen, P. J.: 'The Life, Legacy and Premature Death of Felix Mendelssohn', *Seminars in Neurology* (1999) 19(1).47–52 (p. 50).

196 Neumayr, *Music & Medicine*, vol. 2, 'Mendelssohn', p. 184.

197 O'Shea, John: in *Music and Medicine: Medical Profiles of Great Composers*, 'The Mendelssohn Family', pp. 121–2, J. M. Dent & Sons Ltd, London, 1990.
   Cherington, Smith and Nielsen, 'The Life, Legacy and Premature Death of Felix Mendelssohn', pp. 50–1.

198 Neumayr, *Music & Medicine*, vol. 2, 'Mendelssohn', p. 192.

199 Mercer-Taylor, *The Life of Mendelssohn*, pp. 198–9.

200 Ibid., p. 199.

201 Ibid., p. 200.

202 Cherington, Smith and Nielsen, 'The Life, Legacy and Premature Death of Felix Mendelssohn', p. 50.
   Neumayr, *Music & Medicine*, vol. 2, 'Mendelssohn', pp. 192–3.

203 Cherington, Smith and Nielsen, 'The Life, Legacy and Premature Death of Felix Mendelssohn', p. 50.

204 Hensel, Sebastian: *The Mendelssohn Family 1729–1847 from Letters and Journals* (trans. C. Klingemann), vol. 2, pp. 334, 339, Sampson Low, Marston, Searle and Rivington, London, 1882.

205 Todd, R. Larry: *Mendelssohn: A Life in Music*, pp. 566–7, Oxford University Press, 2003.

206 Mercer-Taylor, *The Life of Mendelssohn*, p. 201.

207 Ibid., p. 201.

208 Neumayr, *Music & Medicine*, vol. 2, 'Mendelssohn', p. 210.

209 Sterndale-Bennett, R.: 'The Death of Mendelssohn', *Music & Letters* (1955) 36.374–6.

210 Neumayr, *Music & Medicine*, vol. 2, 'Mendelssohn', p. 210.

211 Ibid.

212 Sterndale-Bennett, 'The Death of Mendelssohn', p. 375.

213 Kerner, D: 'Mendelssohns Tod', *Deutsche Medizinische Wochenschrift* (1968) 19.454–62.
   Franken, F. H.: *Krankheit und Tod grosser Komponisten*, p. 192, Verlag Gerhard Witzstrock, Baden-Baden, 1979.

214 Schievink, W. J.: 'Genetics of Intracranial Aneurysms', *Neurosurgery* (1997) 40.651–63.

215 Ibid.
   Hamet, P., Pausova, Z., Adarichev, V., et al.: 'Hypertension, Genes and Environment', *Journal of Hypertension* (1998) 16.397–418.

216 Brown, *A Portrait of Mendelssohn*, p. 493.

217 Pollack, Howard: 'Copland, Aaron' in *The New Grove Dictionary of Music and Musicians*, 2nd edn, vol. 6, pp. 399.

218 Pollack, Howard: *Aaron Copland: The Life and Work of an Uncommon Man*, pp. 516–17, Faber & Faber Ltd, London, 2000.

219 Ibid., p. 541.
220 Ibid., p. 546.
221 Ibid., p. 547.

Chapter 8

1 O'Shea, J. G.: 'A Medical History of Franz Liszt', *Medical Journal of Australia* (1986) 145.625–39.

2 Watson, Derek: *Liszt*, The Master Musicians Series, p. 9, J. M. Dent & Sons Ltd, London, 1990.

3 Ibid., p. 9.

4 Ibid., pp. 22–3.

5 Ibid., p. 35.

6 Steen, Michael: *The Lives and Times of the Great Composers*, 'Franz Liszt', p. 435, Icon Books Ltd, London, 2010.

7 Watson, *Liszt*, p. 49.

8 O'Shea, 'A Medical History of Franz Liszt', p. 628.
Watson, *Liszt*, p. 35.

9 O'Shea, John: *Music and Medicine: Medical Profiles of Great Composers*, 'Franz Liszt', p. 157, J. M. Dent & Sons Ltd, London, 1990.

10 O'Shea, 'A Medical History of Franz Liszt', p. 628.

11 O'Shea, J. G.: 'The Abbé and his Alcohol', *Liszt Saeculum* (1987) 40.12–15.
Hilmes, Oliver: *Franz Liszt: Musician, Celebrity, Superstar* (trans. Stewart Spencer), pp. 30–1, 277, Yale University Press, New Haven, 2016.

12 Walker, Alan: *Franz Liszt*, vol. 1, T*he Virtuoso Years, 1811–1847*, p. 296, Faber & Faber, London, 1983.

13 Hilmes, *Franz Liszt*, p. 277.

14 Ibid., pp. 104–12.

15 Ibid., p. 111–12.

16 Walker, Alan: *Franz Liszt*, vol. 2, *The Weimar Years, 1848–1860*, p. 296, Faber & Faber, London, 1989.

17 Watson, *Liszt*, pp. 114–15.

18 Ibid., p. 115.

19 Walker, Alan: *Franz Liszt*, vol. 3, *The Final Years 1861–1886*, p. 511, Faber & Faber, London, 1997.

20 O'Shea, 'The Abbé and his Alcohol', pp. 12–15.
Walker, *Franz Liszt*, vol. 3, p. 5.

21 Litzmann, Berthold: *Clara Schumann* (trans. G. E. Hadow), vol. 1, p. 285, Macmillan & Co. Ltd, London, 1913.

22 O'Shea, 'A Medical History of Franz Liszt', p. 629.

23 O'Shea, *Music and Medicine*, p. 166.

24 O'Shea, 'A Medical History of Franz Liszt', p. 629.

25 Ibid., p. 629.

26 Watson, *Liszt*, pp. 158–9.

27 Hilmes, *Franz Liszt*, p. 280.

28 O'Shea, *Music and Medicine*, p. 163.

29 Hilmes, *Franz Liszt*, p. 295.

30 O'Shea, *Music and Medicine*, p. 158.

31 Ibid., p. 159.

32 Morrison, Bryce: *Franz Liszt*, Illustrated Lives of the Great Composers, p. 108, Omnibus Press, London, 2014.

33 Hilmes, *Franz Liszt*, p. 299.

34 O'Shea, *Music and Medicine*, p. 163.

35 Watson, *Liszt*, p. 160.
    Hilmes, *Franz Liszt*, p. 300.

36 Hilmes, *Franz Liszt*, p. 300.

37 Ibid., p. 303.

38 O'Shea, *Music and Medicine*, p. 164.
    Hilmes, *Franz Liszt*, p. 302.

39 Hilmes, *Franz Liszt*, p. 305.
    Watson, *Liszt*, p. 160.

40 Hilmes, *Franz Liszt*, pp. 303–4.

41 Ibid., p. 304.

42 O'Shea, 'A Medical History of Franz Liszt', p. 630.
    Hilmes, *Franz Liszt*, p. 306.

43 O'Shea, *Music and Medicine*, pp. 159–61.

44 Hilmes, *Franz Liszt*, pp. 307–10.

45 Morrison, *Franz Liszt*, pp. 103–5.

46 Gould, G. M.: 'The Ill-Health of Richard Wagner', *Lancet* (1903) 162.306–13.

47 Gregor-Dellin, Martin: *Richard Wagner: His Life, his Work, his Century* (trans. J. Maxwell Brownjohn), pp. 11–12, Collins, London, 1983.

48 Millington, Barry: *Richard Wagner: The Sorcerer of Bayreuth*, pp. 148–58, Thames & Hudson, London, 2012.

49 Gould, 'The Ill-Health of Richard Wagner', pp. 307–12.
    Göbel, C. H., Göbel, A., and Göbel, H.: '"Compulsive plague! Pain without end!" How Richard Wagner Played out his Migraine in the Opera *Siegfried*', *British Medical Journal* (2013) 347.32–3.

50 Göbel, Göbel and Göbel: '"Compulsive plague! Pain without end!"', pp. 32–3.

51 Ibid., pp. 32–3.

52 Gould, 'The Ill-Health of Richard Wagner', pp. 311–12.

53 Millington, *Richard Wagner*, p. 127.

54 Geck, Martin, *Richard Wagner: A Life in Music* (trans. Stewart Spencer), p. 235, University of Chicago Press, Chicago, 2012.

55 Millington, *Richard Wagner*, p. 127.

56 Gregor-Dellin, *Richard Wagner*, p. 315.

57 Ibid., pp. 432–3.

58 Gould, 'The Ill-Health of Richard Wagner', p. 310.

59 Gregor-Dellin, *Richard Wagner*, pp. 420–1.

60 Millington, *Richard Wagner*, p. 155.

61 Gould, 'The Ill-Health of Richard Wagner', pp. 308–10.

62 Millington, Barry: *Wagner*, The Master Musicians Series, p. 110, J. M. Dent & Sons Ltd, London, 1992.

63 Ibid., p. 111.

64 Millington, *Wagner*, pp. 111–12.
    Westernhagen, Curt von: 'Wagner's Last Day', *Musical Times* (1979) 120.395–7.

65 Gregor-Dellin, *Richard Wagner*, p. 488.
    Millington, *Wagner*, p. 112.

66 Millington, *Wagner*, p. 111.

67 Thiery, J., and Tröhler, U., 'Wagner, Animals and Modern Scientific Medicine' (trans. S. Spencer) in *The Wagner Compendium* (ed. Barry Millington), pp. 174–7, Thames & Hudson, London, 1992.

68 Millington, *Wagner*, p. 112.

69 Ibid., p. 112.

70 Gregor-Dellin, *Richard Wagner*, p. 488.

71 Ibid., p. 496.

72 Stephens, John: Appendix 1, 'Dvořák's Final Illness' in John Clapham, *Dvořák*, pp. 179–81, David & Charles, London, 1979.

73 Steen, *The Lives and Times of the Great Composers*, 'Antonín Dvořák', pp. 708–10, Icon Books, London, 2010.

74 Clapham, *Dvořák*, pp. 147–8.

75 Steen, *The Lives and Times of the Great Composers*, 'Antonín Dvořák', p. 709.

76 Ibid., pp. 710–11.

77 Horton, John: *Grieg*, The Master Musicians Series, p. 111, J. M. Dent & Sons Ltd, London, 1974.

78 Robertson, Alec: *Dvořák*, The Master Musicians Series, p. 77, J. M. Dent & Sons Ltd, London, 1974.

79 Ibid., pp. 206–17.

80 Ibid., p. 142.

81 Clapham, *Dvořák*, p.179.

82 Stephens, 'Dvořák's Final Illness', pp. 179–81.

83 Ibid.

84 Ibid.

85 Kennedy, Michael: *Mahler*, The Master Musicians, p. 42, Oxford University Press, Oxford, 2000.

86 Franklin, Peter: *The Life of Mahler*, p. 94, Cambridge University Press, Cambridge, UK, 1997.

87 Fischer, Jens Malte: *Gustav Mahler* (trans. Stewart Spencer), p. 4, Yale University Press, New Haven and London, 2011.

88 Kennedy, *Mahler*, p. 75.

89 Seckerson, Edward: *Gustav Mahler*, Illustrated Lives of the Great Composers, p. 8, Omnibus Press, London, 2013.

90 Ibid., pp. 8–9.

91 Feder, Stuart: *Gustav Mahler: A Life in Crisis*, pp. 229–30, Yale University Press, New Haven and London, 2004.

92 Ibid., pp. 229–30.
    Jones, Ernest: *Sigmund Freud: Life and Work*, vol. 2, p. 89, Hogarth Press, London, 1955.

93 Levy, D.: 'Gustav Mahler and Emanuel Libman: Bacterial Endocarditis in 1911', *British Medical Journal* (1986) 293.1628–31.
    Kennedy, *Mahler*, pp. 3–4.

94 Fischer, *Gustav Mahler*, p. 5.
    Levy, 'Gustav Mahler and Emanuel Libman: Bacterial Endocarditis in 1911', p. 1628.

95 Fischer, *Gustav Mahler*, p. 68.

96 Kennedy, *Mahler*, p. 15.

97 Ibid., pp. 33–5.

98 Franklin, *The Life of Mahler*, p. 71.

99 Ibid., pp. 85–6.

100 Ekman, Karl: *Jean Sibelius* (trans. Edward Birse), pp. 175–6, Alan Wilmer Ltd, London, 1936.

101 Fischer, *Gustav Mahler*, pp. 325–6.

102 Christy, N. P., Christy, B. M., and Wood, B. G.: 'Gustav Mahler and his Illnesses', *Transactions of the American Clinical and Climatological Association* (1970) 82.200–17.

103 Franklin, *The Life of Mahler*, p. 114.
    Kennedy, *Mahler*, p. 64.

104 Franklin, *The Life of Mahler*, p. 116.
    Kennedy, *Mahler*, p. 70.

105 Neumayr, Anton: *Music & Medicine*, vol. 3, *Chopin, Smetana, Tchaikovsky, Mahler* (English trans. David J. Parent), 'Gustav Mahler', p. 337, Medi-Ed Press, Bloomington, IL, 1997.

106 Ibid., pp. 336–7.

107 Kuehn, J. L.: 'Encounter at Leyden: Gustav Mahler Consults Sigmund Freud', *Psychoanalytic Review* (1965) 52.5–25.

108 Kennedy, *Mahler*, p. 133.

109 Ibid., pp. 133–4.

110 Kennedy, *Mahler*, p. 48.
    Redlich, Hans F.: *Bruckner and Mahler*, The Master Musicians Series, p. 128, J. M. Dent & Sons Ltd, London, 1963.

111 Kennedy, *Mahler*, p. 5.

112 Ibid., pp. 78–9.

113 Lebrecht, Norman: *Why Mahler? How One Man and Ten Symphonies Changed the World*, p. 160, Faber & Faber, London, 2010.

114 Kennedy, *Mahler*, p. 79.

115 Ibid., p. 81.

116 Ibid., p. 80.

117 Ibid., p. 81.

118 Lebrecht, *Why Mahler?*, p. 157.

119 Christy, Christy and Wood, 'Gustav Mahler and his Illnesses', p. 205.

120 Kennedy, *Mahler*, p. 82.

121 Ibid., p. 83.

122 Ibid., p. 100.

123 Feder, *Gustav Mahler*, p. 247.

124 Seckerson, *Gustav Mahler*, p. 120.
    Kennedy, *Mahler*, pp. 93–5.

125 Kennedy, *Mahler*, pp. 93–5.

126 Garcia, E. E.: 'Gustav Mahler's Choice: A Note on Adolescence, Genius and Psychosomatics', *Psychoanalytic Study of the Child* (2000) 55.87–110.

127 Redlich, *Bruckner and Mahler*, p. 219.

128 Kennedy, *Mahler*, p. 171.

129 Franklin, *The Life of Mahler*, p. 189.

130 Kennedy, *Mahler*, p. 97.

131 Ibid..
    Feder, *Gustav Mahler*, p. 190.

132 Kennedy, *Mahler*, pp. 97–9.
    Feder, *Gustav Mahler*, pp. 190–2.

133 Kuehn, 'Encounter at Leyden: Gustav Mahler Consults Sigmund Freud', p. 18.

134 Fischer, *Gustav Mahler*, p. 645.

135 Kennedy, *Mahler*, p. 99.

136 Ibid., pp. 166–79.

137 Cooke, Deryck: *Gustav Mahler: An Introduction to his Music*, 2nd edn, p. 121, Faber Music, London, 1988.

138 Matthews, Colin: 'The Tenth Symphony' in *The Mahler Companion* (ed. Donald Mitchell and Andrew Nicholson), pp. 491, 506–7, Oxford University Press, Oxford, 1999.

139 Redlich, *Bruckner and Mahler*, pp. 218–31.

140 Cooke, *Gustav Mahler*, p. 121.

141 Kuehn, 'Encounter at Leyden: Gustav Mahler Consults Sigmund Freud', pp. 5–25.

142 Seckerson, *Gustav Mahler*, p. 132.

143 Feder, *Gustav Mahler*, p. 233.

144 Ibid., p. 229.

145 Ibid., p. 237.

146 Ibid., p. 237.

147 Neumayr, *Music & Medicine*, vol. 3, 'Gustav Mahler', p. 354.

148 Ibid., p. 349.

149 Feder, *Gustav Mahler*, p. 245.

150 Neumayr, *Music & Medicine*, vol. 3, 'Gustav Mahler', p. 357.

151 Ibid., p. 355.

152 Report in *New York Times*, death of Gustav Mahler, 20 May 1911.
    Mittag Zeitung, 20th May 1911.
    New York Times, 21 May 1911.

153 Roman, Zoltan: *Gustav Mahler's American Years (1907–1911): A Documentary History*, p. 397, Pendragon, NY, 1989.

154 Blaukopf, Kurt: *Gustav Mahler* (trans. Inge Goodwin), p. 233, Allen Lane/Readers Union, London, 1973.

155 Levy, 'Gustav Mahler and Emanuel Libman: Bacterial Endocarditis in 1911', pp. 1629–30.

156 Ibid., p. 1629.

157 Kennedy, *Mahler*, p. 101.

158 Neumayr, *Music & Medicine*, vol. 3, 'Gustav Mahler', p. 358.

159 Redlich, *Bruckner and Mahler*, p. 220.

160 Ibid., p. 219.

161 Kennedy, *Mahler*, p. 101.

162 Levy, 'Gustav Mahler and Emanuel Libman: Bacterial Endocarditis in 1911', p. 1629.

163 Ibid., pp. 1629–30.

164 Kennedy, *Mahler*, p. 102.
    Feder, *Gustav Mahler*, p. 272.

165 Kennedy, *Mahler*, p. 102.

166 Levy, 'Gustav Mahler and Emanuel Libman: Bacterial Endocarditis in 1911', p. 1630.

167 Kennedy, *Mahler*, p. 102.

168 Levy, 'Gustav Mahler and Emanuel Libman: Bacterial Endocarditis in 1911', p. 1630.

169 Report in *New York Times*, 20 May 1911.

170 Neumayr, *Music & Medicine*, vol. 3, 'Gustav Mahler', p. 376.

171 Franklin, *The Life of Mahler*, p. 198.

172 Kennedy, *Mahler*, p. 102.

173 Schonberg, Harold C.: The *Lives of the Great Composers*, 3rd edn, 'Nielsen', p. 451, Abacus, London, 1998.

174 Lawson, Jack: *Carl Nielsen*, Phaidon, London, 1997.
  Schoustoe, Torben: 'Nielsen, Carl (August)' in *The New Grove Dictionary of Music and Musicians* (ed. Stanley Sadie), vol. 13, Macmillan Publishers, London, 1980.
  Simpson, Robert: *Carl Nielsen, Symphonist 1865–1931*, J. M. Dent & Sons Ltd, London, 1952.

175 Lawson, *Carl Nielsen*, p. 205.

176 Ibid., pp. 66–7.

177 Ibid., p. 67.

178 Ibid., p. 105.

179 Ibid., p. 104.

180 Ibid., p. 112.

181 Ibid., p. 129.

182 Schoustoe, 'Nielsen, Carl (August)', pp. 226–7.

183 Lawson, *Carl Nielsen*, pp. 140–1.

184 Schoustoe, 'Nielsen, Carl (August)', pp. 226–7.

185 Lawson, *Carl Nielsen*, p. 153.

186 Ibid., pp. 174–5.

187 Ibid., p. 167.

188 Schoustoe, 'Nielsen, Carl (August)', pp. 226–7.

189 Lawson, *Carl Nielsen*, pp. 178–80.

190 Ibid., pp. 189 and 192.

191 Simpson, *Carl Nielsen, Symphonist*, p. 115.

192 Ibid., p. 191.

193 Lawson, *Carl Nielsen*, p. 194.

194 Ibid., pp. 195–6.

195 Ibid., p. 200.

196 Ibid., p. 205.

197 Ibid., p. 206.

198 Ibid., p. 208.

199 Ibid., p. 210.

200 Ibid., p. 212.

201 Ibid., p. 213.

202 Ibid., p. 203.

203 Ackroyd, Peter: *Albion: The Origins of the English Imagination*, pp. 440–7, Chatto & Windus, London, 2002.

204 Kennedy, Michael: *Benjamin Britten*, The Master Musicians Series, p. 103, J. M. Dent & Sons Ltd, London, 1993.

205 Kennedy, *Benjamin Britten*, pp. 1–4.
  Carpenter, Humphrey: *Benjamin Britten: A Biography*, Chapter 1, pp. 3–25, Faber & Faber, London, 1992.

206 Oliver, Michael: *Benjamin Britten*, p. 213, Phaedon Press, London, 1996.

207 Bridcut, John: *Britten's Children*, pp. 12–13, 90, 118, 170, Faber, London, 2007.

208 Kennedy, *Benjamin Britten*, pp. 60–1.

209 Kildea, Paul: *Benjamin Britten: A Life in the 20th Century*, pp. 160–1, Allen Lane, Penguin Books, London, 2013.

210 Ibid.

211 Kennedy, *Benjamin Britten*, pp. 33, 35.

212 Bridcut, *Britten's Children*, pp. 216–17.

213 Kennedy, Michael and Joyce: personal communications (2013).

214 Kennedy, *Benjamin Britten*, pp. 94–5.

215 Kennedy, personal communications (2013).

216 Tait, Dr Ian: personal communications (March 2012 and February 2013).

217 Ibid.

218 Kildea, *Benjamin Britten*, p. 525.

219 Kennedy, *Benjamin Britten*, p. 237.

220 Britten, Benjamin: medical records from The Red House, Aldeburgh, reviewed by this author, November 2013.

221 Ibid.

222 Kennedy, *Benjamin Britten*, p. 104.

223 Ibid.

224 Ibid.

225 Tait, personal communications (March 2012 and February 2013).
Kennedy, *Benjamin Britten*, p. 104.

226 Kennedy, *Benjamin Britten*, p. 103.

227 Ibid., p. 105.

228 Ibid., p. 103.

229 Tait, personal communications (March 2012 and February 2013).

230 Kennedy, *Benjamin Britten*, pp. 106–9.

231 Ibid., p. 108.

232 Ibid., p. 109.

233 Barnett, Rob: 'Benjamin Britten (1913–1976)', musicweb-international.com/ britten (accessed 2013).

234 Kildea, *Benjamin Britten*, p. 560.

235 Tait, personal communications (March 2012 and February 2013).
Britten, Benjamin: medical records from The Red House.
Petch, Dr Michael: personal communication (2013).

236 Kildea, Paul, 'Benjamin Britten: Death in Aldeburgh', *Sunday Telegraph*, 'Seven', 20 January 2013.

237 Petch, personal communication (2013).

238 Matthews, Colin: personal communication (April 2013).

239 Britten, Benjamin: medical records from The Red House.

240 Tait, personal communications (March 2012 and February 2013).

241 Ibid.

242 Britten, Benjamin: medical records from The Red House.

243 Tait, personal communications (March 2012 and February 2013).
Britten, Benjamin: medical records from The Red House.

244 Britten, Benjamin: medical records from The Red House.

245 Ibid.
Petch, personal communication (2013).

246 Kildea, *Benjamin Britten*, p. 532.

247 Britten, Benjamin: medical records from The Red House.

248 Ibid.

249 Lock, Stephen: personal communication (November 2013).

250 Petch, personal communication (2013).

251 Tait, personal communications (March 2012 and February 2013).
Petch, personal communication (2013).

252 Tait, personal communications (March 2012 and February 2013).

253 Ibid.

Britten, Benjamin: medical records from The Red House.

254 Kildea, 'Benjamin Britten: Death in Aldeburgh'.
Kildea, Paul, *Benjamin Britten*, p. 532.

255 Kildea, Paul, *Benjamin Britten*, p. 532.
Kildea, Paul: 'Yes, the Evidence Does Show that Benjamin Britten Died from Syphilis', *The Guardian*, 30 January 2013.

256 Britten, Benjamin: medical records from The Red House.
Petch, personal communication (2013).

257 Kildea, 'Benjamin Britten', p. 534.

258 Tait, personal communications (March 2012 and February 2013).

259 Higgins, Charlotte: 'On Culture Blog', guardian.co.uk, 25 January 2013.

260 Petch, personal communication (2013).

261 Ibid.

262 Grabau, W., Emanuel, R., Ross, D., et al.: 'Syphilitic Aortic Regurgitation', *British Journal of Venereal Diseases* (1976) 82.366–73.

263 Matthews, personal communication (April 2013).

264 Kildea, 'Benjamin Britten: Death in Aldeburgh'.

265 Davies, Hywel: 'Body of Evidence: Unravelling the Mystery of Benjamin Britten's Death', *New Statesman*, 7–13 June 2013, 48–9.

266 Petch, M. C.: 'The Heart of Benjamin Britten', *Journal of the Royal Society of Medicine* (2014) 107.339–41.

267 Roberts, W. C, Ko, J. M., Moore, T. R., and Jones, W. H.: 'Causes of Pure Aortic Regurgitation in Patients having Isolated Aortic Valve Replacement at a Single US Tertiary Hospital (1993–2005)', *Circulation* (2006) 114.422.

268 Mitchell, Donald: 'Double Portrait: Some Personal Recollections' in *Aldeburgh Anthology* (ed. R. Blythe), pp. 436–7, Snape Maltings Foundation, Snape, 1972.

269 Cole, J. C.: 'Alexander Borodin, the Scientist, the Musician, the Man', *Journal of the American Medical Association* (1969) 208.129–30.

270 O'Neill, D.: '... aber Sonntag ist immer ein Feiertag: Alexander Borodin M.D. 1833–1887', *Journal of the Royal Society of Medicine* (1988) 81.591–3.

271 Cole, 'Alexander Borodin, the Scientist, the Musician, the Man', p. 129.

272 Ibid., p. 130.

273 O'Neill, '... aber Sonntag ist immer ein Feiertag: Alexander Borodin M.D. 1833–1887', p. 593.

274 Ibid., p. 593.

275 Ibid., p. 593.

276 Frolova-Walker, Marina: 'Nikolay Andreyevich Rimsky-Korsakov' in *The New Grove Dictionary of Music and Musicians*, 2nd edn (ed. Stanley Sadie and John Tyrrell), vol. 21, pp. 401–6, Macmillan Publishers, London, 2001.

277 Maes, Francis: *A History of Russian Music* (trans. A. J. Pomerans and E. Pomerans), p. 171, University of California Press, Berkeley, 2002.

278 Frolova-Walker, 'Nikolay Andreyevich Rimsky-Korsakov', pp. 401–6.

279 Abraham, Gerald: *Rimsky-Korsakov: A Short Biography*, p. 80, Duckworth, London, 1945.

280 Rimsky-Korsakov, Nikolai: *Record of My Musical Life (1876–1906)* (trans. and ed. Judah Joffe), 5th edn, p. 309, Ernst Eelenburg Ltd, London, 1974.
Abraham, *Rimsky-Korsakov*, pp. 86–8.

281 Frolova-Walker, 'Nikolay Andreyevich Rimsky-Korsakov', pp. 401–6.

282 Abraham, *Rimsky-Korsakov*, pp. 86–8.

283 Steen, *The Lives and Times of the Great Composers*, 'Nikolai Rimsky-Korsakov', p. 657.

284 Abraham, *Rimsky-Korsakov*, p. 88.

285 Rimsky-Korsakov, *Record of My Musical Life*, p. 315.

286 Ibid., p. 339.

287 Abraham, *Rimsky-Korsakov*, pp. 93–4.

288 Ibid., pp. 125–6.

289 Steen, *The Lives and Times of the Great Composers*, 'Nikolai Rimsky-Korsakov', p. 659.

290 Abraham, *Rimsky-Korsakov*, pp. 125–6.

291 Ibid., p. 126.

292 Rimsky-Korsakov, *Record of My Musical Life*, p. 456.

293 Ivry, Benjamin: *Francis Poulenc*, p. 90, Phaidon Press Ltd, London, 1996.

294 Ibid., p. 74.

295 Schmidt, Carl B.: *Entrancing Muse: A Documented Biography of Francis Poulenc*, pp. 394–5, Pendragon Press, Hillside, NY, 2004.

296 Schmidt, *Entrancing Muse*, p. 397.

297 Ivry, *Francis Poulenc*, p. 218.

298 Schmidt, *Entrancing Muse*, pp. 459–62.

299 Ivry, *Francis Poulenc*, p. 218.

300 Schmidt, *Entrancing Muse*, pp. 459–62.

301 Ivry, *Francis Poulenc*, p. 212.

Chapter 9

1 Warrack, John: *Carl Maria von Weber*, p. 333, Cambridge University Press, Cambridge, UK, 1976.

2 Ibid., pp. 29–30.

3 O'Shea, John: *Music and Medicine: Medical Profiles of Great Composers*, 'Carl Maria von Weber', pp. 97–8, J. M. Dent & Sons Ltd, London, 1990.

4 Warrack, *Carl Maria von Weber*, p. 62.

5 Ibid., pp. 71–2.

6 Ibid., p. 73.

7 Ibid., pp. 124–5.

8 O'Shea, *Music and Medicine*, p. 92.

9 Ibid.

10 Warrack, *Carl Maria von Weber*, pp. 125, 129–30, 299, 301, 306–7.

11 O'Shea, *Music and Medicine*, pp. 93–4.

12 Warrack, *Carl Maria von Weber*, p. 55.

13 Ibid., p. 153.

14 Warrack, John: 'Carl Maria (Friedrich Ernst) von Weber' in *The New Grove Dictionary of Music and Musicians* (ed. Stanley Sadie), vol. 20, p. 245, Macmillan Publishers, London, 1980.

15 O'Shea, *Music and Medicine*, pp. 93–4.

16 Warrack, *Carl Maria von Weber*, p. 244.

17 Ibid., pp. 348–59.

18 Ibid., p. 298.

19 Ibid., p. 304.

20 O'Shea, *Music and Medicine*, pp. 94–5.

21 Ibid., p. 95.

22 Warrack, *Carl Maria von Weber*, p. 301.

23 Ibid., p. 306.
24 Ibid., p. 307.
25 O'Shea, *Music and Medicine*, p. 96.
26 Ibid., p. 97.
27 Warrack, *Carl Maria von Weber*, p. 344.
  O'Shea, *Music and Medicine*, p. 97.
28 Warrack, *Carl Maria von Weber*, p. 345.
  O'Shea, *Music and Medicine*, pp. 97–8.
29 Warrack, *Carl Maria von Weber*, p. 347.
30 Ibid., p. 347.
31 O'Shea, *Music and Medicine*, 'Frédéric Chopin', p. 144.
32 Zamoyski, Adam: *Chopin: Prince of the Romantics*, p. 275, Harper Press, London, 2010.
33 Neumayr, Anton: *Music & Medicine*, vol. 3, *Chopin, Smetana, Tchaikovsky, Mahler* (trans. D. J. Parent), 'Frédéric Chopin', p. 54, Medi-Ed Press, Bloomington, IL, 1997.
34 Jordan, Ruth: *Nocturne: A Life of Chopin*, p. 135, Constable, London, 1978.
35 O'Shea, *Music and Medicine*, p. 141.
36 Jordan, *Nocturne*, p. 38.
37 Hedley, Arthur: *Chopin*, The Master Musicians Series, pp. 125–6, J. M. Dent & Sons Ltd, London, 1974.
38 Neumayr, *Music & Medicine*, vol. 3, 'Frédéric Chopin', pp. 28–9.
39 O'Shea, *Music and Medicine*, p. 143.
40 Neumayr, *Music & Medicine*, vol. 3, 'Frédéric Chopin', p. 30.
41 Jordan, *Nocturne*, p. 52.
42 Hedley, *Chopin*, p. 14.
43 Kuzemko, J. A.: 'Chopin's Illnesses', *Journal of the Royal Society of Medicine* (1994) 87.769–72.
44 Neumayr, *Music & Medicine*, vol. 3, 'Frédéric Chopin', pp. 39–40.
45 Jordan, *Nocturne*, pp. 103–5.
  Neumayr, *Music & Medicine*, vol. 3, 'Frédéric Chopin', p. 46.
46 Neumayr, *Music & Medicine*, vol. 3, 'Frédéric Chopin', p. 46.
47 Brown, Maurice J. E.: *Chopin: An Index of his Works*, p. 74, Macmillan, London, 1972.
48 Hedley, *Chopin*, p. 29.
49 Neumayr, *Music & Medicine*, vol. 3, 'Frédéric Chopin', pp. 129–31.
50 Jordan, *Nocturne*, p. 78.
51 O'Shea, *Music and Medicine*, p. 143.
52 Samson, Jim: *Chopin*, The Master Musicians, pp. 129–32, Oxford University Press, Oxford, 1996.
53 Ibid., p. 132.
54 Hedley, *Chopin*, p. 64.
55 Ibid., p. 63.
56 Samson, *Chopin*, p. 134.
57 Jordan, Ruth: *George Sand: A Biographical Portrait*, p. 168, Constable, London, 1976.
58 Sand, George: *Un hiver á Majorque*, Hippolyte Souverain, Paris, 1842; *Winter in Majorca* (English trans. R. Graves), Cassell & Company Ltd, London, 1956.
59 Jordan, *Nocturne*, pp. 163–4.
60 Orga, Ateş: *Fryderyck Franciszek Chopin*, Lives of Great Composers, p. 101, Omnibus Press, London, 2015.

61 Ibid., p. 101.
62 Hedley, *Chopin*, p. 77.
63 O'Shea, *Music and Medicine*, p. 145.
64 Orga, *Fryderyck Franciszek Chopin*, p. 101.
    Hedley, *Chopin*, pp. 77–8.
65 Hedley, *Chopin*, pp. 78–9.
66 Ibid., p. 79.
67 Ibid., pp. 80–1.
68 Ibid., p. 82.
69 Orga, *Fryderyck Franciszek Chopin*, pp. 110–11.
70 Jordan, *Nocturne*, p. 171.
71 Ibid., pp. 171–2.
    Hedley, *Chopin*, p. 84.
72 Hedley, *Chopin*, p. 84.
    O'Shea, *Music and Medicine*, pp. 141 and 146.
73 Neumayr, *Music & Medicine*, vol. 3, 'Frédéric Chopin', p. 92.
    Jordan, *George Sand*, pp. 217–18
74 Jordan, *Nocturne*, pp. 198–200.
75 Hedley, *Chopin*, p. 94.
76 Ibid., p. 97.
77 Orga, *Fryderyck Franciszek Chopin*, p. 136.
78 Jordan, *Nocturne*, pp. 242 and 256.
79 O'Shea, *Music and Medicine*, pp. 141–2.
80 Orga, *Fryderyck Franciszek Chopin*, pp. 142–3.
81 O'Shea, *Music and Medicine*, p. 146.
82 Neumayr, *Music & Medicine*, vol. 3, 'Frédéric Chopin', p. 100.
83 Abbott, E. C.: 'Composers and Tuberculosis: The Effects on Creativity', *Canadian Medical Association Journal* (1982) 126.534–44.
84 Neumayr, *Music & Medicine*, vol. 3, 'Frédéric Chopin', pp. 102–3.
    Jordan, *Nocturne*, p. 256.
85 Neumayr, *Music & Medicine*, vol. 3, 'Frédéric Chopin', p. 107.
86 Jordan, *Nocturne*, p. 256.
87 O'Shea, *Music and Medicine*, p. 147.
88 Jordan, *Nocturne*, p. 256.
89 Hedley, *Chopin*, p. 116.
90 O'Shea, *Music and Medicine*, pp. 148–9.
91 Ibid., pp. 148–9.
92 Kubba, A. K., and Young, M.: 'The Long Suffering of Frederic Chopin', *Chest* (1998) 113.210–16 (p. 214).
93 O'Shea, J. G.: 'Was Frederic Chopin's Illness Actually Cystic Fibrosis?', *Medical Journal of* Australia (1987) 187.586–9.
    Rietschel, E. T., Rietschel, M., and Beutler, B,: 'How the Mighty have Fallen', *Infectious Disease Clinics of North America* (2004) 18.311–39 (p. 323).
94 Dormandy, Thomas: *The White Death: A History of Tuberculosis*, Hambledon Press, London, 1999.
    Rietschel et al., 'How the Mighty have Fallen', p. 324.
95 O'Shea, *Music and Medicine*, p. 89.
96 Dodge, J. A., Lewis, P. A., Stanton, M., and Wilsher, J.: 'Cystic Fibrosis Mortality and Survival in the UK 1947–2003', *European Respiratory Journal* (2007) 29.522–26.

97 O'Shea, 'Was Frederic Chopin's Illness Actually Cystic Fibrosis?', p. 586.
  O'Shea, *Music and Medicine*, p. 586.
98 Kuzemko, 'Chopin's Illnesses', p. 769.
99 O'Shea, 'Was Frederic Chopin's Illness Actually Cystic Fibrosis?', p. 586.
100 Ibid., p. 586.
101 Dodge et al., 'Cystic Fibrosis Mortality and Survival in the UK 1947–2003'.
102 Quinton, P. M.: 'Cystic Fibrosis Lesions from the Sweat Gland', *Physiology* (2007) 22.212–25.
103 O'Shea, 'Was Frederic Chopin's Illness Actually Cystic Fibrosis?', pp. 586–7.
104 Kubba, A. K., and Young, M.: 'The Long Suffering of Frederic Chopin' pp. 210–16.
105 Zamoyski, *Chopin*, p. 270.
106 Horton, John: *Grieg*, The Master Musicians Series, p. 81, J. M. Dent & Sons Ltd, London, 1974.
107 Ibid., p. 72.
  Poznansky, Alexander: *Tchaikovsky: The Quest for the Inner Man*, p. 485, Lime Tree, London, 1993.
108 Horton, *Grieg*, p. 10.
109 Ibid.
110 O'Shea, *Music and Medicine*, 'Edvard Grieg', p. 174.
111 Ibid., pp. 172–9.
  Monrad-Johansen, David: *Edvard Grieg* (English trans. Madge Robertson), pp. 41, 360–92, Princeton University Press, New York, 1938.
112 Abbott, 'Composers and Tuberculosis: The Effects on Creativity', p. 543.
113 Benestad, Finn, and Schjelderup-Ebbe, Dag: *Edvard Grieg: The Man and the Artist* (trans. W. A. Halverson and L. B. Sateren), pp. 311–13, Allan Sutton Publishing, Gloucester, 1988.
114 O'Shea, *Music and Medicine*, p. 178.
115 Horton, *Grieg*, p. 47.
116 Ibid., p. 45.
117 Ibid., p. 61.
118 Ibid., p. 81.
119 Monrad-Johansen, *Edvard Grieg*, p. 338.
120 Ibid., p. 335.
121 Horton, *Grieg*, pp. 83–4.
122 Benestad and Schjelderup-Ebbe, *Edvard Grieg*, p. 325.
123 Ibid., p. 326.
124 Ibid., p. 347.
125 Ibid., p. 350.
126 Horton, *Grieg*, pp. 102–3.
127 Ibid., p. 103.
128 O'Shea, *Music and Medicine*, p. 175.
129 Ibid., p. 175.
130 Ibid., p. 175.
131 Horton *Grieg*, p. 111.
132 Ibid., pp. 117–18.
133 Ibid., p. 117.
134 Ibid., p. 117.
135 Dahl, Erling: *Edvard Grieg: His Life and Music. A Short Biography*, p. 50, Edvard Grieg Museum, Troldhaugen, 2002.

136 Horton, *Grieg*, p. 118.

137 O'Shea, *Music and Medicine*, p. 178.

138 Ibid., p. 179.

139 Figes, Orlando: *Natasha's Dance: A Cultural History of Russia*, p. 564, Penguin Books, London, 2003.

140 Routh, Francis: *Igor Stravinsky*, The Master Musicians Series, p. 1, J. M. Dent & Sons Ltd, London, 1975.

141 Ibid., p. 14.

142 Walsh, Stephen: *Stravinsky: A Creative Spring. Russia & France 1882–1934*, p. 224, Pimlico, London, 2000.

143 Routh, *Igor Stravinsky*, p. 21.

144 Walsh, Stephen: *Stravinsky: The Second Exile. France and America 1934–71*, pp. 67–8, Pimlico, London, 2007.

145 Routh, *Igor Stravinsky*, p. 44.

146 Walsh, *Stravinsky: The Second Exile*, pp. 66–8.

147 Ibid., pp. 67–8.

148 Routh, *Igor Stravinsky*, pp. 44–5.

149 Ibid., p. 46.

150 Ibid., p. 53.

151 Walsh, *Stravinsky: The Second Exile*, p. 247.

152 Ibid., p. 268.

153 Ibid., pp. 301, 303.

154 Ibid., p. 328.

155 Ibid., pp. 305–7.

156 Cross, Jonathan: *Igor Stravinksy*, Critical Lives, p. 174, Reaktion Books, London, 2015.

157 Walsh, *Stravinsky: The Second Exile*, pp. 282–3.

158 Ibid., p. 318.

159 Ibid., pp. 347–8.

160 Walsh, *Stravinsky: The Second Exile*, pp. 347–8.

161 Craft, Robert: *Stravinsky: Chronicle of a Friendship 1948–71*, pp. 48, 61, Gollancz, London, 1972.

162 Walsh, *Stravinsky: The Second Exile*, p. 348.

163 Ibid., p. 352.

164 Ibid., p. 414.

165 Ibid., p. 414.

166 Figes, Orlando: *Natasha's Dance*, pp. 580–6.

167 Ibid., p. 582.

168 Routh, *Igor Stravinsky*, p. 63.

169 Ibid., p. 64.

170 Walsh, *Stravinsky: The Second Exile*, p. 492.

171 Routh, *Igor Stravinsky*, p. 66.

172 Ibid., p. 66.

173 Walsh, *Stravinsky: The Second Exile*, p. 528.

174 Routh, *Igor Stravinsky*, pp. 67.

175 Walsh, *Stravinsky: The Second Exile*, pp. 528–9.

176 Ibid., p. 531.

177 Ibid., pp. 532–3.

178 Ibid., p. 533.

179 Ibid., p. 538.
180 Ibid., p. 538.
181 Ibid., p. 546.
182 Ibid., p. 546.
183 Ibid., pp. 550–7.
184 Ibid., p. 552.
185 Ibid., pp. 552 and 554.
186 Ibid., p. 555.
187 Ibid., p. 557.
188 Ibid., p. 559.
189 Griffiths, Paul: *Stravinsky*, The Master Musicians Series, p. 192, J. M. Dent & Sons Ltd, London, 1992.
190 Walsh, *Stravinsky: The Second Exile*, pp. 560–1.
191 Heller, Karl: *Antonio Vivaldi: The Red Priest of Venice* (trans. David Marinelli), p. 44, Amadeus Press, Portland, OR, 1997.
192 Berri, P.: 'La malattia di Vivaldi', *Musica d'oggi* (1942) 24.9–13.
193 Travers, Roger-Claude: 'Une mise au point sur la maladie de Vivaldi', *Informazioni e studi Vivaldiani* (1982) 3.52–60.
194 Talbot, Michael: *Vivaldi*, The Dent Master Musicians, 2nd edn, pp. 14–18, J. M. Dent & Sons Ltd, London, 1993.
195 Berri, 'La malattia di Vivaldi', pp. 9–13.
196 Talbot, *Vivaldi*, p. 165.
197 Ibid., p. 67.
198 Heller, *Antonio Vivaldi*, p. 259.
199 Kolneder, Walter: *Antonio Vivaldi: His Life and Work* (trans. Bill Hopkins), p. 21, Faber & Faber, London, 1970.
200 Talbot, *Vivaldi*, p. 68.
201 Ibid., p. 69.
202 Falliers, C. J.: 'Arnold Schoenberg and Alban Berg: The Serial Music and Serious Asthma of Two Leading 20th-Century Composers', *Journal of Asthma* (1986) 23.211–17 (p. 213).
203 Neighbour, O. W.: 'Schoenberg, Arnold (Franz Walter)' in *The New Grove Dictionary of Music and Musicians*, vol. 16, p. 701.
204 Ibid., pp. 702–3.
205 Falliers, 'Arnold Schoenberg and Alban Berg', p. 213.
206 Ibid., p. 213.
207 Ibid., p. 214.
    Neighbour, 'Schoenberg, Arnold (Franz Walter)', p. 705.
208 Neighbour, 'Schoenberg, Arnold (Franz Walter)', p. 705.
    Falliers, 'Arnold Schoenberg and Alban Berg', p. 214.
209 Neighbour, 'Schoenberg, Arnold (Franz Walter)', p. 705.
210 Ibid., pp. 705–6.
211 Falliers, 'Arnold Schoenberg and Alban Berg', p. 214.

Chapter 10

  1 Weinstock, Herbert: *Rossini: A Biography*, Alfred A. Knopf, Inc., New York, 1968.
    Toye, Francis: *Rossini: A Study in Tragi-Comedy*, Arthur Barker, London, 1954.
    Osborne, Richard: *Rossini*, The Dent Master Musicians, J. M. Dent, London, 1993.

2 Schonberg, Harold: *The Lives of the Great Composers*, 3rd edn, 'Rossini', p. 246, Abacus, London, 1998.

3 Ibid., p. 244.

4 Osborne, *Rossini*, p. 11.

5 Weinstock, *Rossini*, pp. 112–13.

6 O'Shea, John: *Music and Medicine: Medical Profiles of Great Composers*, 'Rossini', p. 101, J. M. Dent & Sons Ltd, London, 1990.

7 Osborne, *Rossini*, pp. 94–5.

8 Ibid., p. 121.

9 Ibid., p. 79.

10 Mount Edgcumbe, Earl of: *Musical Reminiscences of an Old Amateur*, p. 126, W. Clarke, London, 1825.

11 Osborne, *Rossini*, p. 61.

12 Weinstock, *Rossini*, p. 234.

13 Toye, *Rossini*, pp. 166–76.

14 Schwartz, D. W.: 'A Psychoanalytical Approach to the Great Renunciation', *Journal of the American Psychoanalytic Association* (1965) 13.551 (p. 569).

15 Osborne, *Rossini*, pp. 79–80.

16 Weinstock, *Rossini*, p. 179.

17 Osborne, *Rossini*, p. 63.

18 Ibid., p. 103.

19 Ibid., p. 80.

20 Weinstock, *Rossini*, pp. 379–81.

21 Ibid., pp. 379–81.

22 Ibid., p. 380.

23 Osborne, *Rossini*, p. 91.

24 Ibid., pp. 95–6.

25 Toye, *Rossini*, p. 212.

26 Osborne, *Rossini*, p. 117.

27 Weinstock, *Rossini*, pp. 230–1.

28 Osborne, *Rossini*, p. 102.

29 Schwartz, 'A Psychoanalytical Approach to the Great Renunciation', p. 567.

30 Ibid., pp. 551–69.

31 Osborne, *Rossini*, pp. 108–9.

32 Schwartz, 'A Psychoanalytical Approach to the Great Renunciation', p. 551.

33 O'Shea, *Music and Medicine*, p. 104.

34 Osborne, *Rossini*, pp. 112–13.

35 Ibid., pp. 116–17.

36 Ibid., p. 122.

37 Ibid., p. 123.
     Weinstock, *Rossini*, p. 362.

38 Weinstock, *Rossini*, p. 362.

39 Ibid., pp. 362–3.

40 Osborne, *Rossini*, p. 123.

41 Weinstock, *Rossini*, p. 363.

42 Lister, J.: 'On the Antiseptic Principle in the Practice of Surgery', *British Medical Journal* 1867, 2 (351).246–8.

43 Toye, *Rossini*, pp. 202–3.

44 Osborne, *Rossini*, p. 123.

45 Shaw, George Bernard: 'Rossini Centenary', *Illustrated London News*, 5 March 1892.
46 Steen, Michael: *The Lives and Times of the Great Composers*, 'Debussy', p. 800, Icon Books Ltd, London, 2010.
47 Howat, Roy: personal communication (May 2013).
48 Roberts, Paul: *Claude Debussy*, p. 93, Phaidon Press, London, 2010.
49 Ibid., pp. 15–17.
50 Ibid., p. 56.
51 Ibid., pp. 49–50.
52 Nichols, Roger: *The Life of Debussy*, Musical Lives, p. 23, Cambridge University Press, Cambridge, UK, 1998.
53 Jensen, Eric, F.: *Debussy*, The Master Musicians, p. 50, Oxford University Press, New York, 2014.
54 Nichols, *The Life of Debussy*, p. 75.
55 Ibid., pp. 78–9.
56 Jensen, *Debussy*, p. 74.
57 Roberts, *Claude Debussy*, p. 145.
58 Ibid., p. 162.
59 Ibid., p. 145.
60 Ibid., p. 103.
61 Nichols, *The Life of Debussy*, p. 93.
62 Jensen, *Debussy*, p. 70.
63 Debussy, Claude: *Debussy Letters* (selected, ed. and trans. François Lesure and Roger Nichols), Faber and Faber, London, 1987.
64 Lockspeiser, Edward: *Debussy*, The Master Musicians, p. 87, J. M. Dent & Sons Ltd, London, 1972.
65 Ibid., p. 87.
66 Nichols, *The Life of Debussy*, pp. 115–16.
67 Ibid., p. 119.
68 Ibid., p. 125.
69 Roberts, *Claude Debussy*, p. 182.
70 Nichols, *The Life of Debussy*, p. 129.
71 Ibid., p. 140.
72 Roberts, *Claude Debussy*, pp. 208–9.
73 Ibid., p. 209.
74 Jensen, *Debussy*, pp. 115–16.
75 Ibid., p. 115.
76 Ibid. pp. 115–16.
77 Lockspeiser, *Debussy*, p. 104.
78 Ibid., p. 105.
79 Roberts, *Claude Debussy*, p. 218.
80 Lockspeiser, *Debussy*, p. 106.
81 Nichols, *The Life of Debussy*, p. 159.
82 Jensen, *Debussy*, pp. 77, 117.
83 Howat, personal communication (May 2013).
84 Cooper, Barry: *Beethoven*, The Master Musicians, p. 350, Oxford University Press, Oxford, 2000.
85 Gal, Hans: *Johannes Brahms: His Work and Personality* (trans. Joseph Stein), pp. 3–4, Alfred A. Knopf, Inc., New York, 1963.
86 Schumann, R.: 'Neue Bahnen', *Neue Zeitschrift für Musik* (1853) 39.185–6.

Neumayr, Anton: *Music & Medicine*, vol. 2, *Hummel, Weber, Mendelssohn, Schumann, Brahms, Bruckner* (English trans. B. C. Clarke), 'Brahms', p. 375, Medi-Ed Press, Bloomington, IL, 1995.

87 Neumayr, *Music & Medicine*, vol. 2, 'Brahms, Johannes', p. 379.

88 Ibid., p. 391.

89 Swafford, Jan: *Johannes Brahms: A Biography*, p. 453, Borzoi Books, Alfred A. Knopf Inc., New York, 1997.

90 MacDonald, Malcolm: *Brahms*, The Master Musicians, p. 412, J. M. Dent & Sons Ltd, London, 1993.

91 MacDonald, Malcolm: *Schoenberg*, The Master Musicians, pp. 35–6, Oxford University Press, Oxford, 2008.

92 Swafford, J.: 'Did the Young Brahms Play Piano in Waterfront Bars?', *19th Century Music* (2001) 24.268–75.
Neumayr, *Music & Medicine*, vol. 2, 'Brahms, Johannes', p. 382.

93 Swafford, 'Did the Young Brahms Play Piano in Waterfront Bars?', p. 268.
MacDonald, *Brahms*, pp. 8–9.

94 Avins, S.: 'The Young Brahms: Biographical Data Reexamined', *19th Century Music* (2001) 24.276–89.
Hoffman, Kurt: *Johannes Brahms und Hamburg*, Reinbeek, 1986 (cited in Wikipedia, accessed March 2013).

95 Swafford, *Johannes Brahms*, pp. 441–2.

96 MacDonald, *Brahms*, pp. 8–9.

97 Swafford, *Johannes Brahms*, p. 547.

98 Ibid., pp. 546–7.

99 Keys, Ivor: *Johannes Brahms*, p. 33, Christopher Helm Ltd, Bromley, 1989.

100 Ibid., p. 215.

101 Swafford, 'Did the Young Brahms Play Piano in Waterfront Bars?', pp. 268–75.
Avins, 'The Young Brahms: Biographical Data Reexamined', pp. 276–89.

102 Avins, 'The Young Brahms: Biographical Data Reexamined', p. 283.

103 May, Florence: *The Life of Johannes Brahms*, 2nd edn, vol. 1, p. 88, William Reeves, London, 1948.

104 Swafford, 'Did the Young Brahms Play Piano in Waterfront Bars?', pp. 270, 275.

105 Keys, *Johannes Brahms*, p. 120.

106 Schumann, Eugenie: *Memoirs of Eugenie Schumann* (trans. Marie Busch, 1927), p. 173, repr. Eulenburg, London, 1985.

107 Gal, *Johannes Brahms*, pp. 41–2.
MacDonald, *Brahms*, pp. 114–15.

108 Swafford, *Johannes Brahms*, p. 606.

109 Ibid., p. 121.

110 Ibid., pp. 529–30.

111 Roses, D. F.: 'Brahms & Billroth', *Surgery, Gynaecology and Obstetrics* (1986) 163.385–98.
Shafar, J.: 'The Brahms-Billroth Friendship', *British Medical Journal* (1981) 282.1775.
Strohl, E. L.: 'The Unique Friendship of Theodor Billroth and Johannes Brahms', *Surgery, Gynaecology and Obstetrics* (1970) 147.757–61.

112 Strohl, 'The Unique Friendship of Theodor Billroth and Johannes Brahms', p. 759.

113 MacDonald, *Brahms*, p. 296.
Neumayr, *Music & Medicine*, vol. 2, 'Brahms, Johannes', p. 429.

114 MacDonald, *Brahms*, p. 296.

115 Ibid., pp. 298–9.

116 Neumayr, *Music & Medicine*, vol. 2, 'Brahms, Johannes', p. 430.
117 MacDonald, *Brahms*, pp. 298–9.
118 Swafford, *Johannes Brahms*, pp. 612–13.
119 Ibid.
120 Ibid., p. 611.
121 MacDonald, *Brahms*, p. 299.
122 Neumayr, *Music & Medicine*, vol. 2, 'Brahms, Johannes', p. 437.
123 Gal, *Johannes Brahms*, p. 154.
124 Swafford, *Johannes Brahms*, p. 613.
125 Ibid., p. 615.
126 Ibid., pp. 614–15.
127 Ibid., p. 615.
128 Swafford, *Johannes Brahms*, p. 615.
129 Neumayr, *Music & Medicine*, vol. 2, 'Brahms, Johannes', p. 439.
130 Ibid. p. 439.
131 Ibid., p. 440.
132 Swafford, *Johannes Brahms*, p. 617.
133 Neumayr, *Music & Medicine*, vol. 2, 'Brahms, Johannes', pp. 440–1.
134 Swafford, *Johannes Brahms*, p. 618.
135 Ibid., p. 618.
136 Neumayr, *Music & Medicine*, vol. 2, 'Brahms, Johannes', pp. 446–7.
137 Ibid., vol. 2, p. 448.
   Swafford, *Johannes Brahms*, p. 615.
138 Ibid., p. 620.
139 Kerner, D.: 'Wie Johannes Brahms starb', *Münchener medizinische Wochenschrift* (1979) 120.565.
140 MacDonald, *Brahms*, pp. 298–9.
   Swafford, *Johannes Brahms*, p. 615.
   Keys, *Johannes Brahms*, p. 154.
141 Neumayr, *Music & Medicine*, vol. 2, 'Brahms, Johannes', pp. 427–8.
142 Keys, *Johannes Brahms*, p. 157.
143 Carner, Mosco: *Puccini: A Critical Biography*, 3rd edn, p. 182, London, 1992.
144 Adami, Giuseppe: *Giacomo Puccini: epistolario* (1928), quoted in Ravenni, Gabriella and Carner, Mosco, in 'Giacomo Puccini (ii)', *The New Grove Dictionary of Music and Musicians* (ed. Stanley Sadie), vol. 15, p. 434, Macmillan Publishers Ltd, London, 1980.
145 Budden, Julian: *Puccini: His Life and Works*, The Master Musicians, pp. 99–100, Oxford University Press, Oxford, 2005.
146 Carner, *Puccini*, pp. 141–2.
147 Ibid., p. 142.
148 Ibid., p. 142.
149 Budden, *Puccini*, p. 239.
150 Carner, *Puccini*, p. 191.
151 Ibid., p. 142.
152 Budden, *Puccini*, pp. 297–9.
153 Carner, *Puccini*, pp. 195–9.
   Budden, *Puccini*, p. 297.
154 Budden, *Puccini*, pp. 297–8.
155 Ibid., pp. 297–8.

156 Carner, *Puccini*, p. 199.

157 Jackson, Stanley: *Monsieur Butterfly: The Story of Puccini*, p. 50, W. H. Allen, London, 1994.
Phillips-Matz, Mary Jane: Puccini: A Biography, pp. 189–98, N. E. University Press, 2002.

158 Carner, *Puccini*, p. 182.

159 Ibid., p. 182.

160 Budden, *Puccini*, p. 442.
Carner, *Puccini*, p. 255.

161 Budden, *Puccini*, pp. 442–3.
Carner, *Puccini*, p. 258.

162 Carner, *Puccini*, p. 258.

163 Ibid., p. 260.

164 Ibid., p. 261.

165 Ibid., p. 224.

166 Ibid., p. 259.

167 Ibid., p. 264.

168 Young, D. A. B.: 'Rachmaninov and Marfan's Syndrome', *British Medical Journal* (1986) 23.1625–6.

169 Palmer, Tony: *The Harvest of Sorrows*, DVD, Voiceprint Records, UK, 2009.

170 Stravinsky, Igor and Craft, Robert: *Conversations with Igor Stravinsky*, p. 41, Faber Music, London, 1959.

171 Norris, Geoffrey: *Rachmaninoff*, The Dent Master Musicians, 2nd edn, p. 22, J. M. Dent & Sons Ltd, London, 1993.

172 Garcia, E. E.: 'Rachmaninoff's Emotional Collapse and Recovery: The First Symphony and Its Aftermath', *Psychoanalytic Review* (2004) 91.221–38.

173 Ibid., p. 222.

174 Ibid., p. 227.

175 Norris, *Rachmaninoff*, p. 23.

176 Ibid., p. 23.

177 Steen, *The Lives and Times of the Great Composers*, 'Rachmaninov', p. 834.

178 Figes, Orlando: *Natasha's Dance: A Cultural History of Russia*, pp. 544–5, Penguin Books Ltd, London, 2003.

179 Ibid., p. 544.

180 Norris, *Rachmaninoff*, pp. 73–4.

181 Harrison, Max: *Rachmaninoff: Life, Works, Recordings*, p. 346, Continuum, London, 2005.

182 Norris, *Rachmaninoff*, pp. 75–6.

183 Ibid., p. 76.

184 Harrison, *Rachmaninoff*, p. 347.

185 Figes, *Natasha's Dance*, p. 542.

186 Stevens, Halsey: *The Life & Music of Béla Bartók*, rev. edn, p. 4, Oxford University Press, New York, 1964.

187 Griffiths, Paul: *Bartók*, in The Master Musicians Series, p. 2, J. M. Dent & Sons Ltd, London, 1984.

188 Stevens, *The Life & Music of Béla Bartók*, p. 11.

189 Griffiths, *Bartók*, p. 7.

190 Stevens, *The Life & Music of Béla Bartók*, pp. 13–14.

191 Ibid., p. 45.

192 Chalmers, Kenneth: *Béla Bartók*, p. 55, Phaidon Press Ltd, London, 1995.
193 Ibid., p. 76.
194 Ibid., p. 74.
195 Griffiths, *Bartók*, p. 54.
196 Ibid., p. 136.
197 Chalmers, *Béla Bartók*, pp. 105–7.
198 Ibid., p. 107.
199 Griffiths, *Bartók*, p. 100.
200 Chalmers, *Béla Bartók*, p. 188.
201 Griffiths, *Bartók*, p. 157.
202 Stevens, *The Life & Music of Béla Bartók*, p. 91.
203 Chalmers, *Béla Bartók*, p. 183.
204 Lempert, Vera, and Somfai, László: 'Bartók, Béla', in *The New Grove Dictionary of Music and Musicians*, vol. 2, p. 205.
205 Stevens, *The Life & Music of Béla Bartók*, pp. 96–101.
206 Ibid., pp. 97–8.
207 Ibid., p. 98.
208 Ibid., pp. 98–9.
209 Cooper, David: *Béla Bartók*, p. 356, Yale University Press, New Haven, 2015. Stevens, *The Life & Music of Béla Bartók*, p. 100.
210 Cooper, *Béla Bartók*, p. 360.
211 Stevens, *The Life & Music of Béla Bartók*, p. 101.
212 Ibid., pp. 103–4.
213 Ibid., pp. 105–6.
214 Griffiths, *Bartók*, p. 181.
215 Chalmers, *Béla Bartók*, p. 214.
216 Marshall, Em: *Music in the Landscape*, p. 214, Robert Hale, London, 2011.
217 McVeagh, Diana: *Gerald Finzi: His Life and Music*, pp. 6, 8 and 15, Boydell Press, Woodbridge, 2010.
218 Ibid., pp. 53, 55.
219 Marshall, *Music in the Landscape*, p. 221.
220 Ibid., pp. 228–9.
221 McVeagh, *Gerald Finzi*, pp. 131–2.
222 Ibid., pp. 131–2.
223 Ibid., p. 198.
224 Finzi, Christopher ('Kiffer') and Hilary: personal communication (July 2013).
225 McVeagh, *Gerald Finzi*, pp. 206 and 211.
226 Ibid., p. 230.
227 Ibid., p. 233.
228 Ibid., pp. 249–50.
229 Banfield, Stephen: *Gerald Finzi: An English Composer*, p. 481, Faber & Faber, London, 1997.
230 McVeagh, *Gerald Finzi*, pp. 249–50. Banfield, *Gerald Finzi*, p. 482.
231 McVeagh, *Gerald Finzi*, pp. 250.
232 Irvine, Demar: *Massenet: A Chronicle of his Life and Times*, Amadeus Press, Portland, OR, 1997.
Harding, James: *Massenet*, J.M. Dent & Sons Ltd, London, 1970.
Macdonald, Hugh: 'Massenet, Jules (Emile Frédéric)' in *The New Grove Dictionary of*

Music and Musicians, 2nd edn (ed. Stanley Sadie and John Tyrrell), vol. 16, pp. 89–93, Macmillan Publishers, London, 2001.

233 Irvine, *Massenet*, p. 46.

234 Ibid., pp. 231–2.

235 Ibid., pp. 284–5.

236 Ibid., p. 285.

237 Ibid., pp. 285–7.

238 Ibid., p. 291.

239 Ibid., p. 295.

240 Ibid., pp. 296–7.

241 Ibid., pp. 296–7.

242 Massenet, Jules: *My Recollections* (trans. H. Villiers Barnett), pp. 302–4, Forgotten Books, Small Maynard & Co., Boston, 2012.

Chapter 11

1 Cooper, Barry: *Beethoven*, The Master Musicians, p. 108, Oxford University Press, Oxford, 2000.

2 Cooper, Martin: *Beethoven: The Last Decade 1817–1827*, p. 417, Oxford University Press, Oxford, 1985.

3 Hood, J. D.: 'Deafness and Musical Appreciation' in *Music and the Brain* (ed. Macdonald Critchley and R. A. Henson), Chapter 18, pp. 337–8, William Heinemann Medical Books Ltd, London, 1977.

4 Swafford, Jan: *Beethoven: Anguish and Triumph. A Biography*, p. 935, Faber & Faber Ltd, London, 2014.

5 B. Cooper, *Beethoven*, p. 260.
Cooper, M.: 'Ludwig van Beethoven', *Proceedings of the Royal Society of Medicine* (1971) 64.5–8 (pp. 497–500).

6 Cooper, Barry: personal communications (September 2014, February and June 2015 and February 2016).

7 B. Cooper, *Beethoven*, p. ix.

8 Larkin, Edward: 'Beethoven's Medical History', in M. Cooper, *Beethoven: The Last Decade*, Appendix A, p. 454, Oxford University Press, Oxford, 1985.

9 Ibid., p. 458.

10 M. Cooper, 'Ludwig van Beethoven', p. 498.

11 Mai, François M: *Diagnosing Genius: The Life and Death of Beethoven*, p. 131–5, McGill–Queen's University Press, Montreal, 2007.
Schwarz, A.: 'Beethoven's Renal Disease, Based on his Autopsy: A Case of Papillary Necrosis', *American Journal of Kidney Diseases* (1993) 21.643–52 (pp. 643–4).
McCabe, B. F.: 'Beethoven's Deafness', *Annals of Otology, Rhinology, and Laryngology* (1958) 67.192–206.

12 McCabe, 'Beethoven's Deafness', p. 197.

13 Newman, Ernest: *The Unconscious Beethoven; An Essay in Musical Psychology*, pp. 45–52, Parsons, London, 1927.
M. Cooper, 'Ludwig van Beethoven', p. 498.

14 M. Cooper, 'Ludwig van Beethoven', p. 499.

15 Larkin, E.: 'Beethoven's Illness: A Likely Diagnosis', *Proceedings of the Royal Society of Medicine* (1971) 64.493–6.

16 Kubba, A. K., and Young, M.: 'Ludwig van Beethoven: A Medical Biography', *Lancet* (1996) 347.167–70.

17 Mai, *Diagnosing Genius*, pp. 165–6.

18 Kubba and Young, 'Ludwig van Beethoven: A Medical Biography', p. 167.

19 Mai, *Diagnosing Genius*, pp. 157–8.

20 Sorsby, M.: 'Beethoven's Deafness', *Journal of Laryngology & Otology* (1930) 45.529–44 (p. 534).

21 Anderson, Emily (ed. and trans.): *The Letters of Beethoven*, vol. 1, p. 59, St Martin's Press, New York, 1961.
Wegeler, Franz G., and Ries, Ferdinand: *Remembering Beethoven: The Biographical Notes of Franz Wegeler and Ferdinand Ries* (trans. Frederick Noonan), p. 28, Andre Deutch Ltd, London, 1988.

22 Ealy, G. T.: 'Of Ear Trumpets and a Resonance Plate: Early Hearing Aids and Beethoven's Hearing Perception', *19th Century Music* (1993–94) 17 (3).262–73.
B. Cooper, *Beethoven*, p. 72.
Liston, S. L., Yanz, J. L., Preves, D., and Jelonek, S.: 'Beethoven's Deafness', *Laryngoscope* (1989) 99.1301–4 (p. 1301).

23 B. Cooper, *Beethoven*, p. 120.

24 B. Cooper, personal communications (September 2014, February and June 2015, and February 2016).
B. Cooper, *Beethoven*, p. 123.

25 Ealy, 'Of Ear Trumpets and a Resonance Plate', p. 263.
Swafford, *Beethoven*, pp. 276–80.

26 Ealy, 'Of Ear Trumpets and a Resonance Plate', p. 264.

27 Wallace, Lady Jane: *Beethoven's Letters*, vol. 1, p. 22, Hurd & Houghton, New York, 1867.

28 Newman, *The Unconscious Beethoven*, pp. 45–52.

29 Donnenberg, M. S., Collins, M. T., Benitez, M., et al.: 'The Sound that Failed: A Clinico-Pathological Conference', *American Journal of Medicine* (2000) 108.475–80 (p. 480).
Mai, *Diagnosing Genius*, p. 51.

30 B. Cooper, *Beethoven*, p. 110.

31 B. Cooper, personal communication (June 2015).

32 London, S. J.: 'Beethoven: Case Report of a Titan's Last Crisis', *Archives of Internal Medicine* (1964) 113.442–8 (p. 443).

33 Mai, *Diagnosing Genius*, p. 121.

34 B. Cooper, *Beethoven*, p. 116.

35 Ibid., p. 120.
Kalischer, A. C.: *Beethoven's Letters* (trans. J. S. Shedlock, ed. A. Eaglefield Hull), p. 38, Dover Publishing Co. Inc., New York, 1972.

36 B. Cooper, *Beethoven*, pp. 120–2.

37 Ibid., pp. 122–3.

38 Ibid., pp. 146–7.

39 B. Cooper, *Beethoven*, pp. 158–9.
Robbins Landon, Howard C.: *Beethoven: His Life, Work and World*, p. 138–9, Thames & Hudson, London, 1992.

40 Robbins Landon, *Beethoven*, p. 139.

41 Swafford, *Beethoven*, pp. 424, 660.

42 Mai, *Diagnosing Genius*, p. 123.

43 B. Cooper, *Beethoven*, p. 175.

44 Keynes, M.: 'The Personality, Deafness and Bad Health of Ludwig van Beethoven'. *Journal of Medical Biography* (2002) 10.46–57 (p. 49).
Palferman, T. G.: 'Classical Notes: Beethoven's Medical History. Variations on a Rheumatological Theme', *Journal of the Royal Society of Medicine* (1990) 83.640–5 (p. 640).

45 Kubba and Young, 'Ludwig van Beethoven: A Medical Biography', p. 168.

46 Mai, *Diagnosing Genius*, p. 109.

47 B. Cooper, *Beethoven*, p. 179.
Swafford, *Beethoven*, p. 483.

48 Ealy, 'Of Ear Trumpets and a Resonance Plate', p. 265.

49 B. Cooper, *Beethoven*, p. 193.

50 Kalischer, *Beethoven's Letters*, pp. 97–8.

51 Swafford, *Beethoven*, pp. 590–4.

52 Ibid., p. 594.

53 Czerny, Carl: 'Recollections of Beethoven', *Dwight's Journal of Music* (1852) 12.185–6.

54 B. Cooper, *Beethoven*, p. 227.

55 Ealy, 'Of Ear Trumpets and a Resonance Plate', p. 267.

56 Ibid., p. 267.

57 Mai, *Diagnosing Genius*, p. 109.

58 B. Cooper, *Beethoven*, p. 276.

59 Bower, H.: 'Beethoven's Creative Illness', *Australian and New Zealand Journal of Psychiatry* (1989) 23.111–16.
Bower, H.: 'Transient Psychosis', *Medical Journal of Australia* (1962) 1.797–800.

60 Ellenberger, Henri, F.: *The Discovery of the Unconscious*, Fontana Press (Harper & Collins), London, 1970.

61 Johnson, Martin: *Art and Scientific Thought*, pp. 39–46, Faber & Faber, London, 1954.

62 B. Cooper, *Beethoven*, p. 254.

63 Robbins Landon, *Beethoven*, p. 178.
Ealy, 'Of Ear Trumpets and a Resonance Plate', p. 270.

64 Ealy, 'Of Ear Trumpets and a Resonance Plate', p. 271.

65 Mai, *Diagnosing Genius*, p. 105.

66 Ealy, 'Of Ear Trumpets and a Resonance Plate', p. 269.
B. Cooper, *Beethoven*, p. 310.

67 B. Cooper, *Beethoven*, p. 310.

68 Keynes, 'The Personality, Deafness and Bad Health', p. 49.

69 B. Cooper, *Beethoven*, p. 317.

70 Czerny, 'Recollections of Beethoven', pp. 185–6.

71 Ealy, 'Of Ear Trumpets and a Resonance Plate', pp. 270 and 272.

72 Swafford, *Beethoven*, pp. 876–7.

73 Palferman, T. G.: 'Beethoven: A Medical Biography', *Journal of Medical Biography* (1993) 1.35–45 (p. 39).
Anderson, *The Letters of Beethoven*, vol. 3, p. 1195.

74 B. Cooper, *Beethoven*, pp. 333–4.

75 Ibid., p. 328.

76 Ibid., p. 335.

77 Ibid., p. 343.

78 Swafford, *Beethoven*, p. 914.

79 Ibid., pp. 915–16.

80 Mai, *Diagnosing Genius*, p. 130.
81 Kubba and Young, 'Ludwig van Beethoven: A Medical Biography', p. 168.
    Mai, *Diagnosing Genius*, p. 130.
82 B. Cooper, *Beethoven*, p. 348.
83 Mai, *Diagnosing Genius*, p. 130.
84 Palferman, 'Beethoven: A Medical Biography', p. 39.
85 Swafford, *Beethoven*, p. 927.
86 Ibid., pp. 916–17.
87 Ibid., p. 922.
88 Ibid., p. 928.
89 Ibid., p. 929.
90 B. Cooper, *Beethoven*, p. 349.
91 Bower, 'Beethoven's Creative Illness', p. 113.
92 Bankl, Hans, and Jesserer, Hans: *Die Krankheiten Ludwig van Beethovens*, pp. 83–7,
    89–95, 103–14, 124–31, 130, Verlag Wilhelm Maudrich, Vienna, 1987.
    Davies, P. J.: 'Beethoven's Deafness: A New Theory', *Medical Journal of Australia*
    (1988), 149.644–9 (p. 646).
93 Martin, Russell: *Beethoven's Hair*, pp. 234–8, Broadway Books, New York, 2000.
94 Meredith, W.: 'The History of Beethoven's Skull Fragments', *Beethoven Journal* (2005)
    20.3–39.
95 Mai, *Diagnosing Genius*, p. 133.
96 Larkin, 'Beethoven's Illness, p. 496.
97 Mai, *Diagnosing Genius*, p. 139.
98 Schwarz, 'Beethoven's Renal Disease', p. 647.
99 Ober, W. B.: 'Beethoven: A Medical View', *The Practitioner* (1970) 205.819–24
    (p. 823).
    Kubba and Young, 'Ludwig van Beethoven: A Medical Biography', p. 168.
100 London, 'Beethoven: Case Report of a Titan's Last Crisis', p. 446.
    Ober, 'Beethoven: A Medical View', pp. 820–1.
    Swafford, *Beethoven*, p. 929 and n. 89.
    Mai, *Diagnosing Genius*, pp. 141–7.
    Schwarz, 'Beethoven's Renal Disease', p. 646.
101 Palferman, 'Beethoven: A Medical Biography', p. 42.
    Adams, P.: 'Historical Hepatology: Ludwig van Beethoven', *Journal of Gastroenterolo-*
    gy and Hepatology (1987) 2.375–9 (p. 378).
102 Mai, *Diagnosing Genius*, p. 130.
103 Palferman, 'Beethoven: A Medical Biography', p. 42.
    Karmody, C. S., and Bachor, E. S.: 'The Deafness of Ludwig van Beethoven: An
    Immunopathy', *Otology and Neurology* (2005) 26.809–14.
    Schindler, Anton: *Beethoven As I Knew Him* (ed. Donald MacArdle), p. 386, Faber &
    Faber, London, 1966.
    Schwarz, 'Beethoven's Renal Disease', p. 646.
104 B. Cooper, *Beethoven*, p. 229.
105 Mai, *Diagnosing Genius*, p. 145.
106 Ibid., p. 144.
107 Palferman, 'Beethoven: A Medical Biography', p. 42.
    Larkin, 'Beethoven's Medical History', pp. 453–5.
108 Mai, *Diagnosing Genius*, p. 144.
109 Keynes, 'The Personality, Deafness and Bad Health', p. 54.

110 Mai, *Diagnosing Genius*, p. 145.

111 Ibid., p. 145.

112 Ibid., p. 146.

113 Adams, Historical Hepatology: Ludwig van Beethoven', p. 378.

114 Broomé, U.: 'Primary Sclerosing Cholangitis may have Caused the Death of Bee-thoven', *Läkartidningen* (2006) 103.2494–6 (p. 2494).

115 Adams, 'Historical Hepatology: Ludwig van Beethoven', p. 378.
Broomé, 'Primary Sclerosing Cholangitis may have Caused the Death of Beethoven' pp. 2494–6.

116 Talwalkar, J. A., and Lindor, K. D.: 'Primary Sclerosing Cholangitis', *Inflammatory Bowel Diseases* (2005) 11.62–72.

117 Collier, J. D., and Webster, G.: 'Liver and Biliary Tract Disease' in *Davidson's Principles and Practice of Medicine* (ed. N. R. Colledge, B. R. Walker and S. H. Ralston), 21st edn, pp. 965–7, Churchill Livingstone/Elsevier, Edinburgh, 2010.

118 London, 'Beethoven: Case Report of a Titan's Last Crisis', p. 447.
Davies, P. J.: 'Beethoven's Nephropathy and Death: Discussion Paper', *Journal of the Royal Society of Medicine* (1993) 86.159–61 (pp. 160–1).

119 Kubba and Young, 'Ludwig van Beethoven: A Medical Biography', p. 170.
Adams, 'Historical Hepatology: Ludwig van Beethoven', p. 377.
Karmody and Bachor, 'The Deafness of Ludwig van Beethoven: An Immunopathy', pp. 809–10.

120 Raj, V., and Lichtenstein, D. R.: 'Hepatobiliary Manifestations of Inflammatory Bowel Disease', *Gastroenterology Clinics of North America* (1999) 28.491–513.

121 Adams, 'Historical Hepatology: Ludwig van Beethoven', p. 375.

122 Shearer, P.: 'The Deafness of Beethoven: An Audiologic and Medical Overview', *American Journal of Otolaryngology* (1990) 11.370–4 (p. 370).

123 McCabe, B. F.: 'Auto-Immune Hearing Loss', *Annals of Otolaryngology* (1979) 88.585–9.

124 Hollanders, D.: 'Sensorineural Deafness: A New Complication of Ulcerative Colitis', *Postgraduate Medicine Journal* (1986) 62.753–5.
Kumar, B. N., Smith, M. S., Walsh, R. M., and Green, J. R.: 'Sensorineural Hearing Loss in Ulcerative Colitis', *Clinical Otolaryngology* (2000) 25.143–5.

125 Bachmeyer, C., Leclerc-Landgraf, N., Laurette, F., et al.: 'Acute Auto-Immune Sensorineural Hearing Loss Associated with Crohn's Disease', *American Journal of Gastroenterology.* (1998) 93.2565–7.

126 Stevens, K. M., and Hemenway, W. G.: 'Beethoven's Deafness', *Journal of the American Medical Association* (1970) 210.434–7.

127 Larkin, 'Beethoven's Illness', p. 496.

128 Ibid., p. 496.
Palferman, 'Beethoven: A Medical Biography', p. 44.

129 B. Cooper, *Beethoven*, p. 333.

130 Palferman, 'Beethoven: A Medical Biography', p. 43.

131 Schwarz, 'Beethoven's Renal Disease', pp. 643–52.

132 Ibid., p. 648.

133 Ibid., p. 647.

134 Davies, P. J.: 'Was Beethoven's Cirrhosis Due to Haemochromatosis?', *Renal Failure* (1995) 17.77–86.

135 Mai, *Diagnosing Genius*, pp. 147–51.

136 Ibid., pp. 147–51.

137 Martin, *Beethoven's Hair*, pp. 234–8.

138 Mai, *Diagnosing Genius*, pp. 147–51.

139 Keynes, 'The Personality, Deafness and Bad Health, p. 53.

140 Drake, M. E.: 'Deafness, Dysaesthesia, Depression, Diarrhoea, Dropsy and Death: The Case for Sarcoidosis in Ludwig van Beethoven', *Neurology* (1994) 44.562–5.

141 Reid, P. T., and Innes, J. A., 'Sarcoidosis' in *Davidson's Principles & Practice of Medicine*, p. 709.

142 Palferman, 'Beethoven: A Medical Biography', p. 44.

143 Drake, 'Deafness, Dysaesthesia, Depression, Diarrhoea, Dropsy and Death: The Case for Sarcoidosis in Ludwig van Beethoven', p. 564.

144 Reid and Innes, *Davidson's Principles & Practice of Medicine*, pp. 708–9.

145 Squires, P.C.: 'The Problem of Beethoven's Deafness', *Journal of Abnormal and Social Psychology* (1937) 32.11–62 (p. 42).

146 McCabe, 'Beethoven's Deafness', p. 205.
Newman, *The Unconscious Beethoven*, pp. 45–52.
Hayden, Deborah: *Pox: Genius and Madness and the Mysteries of Syphilis*, Chapter 8, pp. 71–88, Basic Books, New York, 2003.

147 Frimmel, Theodor, and Jacobsohn, L.: *Beethoven-Handbuch*, vol. 1, p. 38, Breitkopf & Härtel, Leipzig, 1926.
Jacobsohn, L.: 'Beethovens Gehörleiden und letzte Krankheit', *Deutsche Medizinische Wochenschrift* (1927) 53.1610–12.

148 Palferman, T. G.: 'Beethoven: The Case against Syphilis', *Journal of the Royal College of Physicians of* London (1992) 26.112–14.

149 Larkin, 'Beethoven's Medical History', p. 449.

150 Grove, Sir George: *Dictionary of Music and Musicians*, vol. 1, p. 173, Macmillan, London, 1879.

151 Palferman, 'Beethoven: The Case against Syphilis', p. 113.
Hayden, *Pox*, p. 74.

152 Hayden, *Pox*, pp. 71–88.

153 Martin, *Beethoven's Hair*, pp. 234–8.
Keynes, 'The Personality, Deafness and Bad Health', p. 53.

154 Bower, 'Beethoven's Creative Illness', p. 113.

155 Ibid., p. 113.

156 B. Cooper, *Beethoven*, pp. 246–7.

157 Ibid., p. 223.
Sterba, Editha and Richard: *Beethoven and his Nephew*, Pantheon, New York, 1954.

158 Larkin, 'Beethoven's Medical History', p. 451.
Solomon, Maynard: *Beethoven*, 2nd edn, pp. 334–9, Schirmer Books, New York, 1998.

159 B. Cooper, *Beethoven*, pp. 256–7.

160 Larkin, 'Beethoven's Medical History', p. 453.

161 Donnenberg et al., 'The Sound that Failed', p. 478.

162 Karmody and Bachor, 'The Deafness of Ludwig van Beethoven: An Immunopathy', p. 812.

163 Donnenberg et al., 'The Sound that Failed', p. 478.

164 Tramont, E. C.: 'Syphilis: From Beethoven to HIV', *Mount Sinai Journal of Medicine* (1990) 57.192–6.

165 Ibid., p. 193.

166 Hayden, *Pox*, p. 55.

167 Goorney, Dr Benjamin: personal communication (June 2015).

Rees, Dr W. Wynne: personal communication (July 2015).

168 Butz, W. C., Watts, J. C., Rosales-Quintana, S., and Hicklin, M. D.: 'Erosive Gastritis as a Manifestation of Secondary Syphilis', *American Journal of Clinical Pathology* (1975), 63.895–900.

Reisman, T. N., Leverett, L., Hudson, J. R., and Kaiser, M. H.: 'Syphliitic Gastropathy', *Journal of Digestive Diseases* (1975), 20.588–593.

169 Goorney, personal communication (June 2015).

170 Sharma, O. P.: 'Beethoven's Illness: Whipple's Disease rather than Sarcoidosis', *Journal of the Royal Society of Medicine* (1994) 87.283–5.

171 Ealy, 'Of Ear Trumpets and a Resonance Plate', pp. 262–73.

172 Ibid., p. 271.

McCabe, 'Beethoven's Deafness', pp. 201–2.

173 Naiken, V. S.: 'Did Beethoven have Paget's Disease of Bone?', *Annals of Internal Medicine* (1971) 74.995–9.

Naiken, V. S.: 'Paget's Disease and Beethoven's Deafness', *Clinical Orthopaedics and Related Research* (1972) 89.103–5.

174 Neumann, H.: 'Beethovens Gehörleiden', *Wiener Medizinische Wochenschrift* (1927) 77.1015–19.

175 Sparrow, N. L., and Duval, A. J.: 'Hearing Loss and Paget's Disease', *Journal of Laryngology and Otology* (1967) 81.601–11.

176 Ealy, 'Of Ear Trumpets and a Resonance Plate', pp. 262–73.

Karmody and Bachor, 'The Deafness of Ludwig van Beethoven: An Immunopathy', pp. 811–13.

Harrison, P.: 'The Effects of Deafness on Musical Composition', *Journal of the Royal Society of Medicine* (1988) 81.598–601.

Landsberger, M.: 'Beethoven's Medical History from a Physician's Viewpoint', *New York State Journal of Medicine* (1978) 78.676–9 (pp. 677–8).

Stevens and Hemenway, 'Beethoven's Deafness', pp. 434–5.

177 Hood, 'Deafness and Musical Appreciation', pp. 325–6.

178 B. Cooper, *Beethoven*, p. 185.

179 Gutman, A. F., and Kasabach, H.: 'Paget's Disease: Analysis of 116 Cases', *American Journal of the Medical Sciences* (1936) 191.361–80.

180 Ibid., pp. 361–70.

181 Naiken, 'Did Beethoven have Paget's Disease of Bone?', p. 995.

182 Palferman, 'Beethoven: A Medical Biography', pp. 42–3.

183 Bankl, H., and Jesserer, H.: 'Ertaubte Beethoven an einer Pagetschen Krankheit?', *Laryngologie Rhinologie Otologie* (1986) 65.592–7.

184 Shearer, 'The Deafness of Beethoven: An Audiologic and Medical Overview', pp. 370–4.

Stevens and Hemenway, 'Beethoven's Deafness', pp. 434–7.

185 Shearer, 'The Deafness of Beethoven: An Audiologic and Medical Overview', pp. 370–4.

Stevens and Hemenway, 'Beethoven's Deafness', pp. 434–7.

186 Karmody and Bachor, 'The Deafness of Ludwig van Beethoven: An Immunopathy', p. 812.

187 Mai, *Diagnosing Genius*, p. 134.

188 Ealy, 'Of Ear Trumpets and a Resonance Plate', pp. 262–73.

Karmody and Bachor, 'The Deafness of Ludwig van Beethoven: An Immunopathy', p. 811.

B. Cooper, *Beethoven*, p. 335
Mai, *Diagnosing Genius*, pp. 155–6.
189 Squires, 'The Problem of Beethoven's Deafness', p. 49.
190 Seeley, W. W., Matthews, B. R., Crawford, R. K., et al.: 'Unravelling *Bolero*, Progressive Aphasia, Transmodal Creativity and Right Posterior Neocortex', *Brain* (2008) 131.39–49.
191 Harrison, 'The Effects of Deafness on Musical Composition', p. 599.
192 M. Cooper, 'Ludwig van Beethoven', p. 499.
193 Harrison, 'The Effects of Deafness on Musical Composition', p. 599.
194 B. Cooper, *Beethoven*, p. 341.
195 Kerman, Joseph: *The Beethoven Quartets*, p. 76, Oxford University Press, Oxford, 1967.
196 Liston, S. L., Yanz, J. L., Preves, D., and Jelonek, S.: 'Beethoven's Deafness', *Laryngoscope* (1989) 99.1301–4.
197 Ibid., p. 1304.
198 Larkin, 'Beethoven's Illness', pp. 493–6.
199 Kubba and Young, 'Ludwig van Beethoven: A Medical Biography', pp. 167–70.
200 Larkin, 'Beethoven's Illness', p. 496.
201 Adams, 'Historical Hepatology: Ludwig van Beethoven', pp. 375–9.
Broomé, 'Primary Sclerosing Cholangitis may have Caused the Death of Beethoven', pp. 2494–6.
202 Sharma, 'Beethoven's Illness: Whipple's Disease rather than Sarcoidosis', pp. 283–5.
203 Drake, 'Deafness, Dysaesthesia, Depression, Diarrhoea, Dropsy and Death: The Case for Sarcoidosis in Ludwig van Beethoven', pp. 562–5.
204 Adams, 'Historical Hepatology: Ludwig van Beethoven', pp. 375–9.
205 Squires, 'The Problem of Beethoven's Deafness', pp. 11–62.
Hayden, *Pox*, pp. 71–88.
206 Mai, *Diagnosing Genius*, pp. 144–5, 147–51.
207 Davies, 'Beethoven's Nephropathy and Death: Discussion Paper', pp. 159–61.
Schwarz, 'Beethoven's Renal Disease', pp. 643–52.
208 Davies, 'Was Beethoven's Cirrhosis Due to Haemochromatosis?', pp. 77–86.
209 London, 'Beethoven: Case Report of a Titan's Last Crisis', p. 447.
210 Davies, 'Beethoven's Nephropathy and Death: Discussion Paper', pp. 159–61.
211 Shearer, 'The Deafness of Beethoven: An Audiologic and Medical Overview', pp. 370–4.
Stevens and Hemenway, 'Beethoven's Deafness', pp. 434–7.
212 McCabe, 'Auto-Immune Hearing Loss', pp. 585–9.
Hollanders, 'Sensorineural Deafness: A New Complication of Ulcerative Colitis', pp. 753–5.
213 Kubba and Young, 'Ludwig van Beethoven: A Medical Biography', p. 169.
214 Naiken, 'Did Beethoven have Paget's Disease of Bone?', pp. 995–9.
Naiken, 'Paget's Disease and Beethoven's Deafness', pp. 103–5.
215 Squires, 'The Problem of Beethoven's Deafness', pp. 11–62.
Frimmel, *Beethoven-Handbuch*, vol 1, p. 38.
216 McCabe, 'Beethoven's Deafness', p. 193.
217 Ibid., pp. 202–3.
218 Mai, *Diagnosing Genius*, pp. 147–51.
219 Gutt, R. W.: 'Beethoven's Deafness: An Iatrogenic Disease', *Medizinische Klinik* (1970), 65.2294–5.

220 Duchen, Jessica: *Gabriel Fauré*, p. 14, 20th Century Composers, Phaidon Press, London, 2000.

221 Ibid, p. 69.
Orledge, Robert: *Gabriel Fauré*, p. 13, Eulenburg Books, London, 2nd edn 1983.

222 Duchen, *Gabriel Fauré*, p. 66.

223 Ibid., pp. 47–50.

224 Steen, Michael, *The Lives and Times of the Great Composers*, 'Fauré', p. 626, Icon Books, London, 2010.

225 Howat, Roy: personal communications (2013 and 2015).

226 Duchen, *Gabriel Fauré*, p. 108.

227 Ibid., p. 142.

228 Ibid., p. 147.

229 Ibid., p. 140.

230 Howat, personal communications (2013 and 2015).

231 Duchen, *Gabriel Fauré*, p. 142.

232 Jones, J. Barrie (ed. and trans.): *Gabriel Fauré: A Life in Letters*, Letter 116, p. 111, Batsford Books, London, 1989.
Duchen, *Gabriel Fauré*, p. 146.

233 Jones, *Gabriel Fauré*, Letter 111, p. 108.

234 Duchen, *Gabriel Fauré*, p. 146.

235 Orledge, *Gabriel Fauré*, p. 20–1.

236 Duchen, *Gabriel Fauré*, p. 147.

237 Ibid., p. 147.

238 Orledge, *Gabriel Fauré*, p. 21.

239 Howat, personal communications (2013 and 2015).

240 Orledge, *Gabriel Fauré*, p. 29.

241 Jones, *Gabriel Fauré*, Letter 261, p. 184.

242 Ibid., Letter 250, p.180.

243 Orledge, *Gabriel Fauré*, p. 29.
Jones, *Gabriel Fauré*, pp. 201, 203, 205.

244 Nectoux, Jean-Michel: *Gabriel Fauré: A Musical Life* (trans. Roger Nichols), p. 500, Cambridge University Press, Cambridge, UK, 1991.

245 Landormy, P., and Herter, M. D.: 'Gabriel Fauré (1845–1924)', *Musical Quarterly* (1931) 17.293–301.

246 Copland, Aaron: 'Gabriel Fauré: A Neglected Master', *Musical Quarterly* (1923) 10.573–86.

247 Howat, personal communications (2013 and 2015).

248 Duchen, *Gabriel Fauré*, pp. 208–9.

249 Macleod, Donald, and Duchen, Jessica: 'Fauré': *Composer of the Week*, BBC Radio 3, 1 June 2013.

250 Duchen, *Gabriel Fauré*, p. 211.

251 Jones, *Gabriel Fauré*, Letter 312, pp. 205–6.

252 Duchen, *Gabriel Fauré*, p. 212.
Orledge, *Gabriel Fauré*, p. 30.

Epilogue

1 Jack, Adrian: 'Robert Schumann', programme to Prom 10, BBC Proms, 19 July 2013.

2 Ludwig, A. M.: 'Alcohol and Creative Output', *British Journal of Addiction* (1990) 85.953–63.

3 Nicolson, H.: 'The Health of Authors', *Lancet* 1947, 2 (6481), pp. 709–14.

4 Waddell, C.: 'Creativity and Mental Illness – is There a Link?', *Canadian Journal of Psychiatry* (1998) 43.166–72.

5 Juda. A.: 'The Relationship Between Highest Mental Capacity and Psychic Abnormalities', *American Journal of Psychiatry* (1949) 109.296–307.

6 Slater, E., and Meyer, A.: 'Contributions to a Pathography of the Musicians: 2. Organic and Psychotic Disorders', *Confinia Psychiatrica* (1960) 3.65–94.

7 Farnworth, P. R.: 'Musicality and Abnormality', *Confinica Psychiatrica* (1961) 4.158–61.

8 Vernon, Philip E.: *Creativity*, Penguin Books, Harmondsworth, 1970.

9 Post, F.: 'Creativity and Psychopathology: A Study of 291 World-Famous Men', *British Journal of Psychiatry* (1994) 165.22–34.

10 Slater and Meyer, 'Contributions to a Pathography of the Musicians', pp. 65–94.

11 Waddell, 'Creativity and Mental Illness', p. 167.

12 Jamison, Kay R.: *Touched with Fire: Manic-Depressive Illness and the Artistic Temperament*, Free Press Paperbacks, Simon and Schuster, New York, 1993.
Jamison, K. R.: 'Mood Disorders and Patterns of Creativity in British Writers and Artists', *Psychiatry* (1989) 32.125–34.

13 Jamison, *Touched with Fire*.

14 Ludwig, A.: 'Reflections on Creativity and Madness', *American Journal of Psychiatry* (1989) 153.4–14.
Ludwig, A. M.: 'Creative Achievement and Psychopathology: Comparison Among Professions', *American Journal of Psychotherapy* (1992) 46.330–56.

15 Pickering, George: *Creative Malady: Illness in the Lives and Minds of Charles Darwin, Florence Nightingale, Mary Baker Eddy, Sigmund Freud, Marcel Proust, Elizabeth Barrett Browning*, George Allen Unwin Ltd, London, 1972.

16 Ibid., pp. 277–8.

17 Kennedy, Michael: personal communication (June 2013).

18 Toye, Francis: *Rossini: A Study in Tragi-Comedy*, new edn, p. 201, Arthur Barker, London, 1954.

19 Abbott, E. C.: 'Composers and Tuberculosis: The Effects on Creativity', *Canadian Medical Association Journal* (1982) 126.534–44.

20 Reeves, Carol, during Robert Winston's programme on Chopin, BBC Radio 4, 27 March 2012.
Reeves, Dr Carol: personal communication (April 2016).

21 Jamison, 'Mood Disorders and Patterns of Creativity in British Writers and Artists', p. 132.
Jamison, 'Touched with Fire', pp. 13, 264.

22 Harcup, J., and Noble, J: 'Edward Elgar (1857–1934): Moaner or Loner?', *Journal of Medical Biography* (2016) 24.135–8.

23 Nichols, Roger: *The Life of Debussy*, Musical Lives, p. 140, Cambridge University Press, Cambridge, UK, 1998.

24 Garcia, E. E.: 'Gustav Mahler's Choice: A Note on Adolescence, Genius and Psychosomatics', *Psychoanalytic Study of the Child* (2000) 55.87–110.

25 Storr, A.: 'The Sanity of True Genius', unpublished manuscript, quoted by Kay Jamison, *Touched with Fire*, p. 57.

26 White, Michael: 'One Ring to Rule them All', *Daily Telegraph*, 19 July 2013.

27 Owen, David: *In Sickness and in Power: Illness in Heads of Government during the Last 100 Years*, Methuen, London, 2011.

28 Noble, J.: 'Biography, Hagiography or Demonology', *Journal of Medical Biography* (2015) 23.123–4.

Appendix

1 Anthony, James R.: 'Jean Baptiste Lully' in *The New Grove Dictionary of Music and Musicians* (ed. Stanley Sadie), vol. 11, p. 317, Macmillan Publishers, London, 1980.

2 Ibid., p. 317.

3 Kennedy, Michael and Joyce, and Rutherford-Johnson, Tim: *Oxford Dictionary of Music*, 6th edn, 'Baton', p. 62, Oxford University Press, Oxford, 2012.

4 Smith, Ronald: *Alkan: The Enigma*, pp. 73–5, Kahn & Averill, London, 1977

5 Macdonald, H.: 'More on Alkan's Death', *Musical Times* (1988) 129.118–20.

6 MacCullum, S.: 'Alkan: Enigma or Schizophrenia', Alkan Society Bulletin (2007) 75.2–10.

7 Vallas, Léon: *La véritable histoire de César Franck* (trans. Hugo Foss), pp. 229, 234, George G. Harrap & Co. Ltd, London, 1951.

8 Davies, Laurence: *César Franck and his Circle*, p. 242, Barrie & Jenkins, London, 1970.

9 Lockspeiser, Edward: *Debussy: His Life and Mind*, vol. 1, p. 126, Cassell, London, 1965.

10 Grover, Ralph Scott: *Ernest Chausson: The Man and his Music*, p. 56, Athlone Press, London, 1980.

11 La Grange, H. L. de: 'Prometheus Unbound', *Music and Musicians* (1971–72) 20(5).34–43.

12 Bowers, Faubian: *Scriabin: A Biography*, 2nd edn, vol. 2, pp. 256–7, 276–8, Dover Publications, Mineola, NY, 1996.

13 Ibid., pp. 276–8.

14 Barlow, Michael: *Whom the Gods Love: The Life and Music of George Butterworth*, p. 131, Toccata Press, London, 1997.

15 Murphy, Anthony: *Banks of Green Willow*, p. 200, Capella Archive, Great Malvern, 2012.

16 Larrad, Mark: 'Granados y Campiña, Enrique' in *The New Grove Dictionary of Music and Musicians*, 2nd edn (ed. Stanley Sadie and John Tyrrell), vol. 10, p. 278, Macmillan Publishers, London, 2001.

17 Falliers, C. J.: 'Arnold Schoenberg and Alban Berg: The Serial Music and Serious Asthma of Two Leading 20th Century Composers', *Journal of Asthma* (1986) 23.211–17.

18 Carner, Mosco: *Alban Berg: The Man and the Work*, 2nd edn, pp. 85–89, Duckworth, London, 1983.
   Reich, Willi: *The Life and Work of Alban Berg* (trans. Cornelius Cardew), pp. 102–5, Thames & Hudson, London, 1965.
   Falliers, 'Arnold Schoenberg and Alban Berg', p. 216.

19 Falliers, 'Arnold Schoenberg and Alban Berg', p. 216.
   Reich, *The Life and Work of Alban Berg*, p. 105.

20 Moldenhauer, Hans: *Anton Webern: A Chronicle of his Life and Work*, Chapter 36, pp. 626–37, Victor Gallancz, London, 1978.

Bibliography

Books and Book Chapters

Abraham, Gerald: 'Hugo Wolf' in *Lives of Great Composers* (ed. A. L. Bacharach), Victor Gollancz, London, 1935

Abraham, Gerald: *Rimsky-Korsakov: A Short Biography*, Duckworth, London, 1945

Ackroyd, Peter: *Albion: The Origins of the English Imagination*, Chatto & Windus, London, 2002

Adorno, Theodor W.: *Mahler: A Musical Physiognomy*, University of Chicago Press, Chicago, 1996

Anderson, Emily (ed. and trans.): *The Letters of Beethoven*, St Martin's Press, New York, 1961

Anderson, Emily (ed.): *The Letters of Mozart and his Family*, 3rd edn, Macmillan Press, London, 1985

Anderson, Robert: *Elgar*, The Master Musicians, Oxford University Press, Oxford, 1993

Armitage, Merle: *George Gershwin, Man and Legend*, Books for Library Press, Freeport, NY, 1958

Arnold, Denis: *Monteverdi*, The Master Musicians Series, 3rd edn, J. M. Dent & Sons Ltd, London, 1990

Ashbrook, William: *Donizetti and his Operas*, Cambridge University Press, Cambridge, UK, 1982, repr. Cambridge Paperback Library, 2010

Austin, William: *Music in the 20th Century*, 'Prokofiev', pp. 451–71, J. M. Dent & Sons Ltd, London, 1966

Baeck, E.: 'The Longstanding Medical Fascination with "le cas Ravel"' in *Ravel Studies* (ed. Deborah Mawer), pp. 187–208, Cambridge University Press, Cambridge, UK, 2010

Banfield, Stephen: *Gerald Finzi: An English Composer*, Faber & Faber, London, 1997

Bankl, Hans and Jesserer, Hans: *Die Krankheiten Ludwig van Beethovens*, Verlag Wilhelm Maudrich, Vienna, 1987

Bär, Carl, *Mozart: Krankheit – Tod – Begräbnis*, Schriftenreihe der Internationalen Stiftung Mozarteum Salzburg, Bärenreiter, Kassel,1966

Barlow, Michael: *Whom the Gods Love: The Life and Music of George Butterworth*, Toccata Press, London, 1997

Barnett, Andrew: *Sibelius*, Yale University Press, New Haven and London, 2007

Beecham, Thomas: *Frederick Delius*, Hutchinson & Co. Ltd, 1959

Benestad, Finn, and Schjelderup-Ebbe, Dag: *Edvard Grieg: The Man and the Artist* (trans. W. A. Halverson and L. B. Sateren), Allan Sutton Publishing, Gloucester, 1988

Berlioz, Hector: *Selected Letters of Hector Berlioz* (ed. H. Macdonald, English trans. R. Nichols), Faber & Faber, London, 1995

Blaukopf, Kurt: *Gustav Mahler* (trans. Inge Goodwin), Allen Lane/Readers Union, London, 1973

Bloom, Peter: *The Life of Berlioz*, Musical Lives, Cambridge University Press, Cambridge, UK, 1998

Bowers, Faubian: *Scriabin: A Biography*, 2nd edn, Dover Publications, Mineola, NY, 1996

Boyd, Malcolm: *Bach*, Oxford University Press, Oxford, 2000

Boyd, Malcolm: *Bach,* The Master Musicians Series, 2nd edn, J. M. Dent & Sons Ltd, London, 1990

Breuning, Gerhard von: *Memories of Beethoven* (trans. Henry Mins and Maynard Solomon, ed. Maynard Solomon), Cambridge University Press, Cambridge, 1995

Bridcut, John: *Britten's Children*, Faber, London, 2007

Brinkmann, Reinhold: *Late Idyll: The Second Symphony of Johannes Brahms*, Harvard University Press, Cambridge, MA, 1995

Brown, Clive: *A Portrait of Mendelssohn*, Yale University Press, New Haven, 2003

Brown, David: *Musorgsky: His Life and Works*, The Master Musicians, Oxford University Press, 2010

Brown, David: *Tchaikovsky: A Biographical and Critical Study*, vol. 1, *The Early Years 1840–74*, Victor Gollancz Ltd, London, 1978

Brown, David: *Tchaikovsky: A Biographical and Critical Study*, vol. 2, *The Crisis Years 1874–8*, Victor Gollancz Ltd, London, 1982

Brown, David: *Tchaikovsky: A Biographical and Critical Study*, vol. 3, *The Years of Wandering 1878–85*, Victor Gollancz Ltd, London, 1986

Brown, David: *Tchaikovsky: A Biographical and Critical Study*, vol. 4, *The Final Years 1885–93*, Victor Gollancz Ltd, London, 1991

Brown, David: *Tchaikovsky Remembered*, Faber & Faber, London, 1993

Brown, David: *Tchaikovsky: The Man and his Music*, Faber & Faber Ltd, London, 2006

Brown, James A. C.: *Freud and the Post Freudians*, Penguin Books Ltd, Harmondsworth, 1961

Brown, Maurice J. E.: *Chopin: An Index of his Works*, Macmillan, London, 1972

Budden, Julian: *Puccini: His Life and Works*, The Master Musicians, Oxford University Press, Oxford, 2005

Budden, Julian: *Verdi*, The Master Musicians, Oxford University Press, Oxford, 2008

Burk, John, N.: *Clara Schumann: A Romantic Biography*, Random House, New York, 1940

Burney, Charles: *An Eighteenth Century Musical Tour in Central Europe and the Netherlands* (ed. Percy A. Scholes), Dr. Burney's Musical Tours, 2, Oxford University Press, London, 1959

Burrows, Donald: *Handel*, The Master Musicians, Oxford University Press, Oxford, 1996

Burrows, John and Whiffen, Charles: *Classical Music*, Eyewitness Companions Series, Dorling Kindersley Ltd, London, 2005

Burton, Richard D. E.: *Francis Poulenc*, Absolute Press, Bath, 2002

Cairns, David: *Berlioz*, vol. 1, *The Making of an Artist 1803–32*, Sphere Books Ltd, London, 1989

Cairns, David: *Berlioz*, vol. 2, *Servitude and Greatness 1832–1869*, Sphere Books Ltd, London, 1999

Cairns, David (trans. and ed.): *The Memoirs of Hector Berlioz*, Victor Gollancz Ltd, London, 1977

Calvocoressi, M. D.: *Mussorgsky*, The Master Musicians Series (completed and revised by Gerald Abraham in 2nd edn), J. M. Dent & Sons Ltd, London, 1974

Cardus, Neville: *A Composer's Eleven*, Jonathan Cape, London, 1958

Carley, Lionel: *Delius: A Life in Letters (1909–1934)*, Scholar Press, Aldershot, 1988

Carner, Mosco: *Alban Berg: The Man and the Work*, 2nd edn, Duckworth, London, 1983

Carner, Mosco: *Puccini: A Critical Biography*, 3rd edn, Duckworth, London, 1992

Carpenter, Humphrey: *Benjamin Britten: A Biography*, Faber & Faber, London, 1992

Chalmers, Kenneth: *Béla Bartók*, Phaidon Press Ltd, London, 1995

Charness, M. E.: 'Upper Extremity Disorders of Musicians' in *Occupational Disorders of the Upper Extremity* (ed. L. H. Millender, D. S. Louis and B. P. Simmonds), pp. 117–51, Churchill Livingstone, New York, 1992

Chorley, Henry F.: *Modern German Music: Recollections and Criticisms,* Smith, Elder & Co., London, 1854

Clapham, John: *Dvořák*, David and Charles, London, 1979

Clapham, John: *Smetana*, The Master Musicians Series, J. M. Dent and Sons Ltd, London, 1972

Cole, Hugo: *Malcolm Arnold: Introduction to his Music*, Faber Music, London, 1989

Colledge, N. R., Walker, B. R. and Ralston, S. H. (eds.): *Davidson's Principles and Practice of Medicine*, 21st edn, Churchill Livingstone/Elsevier, Edinburgh, 2010

Collier, J. D., and Webster, G.: 'Liver and Biliary Tract Disease' in *Davidson's Principles and Practice of Medicine* (ed. N. R. Colledge, B. R. Walker and S. H. Ralston), 21st edn, pp. 965–7, Churchill Livingstone/Elsevier, Edinburgh, 2010

Collins, Brian: *Peter Warlock: The Composer*, Scholar Press, Aldershot, 1996

Conati, M.: *Interviews and Encounters with Verdi*, Gollancz, London, 1984

Cooke, Deryck: *Gustav Mahler: An Introduction to his Music*, 2nd edn, Faber Music, London, 1988

Cooper, Barry: *Beethoven, The Master Musicians*, Oxford University Press, Oxford, 2000

Cooper, David: *Béla Bartók*, Yale University Press, New Haven, 2015

Cooper, Martin: *Beethoven: The Last Decade 1817–1827*, Oxford University Press, Oxford, 1985

Cooper, Martin: *French Music: From the Death of Berlioz to the Death of Fauré*, Oxford University Press, Oxford, 1951

Cooper, Martin: *Gluck*, Chatto & Windus, London, 1935

Copley, Ian A.: *The Music of Peter Warlock*, Dennis Dobson, London, 1979

Copley, Ian A.: *George Butterworth and his Music: A Centennial Tribute*, Thames Publishing, London, 1985

Craft, Robert: *Stravinsky: Chronicle of a Friendship 1948–71*, Gollancz, London, 1972

Craft, Robert: *Stravinsky in Conversation with Robert Craft*, Penguin, Harmondsworth, 1962

Craft, Robert: 'The Nostalgic Kingdom of Maurice Ravel' in *Current Convictions*, pp. 184–95, Secker and Warburg, London, 1978

Critchley, MacDonald, and Henson R. A (eds.): *Music and the Brain: Studies in the Neurology of Music*, William Heinemann Medical Books Ltd, London, 1977

Crittenden, Camille: *Johann Strauss and Vienna: Operetta and the Politics of Popular Culture*, Cambridge University Press, Cambridge, UK, 2006 (first pub. 2000)

Cross, Jonathan: *Igor Stravinsky, Critical Lives*, Reaktion Books, London, 2015

Curtiss, Mina: *Bizet and his World*, Alfred A. Knopf, New York, 1958

Dahl, Erling: *Edvard Grieg: His Life and Music. A Short Biography*, Edvard Grieg Museum, Troldhaugen, 2002

Davies, Laurence: *César Franck and his Circle*, Barrie & Jenkins, London, 1970

Day, James: *Vaughan Williams,* The Master Musicians Series, J. M. Dent & Sons Ltd, London, 1972

Day, James: *Vaughan Williams,* The Master Musicians, 3rd edn, Oxford University Press, Oxford, 1998

Dean, Winton: *Georges Bizet: His Life and Work*, The Master Musicians Series, J. M. Dent & Sons Ltd, London, 1965

Debussy, Claude: *Debussy Letters* (selected, ed. and trans. François Lesure and Roger Nichols), Faber & Faber, London, 1987

Del Mar, Norman: *Richard Strauss: A Critical Commentary on his Life and Works* (3 vols.), Cornell University Press, Ithaca, NY, 1986

De-la-Noy, Michael: *Elgar the Man*, Allen Lane, Penguin Books Ltd, London, 1983

Deutsch, Otto E.: *Mozart: A Documentary Biography* (trans. E. Blom, P. Branscombe and J. Noble), 2nd edn, Adam & Charles Black, London, 1966

Deutsch, Otto E.: *Schubert: A Documentary Biography* (trans. Eric Blom), J. M. Dent & Sons Ltd, London, 1946

Deutsch, Otto E.: *Schubert: Memoirs by his Friends* (trans. Rosamond Ley and John Nowell), Adam & Charles Black, London, 1958

Dietrich, Albert, and Widmann, J. V.: *Recollections of Johannes Brahms* (trans. Dora E. Hecht), Charles Scribner & Sons, New York, 1899

Dormandy, Thomas: *The White Death: A History of Tuberculosis*, Hambledon Press, London, 1999

Duchen, Jessica: *Gabriel Fauré*, 20th Century Composers, Phaidon Press, London, 2000

Eibl, Joseph H., and Senn, Walter: *Mozarts Bäsle-Briefe*, Bärenreiter-Verlag Karl Vötterle GmbH & Co., K.G., Kassel, 1978

Einstein, Alfred: *Gluck* (trans. E. Blom), The Master Musicians Series, rev. edn, J. M. Dent & Sons Ltd, London, 1964

Eisler, Benita: *Chopin's Funeral*, Abacus, London, 2004

Eismann, G.: *Robert Schumann 1827–1838* (ed. G. Eismann), VEB Deutscher Verlag für Musik, Leipzig, 1971 (originally published 1957)

Ekman, Karl: *Jean Sibelius: His Life and Personality* (trans. Edward Birse), Alan Wilmer Ltd, London, 1936

Ellenberger, Henri F.: *The Discovery of the Unconscious*, Fontana Press (Harper & Collins), London, 1970

Elliot, J. H.: *Berlioz*, The Master Musicians Series, J. M. Dent & Sons Ltd, London, 1967

Emerson, Caryl: *The Life of Musorgsky*, Cambridge University Press, Cambridge, UK, 1999

Engel, Louis: *From Mozart to Mario: Reminiscences of Half a Century*, Richard Bentley and Son, London, 1886

Ewen, David: *A Journey to Greatness: The Life and Music of George Gershwin*, W. H. Allen, London, 1956

Fabbri, Paolo: *Monteverdi* (trans. Tim Carter), Cambridge University Press, Cambridge, 1994

Fay, Laurel, E.: *Shostakovich: A Life*, Oxford University Press, Oxford, 2000

Feder, Stuart: *Gustav Mahler: A Life in Crisis*, Yale University Press, New Haven and London, 2004

Fenby, Eric: *Delius*, The Great Composers Series, Faber & Faber, London, 1971

Fenby, Eric: *Delius As I Knew Him*, Faber & Faber Ltd, London, 1981

Figes, Orlando: *Natasha's Dance, A Cultural History of Russia*, Penguin Books Ltd, London, 2003

Figes, Orlando: *The Whisperers*, Allen Lane, New York and London, 2007

Fischer, Jens Malte: *Gustav Mahler* (trans. Stewart Spencer), Yale University Press, New Haven and London, 2011

Floros, Constantin: *Anton Bruckner: The Man and the Work* (English trans. Ernest Bernhardt-Kabisch), Peter Lang GmbH, Frankfurt am Main, 2nd rev. edn, 2015

Forkel, Johann Nikolaus: *Über Johann Sebastian Bachs Leben, Kunst und Kunstwerke*, Hoffmeister and Kuhne, Leipzig, 1802

Foucault, Michel: *Madness and Civilisation* (trans. Richard Howard), Tavistock Publications, London, 1967

Franken, F. H.: *Krankheit und Tod grosser Komponisten*, Verlag Gerhard Witzstrock, Baden-Baden, 1979

Franken, F. H.: *Die Krankheiten grosser Komponisten*, vol. 4, Florian Noetzel Verlag GmbH, Wilheimshaven, 1997

Franklin, Peter: *The Life of Mahler*, Cambridge University Press, Cambridge, UK, 1997

Freund, Emil: *Selected Letters of Gustav Mahler* (trans. E. Wilkins, E. Kaiser and B. Hopkins, selected by Alma Mahler, ed. Knud Martner), Faber & Faber, London, 1979

Frimmel, Theodor: *Beethoven-Handbuch*, vol. 1, Breitkopf & Härtel, Leipzig, 1926.

Gal, Hans: *Johannes Brahms: His Work and Personality* (trans. Joseph Stein), Alfred A. Knopf, Inc., New York, 1963

Galatopoulos, Stelios: *Bellini: Life, Times, Music*, Sanctuary Publishing Ltd, London, 2002

Garden, Edward: *Tchaikovsky*, The Master Musicians Series, J. M. Dent & Sons Ltd, London, 1973

Garden, Edward, and Gotteri, Nigel: *To My Best Friend: Correspondence between Tchaikovsky and Nadezhda von Meck* (trans. Galina von Meck), Clarendon Press, Oxford, 1993

Gardiner, John Eliot: *Music in the Castle of Heaven: A Portrait of Johann Sebastian Bach*, Allen Lane, London, 2013

Geck, Martin, *Richard Wagner: A Life in Music* (trans. Stewart Spencer), University of Chicago Press, Chicago, 2012

Geiringer, Karl and Irene: *Haydn: A Creative Life in Music*, 3rd edn, George Allen and Unwin, London, 1982

Gilliam, Bryan: *The Life of Richard Strauss*, Musical Lives, Cambridge University Press, Cambridge, UK, 1999

Gillmor, Alan: *Erik Satie*, Macmillan Press Ltd, London, 1988

Glover, Jane: *Mozart's Women: His Family, his Friends, his Music*, Pan Books, London, 2006

Goss, Glenda Dawn: *Sibelius, A Composer's Life and the Awakening of Finland*, University of Chicago Press, Chicago, 2009

Gray, Cecil: *Peter Warlock: A Memoir of Philip Heseltine*, Jonathan Cape, London, 1934

Gray, Cecil, and Heseltine, Philip: *Carlo Gesualdo: Musician and Murderer*, Kegan Paul, Trench, Trubner & Co. Ltd, London, 1926

Greenberg, Rodney: *George Gershwin*, Phaidon Press, London, 1998

Gregor-Dellin, Martin: *Richard Wagner: His Life, his Work, his Century* (trans. J. Maxwell Brownjohn), Collins, London, 1983

Grey, Madeleine: *Mémoires d'une chanteuse française* (ed. Gerard Zwang), L'Harmattan, Paris, 2008

Griffiths, Paul: *Bartók*, The Master Musicians Series, J. M. Dent & Sons Ltd, London, 1984

Griffiths, Paul: *Stravinsky*, The Master Musicians Series, J. M. Dent & Sons Ltd, London, 1992

Grove, Sir George: *Dictionary of Music and Musicians*, vol. 1, Macmillan, London, 1879

Grover, Ralph Scott: *Ernest Chausson: The Man and his Music*, Athlone Press, London, 1980

Gutman, David: *Prokofiev*, The Illustrated Lives of the Great Composers, Omnibus Press, London, 1990

Hadley, Patrick: 'Delius, Frederick', *Oxford Dictionary of National Biography Archive*, Oxford University Press, Oxford, 1949

Halliwell, Ruth: *The Mozart Family*, Clarendon Press, Oxford 1998

Hamburger, Michael: *Beethoven's Letters, Journals and Conversations*, Jonathan Cape, London, 1966

Hanslick, Eduard: *Music Criticisms 1850–1900* (trans. and ed. Henry Pleasants), Penguin Books, London, 1963

Harding, James: *Gounod*, Stein & Day, New York, 1973

Harding, James: *Massenet*, J. M. Dent & Sons Ltd, London, 1970

Harding, James: *Saint-Saëns and his Circle*, Chapman and Hall, London, 1965

Harrison, Max: *Rachmaninoff: Life, Works, Recordings*, Continuum, London, 2005

Hayden, Deborah: *Pox: Genius and Madness and the Mysteries of Syphilis*, Basic Books, New York, 2003

Hedley, Arthur: *Chopin*, The Master Musicians Series, J. M. Dent & Sons Ltd, London, 1974

Hedley, Arthur (ed.): *Selected Correspondence of Chopin*, Heinemann, London, 1962

Heller, Karl: *Antonio Vivaldi: The Red Priest of Venice* (trans. David Marinelli), Amadeus Press, Portland, OR, 1997

Henschel, Sir George: *Musings and Memories of a Musician*, Macmillan and Co. Ltd, London, 1918

Hensel, Sebastian: *The Mendelssohn Family 1729–1847 from Letters and Journals* (trans. C. Klingemann), vols. 1 and 2, Sampson Low, Marston, Searle and Rivington, London, 1882

Hervey, Arthur: *Saint-Saëns*, John Lane, London, 1921

Hilmes, Oliver: *Franz Liszt: Musician, Celebrity, Superstar* (trans. Stewart Spencer), Yale University Press, New Haven, 2016

Holden, Anthony: *Tchaikovsky*, Bantam Press, London, 1995

Hollander, Hans: *Leoš Janáček* (trans. Paul Hamburger), John Calder, London, 1963

Holman, Peter: *Henry Purcell*, Oxford University Press, Oxford, 1994

Holmes, Edward: *The Life of Mozart*, Chapman and Hall, London, 1845, repr. 1932

Holmes, Paul: *Holst*, Omnibus Press, London, 1997

Holoman, D. Kern: *Berlioz*, Faber & Faber, London, 1989

Holst, Imogen: *Gustav Holst: A Biography*, Oxford University Press, London, 1958

Hood, J. D.: 'Deafness and Musical Appreciation' in *Music and the Brain* (ed. Macdonald Critchley and R. A. Henson), pp. 323–43, William Heinemann Medical Books Ltd, London, 1977

Horton, John: *Grieg*, The Master Musicians Series, J. M. Dent & Sons Ltd, London, 1974

Horton, Julian: *Bruckner's Symphonies: Analysis Reception and Cultural Politics*, Cambridge University Press, Cambridge, UK, 2004

Howard, Patricia: *Gluck: An Eighteenth Century Portrait*, Clarendon Press, Oxford, 1995

Hunter, David: *The Lives of George Frideric Handel*, Boydell & Brewer, Woodbridge, 2015

Irvine, Demar: *Massenet, A Chronicle of his Life and Times*, Amadeus Press, Portland, Oregon, 1997

Ivry, Benjamin: *Francis Poulenc*, Phaidon Press Ltd, London, 1996

Jackson, Stanley: *Monsieur Butterfly: The Story of Puccini*, W. H Allen, London, 1994

Jacob, Heinrich E.: *Johann Strauss: A Century of Light Music* (trans. Marguerite Wolff), Hutchinson & Co. Ltd, London, 1940

Jaffé, Daniel: *Sergey Prokofiev*, Phaidon, London, 1998

Jahn, Otto: *Life of Mozart*, 3 vols. (trans. P. D. Townsend), Novello Ewer & Co., London, 1882

Jahoda, Gloria: *The Road to Samarkand: Frederick Delius and his Music*, Charles Scribner, New York, 1969

Jamison, Kay R.: *Touched with Fire: Manic-Depressive Illness and the Artistic Temperament*, Free Press Paperbacks, Simon and Schuster, New York, 1993

Janečková, Zdeňka: *My Life with Janáček* (ed. and trans. John Tyrrell), Faber & Faber, London, 1998

Jefferson, Alan: *Delius*, The Master Musicians Series, J. M. Dent and Sons Ltd, London, 1972

Jensen, Eric, F.: *Debussy*, The Master Musicians, Oxford University Press, New York, 2014

Jensen, Eric, F.: *Schumann*, The Master Musicians, Oxford University Press, Oxford, 2001

Johnson, Martin: *Art and Scientific Thought*, Faber & Faber, London, 1954

Jones, David W.: *The Life of Haydn*, Musical Lives, Cambridge University Press, Cambridge, UK, 2009

Jones, Ernest: *Sigmund Freud: Life and Work*, vol. 2, Hogarth Press, London, 1955

Jones, Henry: *The Life and Extraordinary History of the Chevalier John Taylor (by his Son, John Taylor)*, London, 1761

Jones, J. Barrie (ed. and trans.): *Gabriel Fauré: A Life in Letters*, Batsford Books, London, 1989

Jordan, Rolf: *The Clock of the Years: An Anthology of Writings on Gerald and Joy Finzi*, Chosen Press, Lichfield, 2007

Jordan, Ruth: *George Sand: A Biographical Portrait*, Constable, London, 1976

Jordan, Ruth: *Nocturne: A Life of Chopin*, Constable, London, 1978

Joseph, Charles, M.: *Stravinksy Inside Out*, Yale University Press, New Haven, 2001

Kabalevsky, D.: *A Vivid Personality: Sergei Prokofiev, Autobiography, Articles, Reminiscences*, Foreign Languages Publishing House, Moscow, 1957

Kalischer, A. C.: *Beethoven's Letters* (trans. J. S. Shedlock, ed. A. Eaglefield-Hull), Dover Publishing Co. Inc., New York, 1972

Keates, Jonathan: *Handel: The Man and his Music*, Pimlico, London, 2009

Kennedy, Michael: *Benjamin Britten*, The Dent Master Musicians, J. M. Dent, London, 1993

Kennedy, Michael: *The Life of Elgar*, Musical Lives, Cambridge University Press, Cambridge, UK, 2004

Kennedy, Michael: *Mahler*, The Master Musicians, Oxford University Press, Oxford, 2000

Kennedy, Michael and Joyce, and Rutherford-Johnson, Tim: *Oxford Dictionary of Music*, 6th edn, Oxford University Press, Oxford, 2012

Kennedy, Michael: *Portrait of Elgar*, Clarendon Paperback, 3rd edn, Oxford University Press, Oxford, 1993

Kennedy, Michael: *Richard Strauss*, The Master Musicians Series, J. M. Dent & Sons Ltd, London, 1988

Kennedy, Michael: *Richard Strauss: Man, Musician, Enigma*, Cambridge University Press, Cambridge, UK, 1999

Kennedy, Michael: *The Works of Ralph Vaughan Williams*, Oxford University Press, Oxford, 1964

Kerman, Joseph: *The Beethoven Quartets*, Oxford University Press, Oxford, 1967

Kessel, Neil, and Walton, Henry: *Alcoholism*, Penguin Books, Harmondsworth, 1965

Keys, Ivor: *Johannes Brahms*, Christopher Helm Ltd, Bromley, 1989

Kildea, Paul: *Benjamin Britten: A Life in the 20th Century*, Allen Lane, Penguin Books, London, 2013

King, Robert: *Henry Purcell*, Thames & Hudson Ltd, London, 1994

Kolneder, Walter: *Antonio Vivaldi: His Life and Work* (trans. Bill Hopkins), Faber & Faber, London, 1970

Köppen, Ludwig: *Mozarts Tod*, Köppen Verlag, Cologne, 2004

La Grange, Henry-Louis de: *Mahler*, Vol. 1, Victor Gollancz, London, 1974

La Grange, Henry-Louis de: *Gustav Mahler*, vol. 2, *Vienna: The Years of Challenge (1897–1904)*, Oxford University Press, Oxford, 1995

La Grange, Henry-Louis de: *Gustav Mahler*, vol. 3, *Vienna: Triumph and Disillusion (1904–1907)*, Oxford University Press, Oxford, 1999

La Grange, Henry-Louis de: *Gustav Mahler*, vol. 4, *A New Life Cut Short (1907–1911)*, Oxford University Press, Oxford, 2008

Lambert, Constant: *Music Ho!*, Hogarth Press, London, 1985

Large, Brian: *Smetana*, Duckworth, London, 1970

Larkin, Edward: 'Beethoven's Medical History', in Martin Cooper, *Beethoven: The Last Decade 1817–1827*, Appendix A, Oxford University Press, Oxford, 1985

Lawson, Jack: *Carl Nielsen*, Phaidon, London, 1997

Layton, Robert: *Sibelius*, The Master Musicians Series, 4th edn, J. M. Dent & Sons Ltd, London, 1992

Lebrecht, Norman: *Mahler Remembered*, Faber & Faber, London, 1987

Lebrecht, Norman: *Why Mahler? How One Man and Ten Symphonies Changed the World*, Faber & Faber, London, 2010

Lee-Browne, Martin, and Guinery, Paul: *Delius and his Music*, Boydell Press, Woodbridge, 2014

Leontaridi, R.: *Alcohol Misuse: How Much Does it Cost?*, Cabinet Office Strategy Unit, September 2003

Lesser, Wendy: *Music for Silenced Voices: Shostakovich and his Fifteen Quartets*, Yale University Press, New Haven and London, 2011

Levas, Santeri: *Sibelius: A Personal Portrait*, J. M. Dent & Sons Ltd, London, 1972

Levin, Ernst: 'Smetana's Post Mortem', Appx. E, in John Clapham, *Smetana*, The Master Musicians Series, J. M. Dent and Sons Ltd, London, 1972pp. 150–2

Litzmann, Berthold: *Clara Schumann* (trans. G. E. Hadow), Macmillan & Co. Ltd, London, 1913

Lloyd, Stephen: *Constant Lambert: Beyond the Rio Grande*, Boydell Press, Woodbridge, 2014

Lock, Stephen: 'Janáček's Illnesses' in John Tyrrell, *Janáček: Years of a Life*, vol. 1, *(1854–1914): The Lonely Blackbird*, Chapter 64, pp. 245–7, Faber & Faber, London, 2006.

Lockspeiser, Edward: *Debussy*, The Master Musicians Series, J. M. Dent & Sons Ltd, London, 1972

Lockspeiser, Edward: *Debussy: His Life and Mind*, vols. 1 and 2, Cassell, London, 1965

Long, Marguerite: *Au piano avec Maurice Ravel*, Juillard, Paris, 1971

Macdonald, Hugh: *Berlioz*, The Master Musicians, Oxford University Press, Oxford, 2000

Macdonald, Hugh: *Bizet*, The Master Musicians, Oxford University Press, Oxford, 2014

MacDonald, Ian: *The New Shostakovich*, Fourth Estate, London, 1990

MacDonald, Malcolm: *Brahms*, The Master Musicians, J. M. Dent, London, 1993

MacDonald, Malcolm: *Schoenberg*, The Master Musicians, Oxford University Press, Oxford, 2008

Maes, Francis: *A History of Russian Music* (trans. A. J. Pomerans and E. Pomerans), University of California Press, Berkeley, 2006

Mahler, Alma: *Gustav Mahler: Memories and Letters* (trans. Basil Creighton, ed. Donald Mitchell), John Murray, London, 1968

Mai, François M.: *Diagnosing Genius: The Life and Death of Beethoven*, McGill–Queen's University Press, Montreal, 2007

Mainwaring, John: *Memoirs of the Life of the Late George Frederic Handel*, Dodsley, London, 1760

Marek, George R.: *Chopin: A Biography*, Harper & Row, New York, 1978

Marek, George R.: *Gentle Genius: The Story of Felix Mendelssohn*, Funk & Wagnalls, New York, 1972

Marshall, Em: *Music in the Landscape*, Robert Hale, London, 2011

Martin, Russell: *Beethoven's Hair*, Broadway Books, New York, 2000

Massenet, Jules: *My Recollections* (trans. H. Villiers Barnett), Forgotten Books, Small Maynard & Co., Boston, 2012

Matthews, Colin: 'The Tenth Symphony' in *The Mahler Companion* (ed. Donald Mitchell and Andrew Nicholson), pp. 491–507, Oxford University Press, Oxford, 1999

Matthews, Denis: *Beethoven*, The Master Musicians Series, J. M. Dent & Sons Ltd, London, 1985

May, Florence: *The Life of Johannes Brahms*, Vol. 1, 2nd edn, William Reeves, London, 1948

McBurney, Gerard: 'Whose Shostakovich?' in *A Shostakovich Casebook* (ed. M. Hamrick-Brown), pp. 283–302, Indiana University Press, Bloomington, 2002

McKay, Elizabeth Norman: *Franz Schubert: A Biography*, Clarendon Press, Oxford, 1997

McVeagh, Diana: 'Delius, Frederick Theodor Albert (1862–1934)' in Oxford Dictionary of National Biography, Oxford University Press Oxford, 2004

McVeagh, Diana: *Gerald Finzi: His Life and Music*, Boydell Press, Woodbridge, 2010

McVeagh, Diana M.: *Elgar: His Life and Music*, J. M. Dent & Sons Ltd, London, 1955

Mercer-Taylor, Peter: *The Life of Mendelssohn*, Musical Lives, Cambridge University Press, 2000

Meredith, Anthony and Harris, Paul: *Malcolm Arnold: Rogue Genius*, Thames/Elkin, London, 2004

Millington, Barry: *Richard Wagner: The Sorcerer of Bayreuth,* Thames & Hudson, London, 2012

Millington, Barry: *Wagner*, The Master Musicians Series, J. M. Dent & Sons Ltd, London, 1992

Millington, Barry (ed): *The Wagner Compendium*, Thames & Hudson, London, 1992

Mitchell, Donald: ' ' in *Aldeburgh Anthology* (ed. R. Blythe), Snape Maltings Foundation, Snape, 1972

Mitchell, Donald: *Gustav Mahler: The Early Years*, Faber & Faber, London, 1980

Mitchell, Donald, and Nicholson, Andrew (eds.), *The Mahler Companion*, Oxford University Press, Oxford, 1999

Moldenhauer, Hans: *Anton Webern: A Chronicle of his Life and Work*, Victor Gollancz, London, 1978

Moldenhauer, Hans: *The Death of Anton Webern: A Drama in Documents*, Philosophical Library, New York, 1961

Monrad-Johansen, David: *Edvard Grieg* (English transl. Madge Robertson), Princeton University Press, New York, 1938

Morrison, Bryce: *Franz Liszt*, Illustrated Lives of the Great Composers, Omnibus Press, London, 2014

Morrison, Simon: *The Love and Wars of Lina Prokofiev*, Harvill Secker, London, 2013

Mount Edgcumbe, Earl of: *Musical Reminiscences of an Old Amateur*, W. Clarke, London, 1824

Mozarteum Foundation, Salzburg: *Next to Mozart: Answers to the III Most Common Questions* (ed. S. Greger-Amanshauser, C. Grosspietsch and G. Ramsauer, trans. K. Kopp), Verlag Anton Pustet, Salzburg, 2011

Murdoch, W. D.: *Chopin: His Life*, Macmillan Company, London, 1935

Murphy, Anthony: *Banks of Green Willow*, Capella Archive, Great Malvern, 2012

Musgrave, Michael: *The Life of Schumann*, Musical Lives, Cambridge University Press, Cambridge, UK, 2011

Nabokov, Nicolas: *Old Friends and New Music*, Hamish Hamilton, London, 1951

Nectoux, Jean-Michel: *Gabriel Fauré: A Musical Life* (trans. Roger Nichols), Cambridge University Press, Cambridge, UK, 1991

Neumayr, Anton: *Music and Medicine*, vol. 1, *Haydn, Mozart, Beethoven, Schubert* (English trans. B. C. Clarke), Bloomington, IL, 1994

Neumayr, Anton: *Music and Medicine*, vol. 2, *Hummel, Weber, Mendelssohn, Schumann, Brahms, Bruckner* (English trans. B. C. Clarke), Medi-Ed Press, Bloomington, IL, 1995

Neumayr, Anton: *Music and Medicine*, vol. 3, *Chopin, Smetana, Tchaikovsky, Mahler* (English trans. D. J. Parent), Medi-Ed Press, Bloomington, IL, 1997

The New Grove Dictionary of Music and Musicians (ed. Stanley Sadie), 20 vols., Macmillan Publishers, London, 1980

The New Grove Dictionary of Music and Musicians, 2nd edn (ed. Stanley Sadie and John Tyrrell), 29 vols., Macmillan Publishers, London, 2001

Newbould, Brian: *Schubert and the Symphony: A New Perspective*, Toccata Press, London, 1992

Newbould, Brian: *Schubert: The Music and the Man*, Victor Gollancz, London, 1999

Newman, Ernest: *Hugo Wolf*, Dover Publications, New York, 1966

Newman, Ernest: *The Unconscious Beethoven: An Essay in Musical Biography*, Parsons, London, 1927

Newmarch, Rosa: *The Music of Czechoslovakia*, Oxford University Press, Oxford, 1942

Nice, David: *Prokofiev: From Russia to the West 1891–1935*, Yale University Press, New Haven and London, 2003

Nichols, Roger: *The Life of Debussy*, Musical Lives, Cambridge University Press, Cambridge, UK, 1998

Nichols, Roger: *Ravel*, Yale University Press, New Haven and London, 2011

Niemetschek, F.: *Leben des k.k. Kapellmeisters Wolfgang Gottlieb Mozart, nach Originalquellen beschrieben*, Herrlische Buchhandlung, Prague, 1798

Nissen, Georg N. von: *Biographie W. A. Mozarts nach Originalbriefen 1828*, Georg Olms Verlag, Leipzig, 1984

Norris, Christopher (ed.): *Shostakovich: The Man and his Music*, Lawrence and Wishart, London, 1982

Norris, Geoffrey: *Rachmaninoff*, The Dent Master Musicians, 2nd edn, J. M. Dent, London, 1993

Northrop Moore, Jerrold: *Edward Elgar: A Creative Life*, Oxford University Press, Oxford, 1984

Northrop Moore, Jerrold: *Edward Elgar: Letters of a Lifetime*, 2nd edn, vols. 1 and 2, Oxford University Press, Oxford, 2012

Northrop Moore, Jerrold: *Spirit of England: Edward Elgar in his World*, Heinemann, London, 1984

Novello, Mary and Vincent: *A Mozart Pilgrimage, Being the Travel Diaries of Vincent and Mary Novello in the Year 1829* (transcribed and compiled by Nerina Medici di Marignano and Rosemary Hughes), London, 1955

O'Shea, John: *Music and Medicine: Medical Profiles of Great Composers*, J. M. Dent and Sons Ltd, London, 1990

Oliver, Michael: *Benjamin Britten*, Phaedon Press, London, 1996

Oliver, Michael: *Igor Stravinsky*, Phaedon Press, London, 1995

Orenstein, Arbie: *Ravel – Man and Musician*, Dover Publications, New York, 1991

Orga, Ateş: *Fryderyck Franciszek Chopin*, Illustrated Lives of Great Composers, Omnibus Press, London, 2015

Orledge, Robert: *Gabriel Fauré*, 2nd edn, Eulenburg Books, London, 1983

Orledge, Robert: *Satie Remembered* (trans. Roger Nichols), Faber & Faber, London, 1995

Orledge, Robert: *Satie the Composer*, Music in the Twentieth Century, Cambridge University Press, Cambridge, UK, 1990

Orlova, Alexandra: *Tchaikovsky: A Self-Portrait*, Oxford University Press, Oxford, 1990

Orrey, Leslie: *Bellini*, The Master Musicians Series, J. M. Dent & Sons Ltd, London, 1969

Osborne, Charles: *Schubert and his Vienna*, Weidenfeld and Nicolson, London, 1985

Osborne, Richard: *Rossini*, The Dent Master Musicians, J. M. Dent, London 1993

Osborne, Richard: *Rossini: His Life and Works*, The Master Musicians, 2nd edn, Oxford University Press, Oxford, 2007

Ostwald, Peter F.: *Schumann: Music and Madness*, Victor Gollancz Ltd, London, 1985

Owen, David: *In Sickness and in Power: Illness in Heads of Government during the Last 100 Years*, Methuen, London, 2011

Pesce, Dolores: *Liszt's Final Decade*, University of Rochester Press, Rochester, NY, 2014

Peyser, Joan: *The Memory of All That*, Simon & Schuster, New York, 1993

Phillips-Matz, Mary Jane: *Puccini: A Biography*, Northeastern University Press, Boston, 2002

Phillips-Matz, Mary Jane: *Verdi: A Biography*, Oxford University Press, Oxford and New York, 1993

Pickering, George: *Creative Malady: Illness in the Lives and Minds of Charles Darwin, Florence Nightingale, Mary Baker Eddy, Sigmund Freud, Marcel Proust, Elizabeth Barrett Browning*, George Allen Unwin Ltd, London, 1972

Piggott, Patrick: *The Life and Music of John Field (1782–1837), Creator of the Nocturne*, University of California Press, Berkeley and Los Angeles,1973

Pollack, Howard: *Aaron Copland: The Life and Work of an Uncommon Man*, Faber & Faber Ltd, London, 2000

Potter, Caroline: *Erik Satie: A Parisian Composer and his World*, Boydell & Brewer, Woodbridge, 2016

Poulenc, Francis: *Emmanuel Chabrier*, La Palatine, Paris, 1961

Poznansky, Alexander: *Tchaikovsky's Last Days, A Documentary Study*, Clarendon Press, Oxford, 1996

Poznansky, Alexander: *Tchaikovsky: The Quest for the Inner Man*, Lime Tree, London, 1993

Radcliffe, Philip: *Mendelssohn*, The Master Musicians Series, 3rd edn, J. M. Dent & Sons Ltd, London, 1990

Ramba, J.: *Famous Czech Skulls*, 2nd edn, Galen, Prague, 2009

Redlich, Hans F.: *Bruckner and Mahler*, The Master Musicians Series, J. M. Dent & Sons Ltd, London, 1963

Redlich, Hans, F.: *Claudio Monteverdi: Life and Works* (trans. K. Dale), Oxford University Press, Oxford, 1952

Redwood, Christopher (ed.): *A Delius Companion*, John Calder, London, 1976

Reed, John: *Schubert: The Final Years*, Faber & Faber, London, 1972

Reed, John: *Schubert*, The Master Musicians, Oxford University Press, Oxford, 1997

Reed, William H.: *Elgar As I Knew Him*, Victor Gollancz Ltd, London 1936

Rees, Brian: *Camille Saint-Saëns*, Chatto and Windus, London, 1999

Reich, Willi: *The Life and Work of Alban Berg* (trans. Cornelius Cardew), Thames & Hudson, London, 1965

Reid, P. T., and Innes, J. A.: 'Sarcoidosis' in *Davidson's Principles & Practice of Medicine*, p. 709, Churchill Livingstone/Elsevier, Edinburgh, 2010.

Rimsky-Korsakov Nikolai: *Record of My Musical Life (1876–1906)* (trans. and ed. Judah Joffe), 5th edn, Ernst Eueenburg Ltd, London, 1974

Robbins Landon, Howard C.: *1791, Mozart's Last Year*, Thames & Hudson, London, 1999

Robbins Landon, Howard C.: *Beethoven: His Life, Work and World*, Thames & Hudson, London, 1992

Robbins Landon, Howard C.: *Haydn*, Faber & Faber, London, 1972

Robbins Landon, Howard C.: *The Mozart Compendium: A Guide to Mozart's Life and Music*, Thames & Hudson, London, 1990

Robbins Landon, Howard C.: *Vivaldi: Voice of the Baroque*, University of Chicago Press, Chicago, 1996

Roberts, Paul: *Claude Debussy*, Phaidon Press, London, 2010

Roberts, Warren: *Rossini and Post-Napoleonic Europe*, Boydell & Brewer, Woodbridge, 2015

Robertson, Alec: *Dvořák*, The Master Musicians Series, J. M. Dent & Sons Ltd, London, 1974

Robinson, Harlow: *Sergei Prokofiev*, Robert Hale, London, 1987

Rockstro, William S.: *The Life of George Frederick Handel*, Macmillan, London, 1883

Roller, Alfred: *A Portrait of Mahler in the Mahler Album* (ed. Gilbert Kaplan), Kaplan Foundation, New York, 1995

Roman, Zoltan: *Gustav Mahler's American Years (1907–1911): A Documentary History*, Pendragon, Stuyvesant, NY, 1989

Rosselli, John: *The Life of Bellini*, Musical Lives, Cambridge University Press, Cambridge, UK, 1996

Rosselli, John: *The Life of Mozart*, Musical Lives, Cambridge University Press, Cambridge, UK, 1998

Rosselli, John: *The Life of Verdi*, Musical Lives, Cambridge University Press, Cambridge, UK, 2000

Routh, Francis: *Igor Stravinsky*, The Master Musicians Series, J. M. Dent & Sons Ltd, London, 1975

Sacks, Oliver: *Musicophilia: Tales of Music and the Brain*, Picador, London, 2008

Samson, Jim: *Chopin*, The Master Musicians, Oxford University Press, Oxford, 1996

Samuel, Claude: *Prokofiev*, Calder & Boyars, London, 1971

Sand, George: *My Life* (trans. D. Hofstadter), Harper & Row, New York, 1979

Sand, George: *Un hiver à Majorque*, Hippolyte Souverain, Paris, 1842; as *Winter in Majorca* (English trans. R. Graves), Cassell & Company Ltd, London, 1956

Schauffler, Robert, H.: *The Unknown Brahms, his Life, Character and Works: Based on New Material*, Dodd, Mead & Co., New York, 1933

Schindler, Anton F.: *Beethoven As I Knew Him* (ed. Donald MacArdle), Faber & Faber, London, 1966

Schmalhausen, Lina: *The Death of Franz Liszt: Based on the Unpublished Diary of his Pupil, Lina Schmalhausen* (trans. and ed. Alan Walker), Cornell University Press, Ithaca, NY, 2011

Schmidt, Carl B.: *Entrancing Muse: A Documented Biography of Francis Poulenc*, Pendragon Press, Hillside, NY, 2001

Schoenberg, Arnold: 'Brahms the Progressive' in *Style and Idea: Selected Writings of Arnold Schoenberg* (ed. L. Stein, trans. L. Black, 1975), pp. 398–441, University of California Press, Los Angeles, 1984

Schonberg, Harold, C.: *The Lives of the Great Composers*, 3rd edn, Abacus, London, 1998

Schrade, Leo: *Monteverdi: Creator of Modern Music*, Victor Gollancz, London, 1979

Schumann, Eugenie: *Memoirs of Eugenie Schumann* (trans. Marie Busch, 1927), repr. Eulenburg, London, 1985

Schumann, Eugenie: *The Schumanns and Johannes Brahms* (trans. Marie Busch), repr. Books for Libraries Press, Freeport, NY, 1970

Seckerson, Edward: *Gustav Mahler*, Illustrated Lives of the Great Composers, Omnibus Press, London, 2013

Seroff, Victor: *Modest Moussorgsky*, Funk & Wagnalls, New York, 1968

Seroff, Victor: *Sergei Prokofiev: A Soviet Tragedy*, Leslie Frewin, London, 1969

Shead, Richard: *Constant Lambert*, Simon Publications, London, 1973

Short, Michael: *Gustav Holst: The Man and His Music*, Circaidy Gregory Press, Hastings, 2014

Shostakovich, Dmitri: *Shostakovich about Himself and his Times* (compiled Grigoryev, L. and Platek, Y., trans. Angus and Neilian Roxburgh), Progress Publishers, Moscow, 1981

Simkin, Benjamin: *Medical and Musical Byways of Mozartiana*, Fithian Press, Santa Barbara, CA, 2001

Simpson, Robert: *Carl Nielsen, Symphonist, 1865–1931*, J. M. Dent & Sons Ltd, London, 1952

Slater, Eliot: 'Schumann's Illness' in *Robert Schumann: The Man and his Music* (ed. Alan Walker), pp. 406–17, Barrie and Jenkins Ltd, London, 1972

Smith, Barry: *Peter Warlock: The Life of Philip Heseltine*, Oxford University Press, Oxford, 1994

Smith, Ronald: *Alkan: The Enigma*, Kahn & Averill, London, 1977

Solomon, Maynard: *Beethoven*, 2nd edn, Schirmer Books, New York, 1998

Stafford, William: *The Mozart Myths: A Critical Reassessment*, Stanford University Press, Stanford, 1991

Steen, Michael: *The Lives and Times of the Great Composers*, Icon Books Ltd, London, 2010

Stengel, Erwin: *Suicide and Attempted Suicide*, Pelican, Penguin Books Ltd, Harmondsworth, 1964

Stephens, John: Appendix 1, 'Dvořák's Final Illness' in John Clapham, *Dvořák*, pp. 179–81, David & Charles, London, 1979

Sterba, Editha and Richard: *Beethoven and his Nephew*, Pantheon, New York, 1954

Stevens, Halsey: *The Life and Music of Béla Bartók*, rev. edn, Oxford University Press, New York, 1964

Stove, R. J.: *César Franck: His Life and Times*, Scarecrow Press, Inc., Lanham, 2012

Stradling, R.: 'Shostakovich and the Soviet System 1925–75' in *Shostakovich: The Man and his Music* (ed. C. Norris), pp. 189–218, Lawrence and Wishart, London, 1982

Stravinsky, Igor, and Craft, Robert: *Conversations with Igor Stravinsky*, Faber & Faber, London, 1959

Stravinsky, Theodore: *Catherine and Igor Stravinsky: A Family Album*, Boosey & Hawkes, London, 1973

Swafford, Jan: *Beethoven: Anguish and Triumph, A Biography*, Faber & Faber, London, 2014

Swafford, Jan: *Johannes Brahms: A Biography*, Borzoi Books, Alfred A. Knopf Inc., New York, 1998

Talbot, Michael: *Vivaldi*, The Dent Master Musicians, 2nd edn, J. M. Dent & Sons Ltd, London, 1993

Taruskin, Richard: *On Russian Music*, University of California Press, 2009

Taylor, John: *The History of the Travels and Adventures of the Chevalier Taylor, Opthalmiater*, vol. 1, London, 1761

Taylor, Ronald: *Robert Schumann: His Life and Work*, Granada Publishing, London, 1982

Terry, Charles S.: *Bach*, Oxford University Press, Oxford, 1928

Thayer, Alexander W.: *Life of Beethoven* (rev. and ed. Elliot Forbes), Princeton University Press, Princeton, NJ, 1967

Thiery, J., and Tröhler, U., 'Wagner, Animals and Modern Scientific Medicine' (trans. S. Spencer) in *The Wagner Compendium* (ed. Barry Millington), pp. 174–7, Thames & Hudson, London, 1992

Thompson, Oscar: *Debussy: Man and Artist*, Tudor Publishing Co., New York, 1940

Tillard, Françoise: *Fanny Mendelssohn* (trans. Camille Naish), Amadeus Press, Portland, OR, 1996

Todd, R. Larry: *Mendelssohn: A Life in Music*, Oxford University Press, Oxford, 2003

Toye, Francis: *Rossini: A Study in Tragi-Comedy*, new edn, Arthur Barker, London, 1954

Treitler, Leo: *Music and the Historical Imagination*, Harvard University Press, Cambridge, MA, 1989

Turner, Walter J.: *Mozart, The Man and his Works*, Victor Gollancz Ltd, London, 1938

Vallas, Léon: *La véritable histoire de César Franck* (trans. Hugo Foss), George G. Harrap & Co. Ltd, London, 1951

Vaughan Williams, Ursula: *A Biography of Ralph Vaughan Williams*, Oxford University Press, Oxford, 1964

Venturini, Donald J.: *Alexander Glazounov, 1865–1936: His Life and Works*, Aero Printing, Delphos, Ohio, 1992

Vernon, P. E.: *Creativity*, Penguin Books, Harmondsworth, 1970

Vishnevskaya, Galina: *Galina: A Russian Story*, Sceptre, London, 1986

Volkov, Solomon (ed.): *Testimony: The Memoirs of Dmitri Shostakovich* (trans. Antonina W. Bouis), Hamish Hamilton, London, 1979

Von Lenz, Wilhelm: *The Great Piano Virtuosos of Our Time* (German original 1872, English trans. P. Reder), Kahn & Averill, London, 1983

Wagner, Cosima: *Diaries* (trans., abridged and ed. G. Skelton), Pimlico, London, 1994

Wagner, Cosima: *Diaries*, vol. 1 (ed. M. Gregor-Dellin and D. Mack, trans. Geoffrey Skelton), London 1978–80

Walker, Alan: *Franz Liszt*, vol. 1: *The Virtuoso Years, 1811–1847*, Faber & Faber, London, 1983

Walker, Alan: *Franz Liszt*, vol. 2: *The Weimar Years, 1848–1860*, Faber & Faber, London, 1989

Walker, Alan: *Franz Liszt*, vol. 3: *The Final Years, 1861–1886*, Faber & Faber, London, 1997

Walker, Alan: *Robert Schumann: The Man and his Music*, Barrie & Jenkins, London, 1972

Walker, Frank: *The Man Verdi*, J. M. Dent & Sons Ltd, London, 1962

Walker, Frank: *Hugo Wolf*, J. M. Dent & Sons Ltd, London, 1951

Walker, Robert: *Rachmaninoff: His Life and Times*, Midas, Tunbridge Wells, 1980

Wallace, Lady Jane: *Beethoven's Letters 1790–1826*, vols. 1 and 2, Hurd & Houghton, New York, 1867

Walsh, Stephen: *Stravinsky: A Creative Spring. Russia and France 1882–1934*, Pimlico, London, 2000

Walsh, Stephen: *Stravinsky: The Second Exile. France and America, 1934–71*, Pimlico, London, 2007

Walter Bruno: *Gustav Mahler* (2nd English trans. by L. W. Lindt), Hamish Hamilton, London, 1958

Walter, Bruno: *Theme and Variations: An Autobiography* (English transl. J. Galston), Hamish Hamilton, London, 1947

Warlock, Peter: *Frederick Delius,* The Bodley Head, London, 1923 (rev. 1952 by Hugo Foss)

Warrack, John: *Carl Maria von Weber*, Cambridge University Press, Cambridge, UK, 1976

Warrack, John: *Tchaikovsky*, Hamish Hamilton, London, 1973

Wasserman, E., Sagel, I., and Bingol, N.: 'Renal Disease, Polycystic Adult Type' in *Birth Defects Compendium* (ed. D. Bergsma), pp. 925–6, Macmillan, London, 1979

Watkins, Glenn: *Gesualdo: The Man and the Music*, 2nd edn, Clarendon Press, Oxford, 1991

Watson, Derek: *Bruckner*, The Master Musicians, 2nd edn, Oxford University Press, Oxford, 1997

Watson, Derek: *Liszt*, The Master Musicians Series, J. M. Dent & Sons Ltd, London, 1990

Watson, Lyle: *Camille Saint-Saëns: His Life and Art*, Kegan Paul, London, 1923

Wegeler, Franz G., and Ries, Ferdinand: *Remembering Beethoven. The Biographical Notes of Franz Wegeler and Ferdinand* Ries (trans. Frederick Noonan), Andre Deutsch Ltd, London, 1988

Weinstock, Herbert: *Donizetti and the World of Opera in Italy, Paris and Vienna, in the First Half of the 19th Century*, Methuen & Co., London, 1964

Weinstock, Herbert: *Rossini: A Biography*, Methuen, London, 1974

Westrup, Jack A.: *Purcell*, The Master Musicians Series, J. M. Dent & Sons Ltd, London, 1980

Whenham, John, and Weistrich, Richard (eds.): *Cambridge Companion to Monteverdi*, Cambridge University Press, Cambridge, UK, 2007

White, Eric W.: *Stravinsky: The Composer and his Works*, 2nd edn, University of California Press, Berkeley and Los Angeles, 1979

Whiting, Stephen M.: *Satie the Bohemian: From Cabaret to Concert Hall*, Clarendon Press, Oxford, 1999

Wiley, Roland J.: *Tchaikovsky*, The Master Musicians, Oxford University Press, Oxford, 2009

Williams, Adrian: *Portrait of Liszt: By Himself and his Contemporaries*, Clarendon Press, Oxford, 1990

Williams, Peter: *J. S. Bach. A Life in Music*, Cambridge University Press, Cambridge, UK, 2007

Williams, Peter: *The Life of Bach*, Cambridge University Press, Cambridge, UK, 2004

Wilson, Elizabeth: *Shostakovich: A Life Remembered*, rev. edn, Faber & Faber, London, 2006

Wolff, Christopher: *Johann Sebastian Bach: The Learned Musician*, Oxford University Press, Oxford, 2000

World Health Organization: *Problems Related to Alcohol Consumption*, WHO Technical Report Series, No. 650, Geneva, World Health Organization, 1980

Worthen, John: *Robert Schumann: Life and Death of a Musician*, Yale University Press, London, 2010

Youmans, Charles: *The Cambridge Companion to Richard Strauss*, Cambridge University Press, Cambridge, UK, 2010

Young, Percy, M.: *Handel*, The Master Musicians Series, J. M. Dent & Sons Ltd, London, 1979

Young, Percy: *Haydn*, Masters of Music, Ernest Benn Ltd, London, 1969

Zamoyski, Adam: *Chopin: Prince of the Romantics*, Harper Press, London, 2010

Zemanová, Mirka: *Janáček: A Composer's Life*, John Murray, London, 2002

Zimmerman, Franklin B.: *Henry Purcell 1659–1695: His Life and Times*, University of Pennsylvania Press, PA, 1983

Articles

Abbott, E. C.: 'Composers and Tuberculosis: The Effects on Creativity', *Canadian Medical Association Journal* (1982) 126.534–44

Adams, P.: 'Historical Hepatology: Ludwig van Beethoven', *Journal of Gastroenterology and Hepatology* (1987) 2.375–9

Alajouanine, T.: 'Aphasia and Artistic Realisation', *Brain* (1948) 71.229–41

Allberger, F.: 'Julius Wagner-Jauregg (1857–1940)', *Journal of Neurology, Neurosurgery and Psychiatry* (1997) 62.221

Alonso, R. J., and Pascuzzi, R. M.: 'Ravel's Neurological Illness', *Seminars in Neurology* (1991) 19 (Suppl. 1).53–7

Amaducci, L., Grassi, E., and Boller, F.: 'Maurice Ravel and Right Hemisphere Musical Creativity: Influence of Disease on his Last Musical Works', *European Journal of Neurology* (2002) 9.75–82

Ashoori, A., and Jankovic, J.: 'Mozart's Movements and Behaviour, a Case of Tourette's Syndrome', *Journal of Neurology, Neurosurgery and Psychiatry* (2007) 78.1171–5

Avins, S.: 'The Young Brahms: Biographical Data Re-Examined', *19th Century Music* (2001) 24.276–89

Bachmeyer, C., Leclerc-Landgraf, N., Laurette, F., et al,: 'Acute Auto-Immune Sensorineural Hearing Loss Associated with Crohn's Disease', *American Journal of Gastroenterology* (1998) 93.2565–7

Baeck, E.: 'Maurice Ravel and Right Hemisphere Activity', *European Journal of Neurology* (2002) 9.321

Baeck, E.: 'La mort de Maurice Ravel', *Cahiers Maurice Ravel* (2008) 11.56–62

Baeck, E.: 'The Terminal Illness and Last Compositions of Maurice Ravel', *Neurology Neuroscience* (2005) 19.132–40

Baeck, E.: 'Was Maurice Ravel's Illness a Cortico-Basal Degeneration?', *Clinical Neurology and Neurosurgery* (1996) 98.57–61

Baer, K. A.: 'Johann Sebastian Bach (1685–1750) in Medical History', *Bulletin of the Medical Library Association* (1951) 39.206–11

Baker, T.: 'Pauline Viardot to Julius Rietz, Letters of Friendship', *Musical Quarterly* (1916) 2.42–5

Bankl, H., and Jesserer, H.: 'Ertaubte Beethoven an einer Pagetschen Krankheit?', *Laryngologie Rhinologie Otologie* (1986) 65.592–7

Barton, N. J., Hooper, G., Noble, J., and Steel, W. M.: 'Occupational Causes of Disorders in the Upper Limb', *British Medical Journal* (1992) 304.309–11

Berberova, N., Brown, M., and Karlinsky, S.: 'Tchaikovsky's Suicide Reconsidered: A Rebuttal', *High Fidelity* (1981) 31, pp. 49–51

Berri, P.: 'La malattia di Vivaldi', *Musica d'oggi* (1942) 24.9–13

Bower, H.: 'Beethoven's Creative Illness', *Australian and New Zealand Journal of Psychiatry* (1989) 23.111–116

Bower, H.: 'Transient Psychosis', *Medical Journal of Australia* (1962) 1.797–800

Breitenfeld, D., Mikula, I., Breitenfeld, T., et al,: 'Wolfgang Amadeus Mozart (1756–1791): Pathography, Sociopsychosomatic Factors that Precipitated Mozart's Final Illness', *Alcoholism* (1992) 28.107–10

Brooks, Richard: 'Sewell's Father was Sex Sadist Composer', *Sunday Times*, 13 Nov 2011

Broomé, U.: 'Primary Sclerosing Cholangitis may have Caused the Death of Beethoven', *Läkartidningen* (2006) 103.2494–6

Butz, W. C., Watts, J. C., Rosales-Quintana, S., and Hicklin, M. D.: 'Erosive Gastritis as a Manifestation of Secondary Syphilis', *American Journal of Clinical Pathology* (1975) 63.895–900

Bywaters, E. G. L., Isdale, I., and Kempton, J. J.: 'Schönlein-Henoch Purpura: Evidence for a Group A β Haemolytic Streptococcal Aetiology', *Quarterly Journal of Medicine* (1957) 26.161–75

Cabinet Office Strategy Unit: 'Alcohol Misuse: How Much Does it Cost?', September 2003

Carerj, L.: 'Le mano invalida di Robert Schumann', *Nuova rivista musicale italiana* (1979) 13.609–19

Carp, L.: 'George Gershwin – Illustrious American Composer: His Fatal Glioblastoma', *American Journal of Surgical Pathology* (1979) 3.473–8

Carp, L.: 'Mozart: His Tragic Life and Controversial Death', *Bulletin of the New York Academy of Medicine* (1970) 46.267–79

Cavallera, G. M., Guidici, S., and Tommassi, L.: 'Shadows and Darkness in the Brain of a Genius: Aspects of Neuropsychological Literature about the Final Illness of Maurice Ravel (1875–1937)', *Medical Science Monitor* (2012) 18.1–8

Cherington, M., Smith, R., and Nielsen, P. J.: 'The Life, Legacy and Premature Death of Felix Mendelssohn', *Seminars in Neurology* (1999) 19(1).47–52

Christy, N. P., Christy, B. M., and Wood, B. G.: 'Gustav Mahler and his Illnesses', *Transactions of the American Clinical and Climatological Association* (1970) 82.200–17

Cole, J. C.: 'Alexander Borodin, the Scientist, the Musician, the Man', *Journal of the American Medical Association* (1969) 208.129–30

Cooke, D.: 'The Bruckner Problem Simplified', *Musical Times* (January–May 1969) 110, 59–62

Cooper, M.: 'Ludwig van Beethoven', *Proceedings of the Royal Society of Medicine* (1971) 64.5–83

Copland, A.: 'Gabriel Fauré: A Neglected Master', *Musical Quarterly* (1923) 10.573–86

Cybulska, E. M.: 'Bolero Unravelled: A Case of Musical Perseveration', *Psychiatric Bulletin* (1997) 21.567–76

Czerny, C.: 'Recollections of Beethoven', *Dwight's Journal of Music* (1852) 12.185–6

Dalessio, D. J.: 'Maurice Ravel and Alzheimer's Disease', *Journal of the American Medical Association.* (1984) 252.3412–13

Dandy, W. E.: 'Roentgenography of the Brain after the Injection of Air into the Spinal Canal', *Annals of Surgery* (1919) 70.397–403

Davies, H.: 'Body of Evidence: Unravelling the Mystery of Benjamin Britten's Death', *New Statesman*, 7–13 June 2013, 48–9

Davies, P. J.: 'Beethoven's Deafness: A New Theory', *Medical Journal of Australia* (1988) 149.644–649

Davies, P. J.: 'Beethoven's Nephropathy and Death: Discussion Paper', *Journal of the Royal Society of Medicine* (1993) 86.159–161

Davies, P. J.: 'Mozart's Death: A Rebuttal of Karhausen, Further Evidence for Schönlein-Henoch Purpura', *Journal of the Royal Society of Medicine*(1991) 84.737–40

Davies, P. J.: 'Mozart's Illnesses and Death', *Journal of the Royal Society of Medicine* (1983) 76.776–85

Davies, P. J.: 'Mozart's Illnesses and Death – 1, The Illnesses 1756–1790', *Musical Times* (1984) 125.437–42

Davies, P. J.: 'Mozart's Illnesses and Death – 2. The Last Year and the Fatal Illness', *Musical Times* (1984) 125.554–61

Davies, P. J.: 'Mozart's Left Ear, Nephropathy and Death', *Medical Journal of Australia* (1987) 147.581–5

Davies, P. J.: 'Mozart's Manic-Depressive Tendencies – 1', *Musical Times* (1987) 128.123–6

Davies, P. J.: 'Mozart's Manic-Depressive Tendencies – 2', *Musical Times* (1987) 128.191–6

Davies, P. J.: 'Mozart's Scatological Disorder', *British Medical Journal* (1993) 306.521–2

Davies, P. J.: 'Was Beethoven's Cirrhosis Due to Haemochromatosis?', *Renal Failure* (1995) 17.77–86

Delage, R.: 'Ravel and Chabrier', *Musical Quarterly* (1975) 61.4

Dodge, J. A., Lewis, P. A., Stanton, M., and Wilsher, J.: 'Cystic Fibrosis Mortality and Survival in the UK 1947–2003', *European Respiratory Journal* (2007) 29.522–6

Donnenberg, M. S., Collins, M. T., Benitez, M., et al,: 'The Sound that Failed: A Clinico-Pathological Conference', *American Journal of Medicine* (2000) 108.475–80

Drake, M. E.: 'Deafness, Dysaesthesia, Depression, Diarrhoea, Dropsy and Death: The Case for Sarcoidosis in Ludwig van Beethoven', *Neurology* (1994) 44.562–5

Ealy, G. T.: 'Of Ear Trumpets and a Resonance Plate: Early Hearing Aids and Beethoven's Hearing Perception', *19th Century Music* (1993–44) 17.262–73

Elgar, Sir Edward: 'My visit to Delius', *Daily Telegraph*, 1 July 1933

Evans, R. W.: 'Complications of Lumbar Puncture', *Neurologic Clinics* (1998) 16.83–103

Eybler, J., Selbstbiographie', *Allgemeine musikalische Zeitung*, Leipzig, 24 May 1826

Fabricant, N. D.: 'George Gershwin's Fatal Headache', *Eye, Ear, Nose and Throat Monthly* (1958) 37.332–4

Falliers, C. J.: 'Arnold Schoenberg and Alban Berg: The Serial Music and Serious Asthma of Two Leading 20th Century Composers', *Journal of Asthma* (1986) 23.211–17

Farley, T. A., Gillespie, S., Rasoulpour, M., et al.: 'Epidemiology of a Cluster of Henoch-Schönlein Purpura', *American Journal of Diseases of Children* (1989) 143,798–803

Farnworth, P. R.: 'Musicality and Abnormality', *Confinica Psychiatrica* (1961) 4.158–61

Fay, Laurel E.: 'Shostakovich vs Volkov: Whose Testimony?' *Russian View* (October 1980) 484–93

Feldmann, H.: 'The Otological Aspects of Bedrich Smetana's Disease' (transl. E. Levin), *Music Review* (1971) 32.233–47

Fluker, J. L.: 'Mozart: His Health and Death', *The Practitioner* (1972): 209.841–5

Fog, R., and Regeur, L.: 'Did W. A. Mozart Suffer from Tourette's Syndrome?', Proceedings of World Congress of Psychiatry, Vienna, 1985

Foss, H.: 'The Instrumental Music of Frederick Delius', *Tempo* (1952–53) 26.30–7

Franzen, C.: 'Syphilis in Composers and Musicians – Mozart, Beethoven, Paganini, Schubert, Schumann, Smetana', *European Journal of Clinical Microbiology and Infectious Diseases* (2008) 27.1151–7

Frosch, W. A.: 'The Case of George Frideric Handel', *New England Journal of Medicine* (1989) 321.765

Frosch, W. A.: 'Madness and Music', *Comprehensive Psychiatry* (1987) 28.315–22

Garcia, E. E.: 'Gustav Mahler's Choice: A Note on Adolescence, Genius and Psychosomatics', *Psychoanalytic Study of the Child* (2000) 55.87–110

Garcia, E. E.: 'Rachmaninoff's Emotional Collapse and Recovery: The First Symphony and its Aftermath', *Psychoanalytic Review* (2004) 91.221–38

Gelma E.: 'La mort du musicien Georges Bizet', *Cahiers de psychiatrie* (Strasbourg 1948)

Gelma, E.: 'Quelques souvenirs sur Georges Bizet', *L'Alsace française*, 10 December 1938

Gerber, P. H.: 'Mozarts Ohr', *Deutsche Medizinische Wochenschrift* (1898) 24.351–2

Gibbs, F. A., Davis, H., and Lennox, W. G.: 'The EEG in Epilepsy and in Conditions of Impaired Consciousness', *Archives of Neurology and Psychiatry* (1935) 34.1133–48

Gjestland, T.: 'An Epidemiological Investigation of the Natural Course of the Syphilitic Infection, Based upon a Re-Study of the Boeck-Bruusgard Material', *Acta Derm-Venerologica* (Stockholm) (1955) 35 (Suppl. 34)

Göbel, C. H., Göbel, A., and Göbel, H.: '"Compulsive plague! Pain without end!" How Richard Wagner Played out his Migraine in the Opera *Siegfried*', *British Medical Journal* (2013) 347.32–3

Gould, G. M.: 'The Ill-Health of Richard Wagner', *Lancet* (1903) 162.306–13

Grabau, W., Emanuel, R., Ross, D., et al.: 'Syphilitic Aortic Regurgitation', *British Journal of Venereal Diseases* (1976) 82.366–73

Greither, A., 'Die Todeskrankheit Mozarts'. *Deutsche Medizinische Wochenschrift* (1967) 92.723–5.

Grühle, H.: 'Brief über Robert Schumanns Krankheit an P. J. Möbius, *Zentralblatt fur Nervenheilkunde* (1906) 29.805–10

Guillery, E. N.: 'Did Mozart Die of Kidney Disease? A Review from the Bicentennial of his Death', *Journal of the American. Society of Nephrology* (1992) 2.1671–6

Gutman, A. F., and Kasabach, H.: 'Paget's Disease: Analysis of 116 Cases', *American Journal of the Medical Sciences* (1936) 191.361–80

Gutt, R. W.: 'Beethoven's Deafness: An Iatrogenic Disease', *Medizinische Klinik* (1970) 65.2294–5

Hamet, P., Pausova, Z., Adarichev, V., et al.: 'Hypertension, Genes and Environment', *Journal of Hypertension* (1998) 16.397–418

Harcup, J.: 'Edward Elgar – a Medical Enigma?' *Elgar Society Journal* (2012) 17.16–31

Harcup, J., and Noble, J.: 'Edward Elgar (1857–1934): Moaner or Loner?', *Journal of Medical Biography* (2016) 24.135–8

Harrison, P.: 'The Effects of Deafness on Musical Composition', *Journal of the Royal Society of Medicine.* (1988) 81.598–601

Henson, R. A.: 'Maurice Ravel's Illness: A Tragedy of Lost Creativity', *British Medical Journal* (1988) 296.1585–8

Henson, R. A., and Urich, H.: 'Schumann's Hand Injury', *British Medical Journal* (1978) 1.900–3

Hilson, D.: 'Malformation of Ears as a Sign of Malformation of Genito-Urinary Tract', *British Medical Journal* (October 1957) 785–9

Hindemarsh, J. T.: 'Caveats in Hair Analysis in Chronic Arsenic Poisoning', *Clinical Biochemistry* (2002) 35.1–11

Hingtgen, C. M.: 'The Painful Perils of a Pair of Pianists: The Chronic Pain of Clara Schumann and Sergei Rachmaninov', *Seminars in Neurology* (1999) 19 (Suppl. 1).29–34

Hingtgen, C. M.: 'The Tragedy of Sergei Prokofiev', *Seminars in Neurology* (1999) 19(1).59–61

Hirschmann, J. V.: 'What Killed Mozart?' *Archives of Internal Medicine* (2001) 161.1381–9

Hollanders, D.: 'Sensorineural Deafness: A New Complication of Ulcerative Colitis', *Postgraduate Medicine Journal* (1986) 62.753–5

Hunter, D.: 'Handel's Illnesses, the Narrative Tradition of Heroic Strength and the Oratorio Turn', *Eighteenth Century Music* (2006) 3.253–67

Jack, Adrian: 'Robert Schumann', Programme to Prom 10, BBC Proms, 19 July 2013

Jacobsohn, L.: 'Beethovens Gehörleiden und letzte Krankheit', *Deutsche medizinische Wochenschrift* (1927) 53.1610–12

Jamison, K. R.: 'Mood Disorders and Patterns of Creativity in British Writers and Artists', *Psychiatry* (1989) 32.125–34

Jänisch, W., and Nauhaus. G.: 'Autopsy Report of the Corpse of the Composer Robert Schumann: Publication and Interpretation of a Rediscovered Document', *Zentralblatt Fur Allgemeine Pathologie und Pathologische Anatomie* (1986) 132.129–36

Jenkins, J. S.: 'The Medical History and Death of Mozart', *Journal of the Royal College of Physicians of London* (1991): 25.351–3

Jenkins, J. S.: 'Mozart's Last Months and Controversial Death', *Journal of Medical Biography* (1994) 2.185–6

Juda, A.: 'The Relationship between Highest Mental Capacity and Psychic Abnormalities', *American Journal of Psychiatry* (1949) 106.296–307

Kammer, T.: 'Mozart in the Neurological Department – Who Had the Tic?' *Neurology and Neurosciences* (2007) 22.184–92

Kanat, A., Kayaci, S., Yazar, U., and Yilmaz, A.: 'What Makes Ravel's Deadly Craniotomy Interesting? Concerns of One of the Famous Craniotomies in History', *Acta Neurochirurgica* (2010) 152.737–42

Karhausen, L. R.: 'Contra-Davies: Mozart's Terminal Illness', *Journal of the Royal Society of Medicine* (1991) 84.734–6

Karhausen, L. R.: 'Did Mozart Have Tourette's Syndrome?' *Perspectives in Biology and Medicine*(1995) 39.152–5

Karhausen, L. R.: 'Mozart Ear and Mozart Death', *British Medical Journal* (1987) 294.511–12

Karhausen, L. R.: 'Mozart's Scatological Disorder', *British Medical Journal* (1993) 306.522

Karhausen, L. R.: 'Mozart's Terminal Illness: Unravelling the Clinical Evidence', *Journal of Medical Biography* (2001) 9.34–48

Karhausen, L. R.: 'The Myth of Mozart's Poor Health and Weak Constitution', *Journal of Medical Biography* (1999) 7.111–17

Karhausen, L. R.: 'Weeding Mozart's Medical History', *Journal of the Royal Society of Medicine* (1998) 91.546–50

Karmody, C. S., and Bachor, E. S.: 'The Deafness of Ludwig van Beethoven: An Immunopathy', *Otology and Neurology* (2005) 26.809–814

Katz, D.: 'Smetana's First String Quartet: Voice of Madness or Triumph of Spirit?', *Musical Quarterly* (1997) 81.516–36

Kerner, D.: 'Mendelssohns Tod', *Deutsch. med. J.* (1968) 19.454–62

Kerner, D.: 'Mozarts Tod bei Alexander Puschkin', *Deutsches medizinisches Journal* (1969) 26.743–7

Kerner, D.: 'Ravels Tod', *Münchener medizinische Wochenschrift* (1975) 117. 591–6

Kerner, D.: 'Wie Johannes Brahms starb', *Münchener medizinische Wochenschrift* (1979) 120.565

Keynes, M.: 'Handel and his Illnesses'. *Musical Times* (1982) 123.613–14

Keynes, M.: 'Handel's Illnesses', *Lancet* (December 1980) 1354–5

Keynes, M.: 'The Personality and Illnesses of Wolfgang Amadeus Mozart', *Journal of Medical Biography* (1994) 2.217–32

Keynes, M.: 'The Personality, Deafness and Bad Health of Ludwig von Beethoven', *Journal of Medical Biography* (2002) 10.46–57

Kildea, Paul: 'Benjamin Britten: Death in Aldeburgh', *Sunday Telegraph*, 'Seven', 20 January 2013

Kildea, Paul: 'Yes, the Evidence Does Show that Benjamin Britten Died from Syphilis', *The Guardian*, 30 January 2013

Kingston, R. L., Hall, S., and Sioris., L.: 'Clinical Observations and Medical Outcome in 149 Cases of Arsenate Ant Killer Ingestion', *Clinical Toxicology* (1993) 31.581–91

Kranemann, Detlef: 'Johann Sebastian Bachs Krankheit und Todesursache – Versuch einer Deutung', *Bach-Jahrbuch* (1990) 53–64

Kubba, A. K., and Young, M.: 'The Long Suffering of Frederic Chopin', *Chest* (1998) 113.210–16

Kubba, A. K., and Young, M.: 'Ludwig van Beethoven: A Medical Biography', *Lancet* (1996) 347.167–70

Kuehn, J. L.: 'Encounter at Leyden: Gustav Mahler Consults Sigmund Freud', *Psychoanalytic Review* (1965) 52.5–25

Kumar, B. N., Smith, M. S., Walsh, R. M., and Green, J. R.: 'Sensorineural Hearing Loss in Ulcerative Colitis', *Clinical Otolaryngology* (2000) 25.143–45

Kuzemko, J. A.: 'Chopin's Illnesses', *Journal of the Royal Society of Medicine* (1994) 87.769–72

La Grange, H. L. de: 'Prometheus Unbound', *Music and Musicians* (1971–72) 20(5).34–43

Landormy, P., and Herter, M. D.: 'Gabriel Fauré (1845–1924)', *Musical Quarterly* (1931) 17.293–301

Landsberger, M.: 'Beethoven's Medical History from a Physician's Viewpoint', *New York State Journal of Medicine*(1978) 78.676–9

Langham-Smith, R.: 'The Ooze of the Erotic Priest', programme notes for *Faust*, Royal Opera House, Covent Garden, 2012

Larkin, E.: 'Beethoven's Illness: A Likely Diagnosis', *Proceedings of the Royal Society of Medicine* (1971) 64.1–4

Lederman, R. J.: 'Robert Schumann', *Seminars in Neurology* (1999) 19 (Suppl. 1).17–24

Levy, D.: 'Gustav Mahler and Emanuel Libman: Bacterial Endocarditis in 1911', *British Medical Journal* (1986) 293.1628–31

Lister, J.: 'On the Antiseptic Principle in the Practice of Surgery', *British Medical Journal* 1867, 2 (351).246–8

Liston, S. L., Yanz, J. L., Preves, D., and Jelonek, S.: 'Beethoven's Deafness', *Laryngoscope* (1989) 99.1301–4

Ljunggren, B.: 'The Case of George Gershwin', *Neurosurgery* (1982) 10.733–6

Lombroso, P. J., and Scahill, L., 'Tourette Syndrome and Obsessive-Compulsive Disorder'. *Brain and Development* (2008) 30.231–7

London, S. J.: 'Beethoven: Case Report of a Titan's Last Crisis', *Archives of Internal Medicine* (1964) 113.442–8

Ludwig, A. M.: 'Alcohol and Creative Output', *British Journal of Addiction* (1990) 85.953–63

Ludwig, A. M.: 'Creative Achievement and Psychopathology: Comparison Among Professions', *American Journal of Psychotherapy* (1992) 46.330–56

Ludwig, A. M.: 'Reflections on Creativity and Madness', *American Journal of Psychotherapy* (1989) 153.4–14

Macdonald, H.: 'The Death of Alkan', *Musical Times* (1973) 114.25

Macdonald, H.: 'More on Alkan's Death', *Musical Times* (1988) 129.118–20

Macleod, Donald and Duchen, Jessica: Fauré: Composer of the Week, BBC Radio Three, 1 June 2013

Mari, F., Polletini, A., Lippi, D., and Bertol, E.: 'The Mysterious Death of Francesco I de'Medici and Bianca Capello', *British Medical Journal* (2006) 331.1299–1301

Marins, E. M.: 'Maurice Ravel and Right Hemisphere Activity', *European Journal of Neurology* (2002) 9.320–1

Martin, R.: *Beethoven's Hair*', Broadway Books, New York, 2000

McCabe, B. F.: 'Auto-Immune Hearing Loss', *Annals of Otolaryngology* (1979) 88.585–9

McCabe, B. F.: 'Beethoven's Deafness', *Annals of Otology, Rhinology, and Laryngology* (1958) 67.192–206

Meredith, W.: 'The History of Beethoven's Skull Fragments', *Beethoven Journal* (2005) 20.3–39

Miller, B., Ponton, M., et al.: 'Enhanced Artistic Creativity with Temporal Lobe Degeneration', *Lancet* (1996) 348.1744–5

'Mittag Zeitung, 20th May 1911', *New York Times*, 21 May 1911

Mizler, L. C.: obituary of J. S. Bach, *Musikalische Bibliothek* (Leipzig, 1752) 3

Naiken, V. S.: 'Did Beethoven have Paget's Disease of Bone?', *Annals of Internal Medicine.* (1971) 74.995–9

Naiken, V. S.: 'Paget's Disease and Beethoven's Deafness', *Clinical Orthopaedics and Related Research* (1972) 89.103–5

Neumann, H.: 'Beethovens Gehörleiden', *Wiener medizinische Wochenschrift* (1927) 77.1015–19

Newman, Ernest: *The Sunday Times*, 20 October 1955

Newman, Ernest: Letter to Gerald Abraham, published in *The Sunday Times*, 6 November 1955, and quoted again in *The Listener*, 23 July 1959

Nichols, R.: 'Ravel', *BBC Music Magazine*, September 2014

Nicolson, H.: 'The Health of Authors', *Lancet* (15 November 1947), pp. 709–14

Nielsen, H. E.: 'Epidemiology of Schönlein-Henoch Purpura', *Acta Paediatrica Scandinavica* (1988) 77.125–31

Noble, J.: 'Biography, Hagiography or Demonology', *Journal of Medical. Biography* (2015) 23.123–4

Noble, J.: 'Malady Makers', *BBC Music Magazine*, August 2014

Noble, J.: 'Ravel Response (to Roger Nichols)', *BBC Music Magazine*, October 2014

O'Neill, D.: '... aber Sonntag ist immer ein Feiertag', Alexander Borodin M.D. 1833–1887', *Journal of the Royal Society of Medicine* (1988) 81.591–2

O'Shea, J. G.: 'A Medical History of Franz Liszt', *Medical Journal of Australia* (1986) 145.625–39

O'Shea, J. G.: 'The Abbé and his Alcohol', *Liszt Saeculum* (1987) 40.12–15

O'Shea, J. G.: '"Two minutes with Venus, two years with mercury" – Mercury as an Anti-Syphilitic Chemotherapeutic Agent', *Journal of the Royal Society of Medicine* (1990) 83.392–5

O'Shea, J. G.: 'Was Frederic Chopin's Illness Actually Cystic Fibrosis?', *Medical Journal of Australia* (1987) 187.586–9

Ober, W. B.: 'Bach, Handel and "Chevalier" John Taylor M.D., Opthalmiater', *New York State Journal of Medicine* (1969) 69.1797–1807

Ober, W. B.: 'Beethoven: A Medical View', *The Practitioner* (1970) 205.819–924

Ober, W. B.: 'Carlo Gesualdo, Prince of Venosa: Murder, Madrigals and Masochism', *Bulletin of the New York Academy of Medicine* (1973) 7 634–45

Ostwald, P. F.: 'Florestan, Eusebius, Clara, and Schumann's Right Hand', *19th Century Music* (1980) 4, 17–31

Ostwald, P. F.: 'Robert Schumann and his Doctors', *American Journal of Social Psychiatry* (1983) 3.5–14

Otte, A., De Bondt, P., Van de Wiele, C., et al.: 'The Exceptional Brain of Maurice Ravel', *Medical Science Monitor* (2003) 9.RA 154–9

Otte, A., Juengling, F. D. and Nizsche, E. U.: 'Rethinking Mild Head Injury', *Journal of Vascular Investigation* (1998) 4.45–6

Palferman, T. G.: 'Beethoven: A Medical Biography', *Journal of Medical Biography* (1993) 1.35–45

Palferman, T. G.: 'Beethoven: The Case against Syphilis', *Journal of the Royal College of Physicians of London* (1992) 26.112–14

Palferman, T. G.: 'Classical Notes: Beethoven's Medical History, Variations on a Rheumatological Theme', *Journal of the Royal Society of Medicine*(1990) 83.640–5

Palmer, Christopher: 'Constant Lambert: A Postscript' *Music & Letters* (1971) 52.173–6

Pascuzzi, R. M.: 'Shostakovich and Amyotrophic Lateral Sclerosis', *Seminars in Neurology* (1999) 19(1).63–6

Paton, A., Pahor, A. L., and Graham, G. R.: 'Looking for Mozart's Ears', *British Medical Journal* (1986): 293,1622–4

Payne, A., and Anderson, R.: 'Delius, Frederick', Grove Online, acessed 20 April 2010

Petch, M. C.: 'The Heart of Benjamin Britten', *Journal of the Royal Society of Medicine* (2014) 107.339–41

Post, F.: 'Creativity and Psychopathology: A Study of 291 World-Famous Men', *British Journal of Psychiatry* (1994) 165.22–34

Poznansky, A.: 'Tchaikovsky's Suicide: Myth or Reality', *19th Century Music* (1988) 11.199–220

Poznansky, A.: 'Tchaikovsky: The Man Behind the Myth', *Musical Times* (1992) 13.175–82

Puech, P. F.: 'Apartenne proprio a Mozart il cranio esposto a Salisburgo', *La stampa*, 21 October 1987

Puech, B., Puech, P. F., Dhellemes, P., et al.: 'Did Mozart have a Chronic Extra-Dural Haematoma?', *Injury* (1989): 20.327–30

Puech, P. F, Puech, B., and Tichy. G.: 'Identification of the Cranium of W. A. Mozart', *Forensic Science International* (1989): 41.101–10

Puech, B., Puech, P. F., Tichy, G., et al.: 'Craniofacial Dysmorphism in Mozart's Skull', *Journal of Forensic Sciences.* (1989) 34.487–90

Quinton, P. M.: 'Cystic Fibrosis Lesions from the Sweat Gland', *Physiology* (2007) 22.212–25

Raj, V., and Lichtenstein, D. R.: 'Hepatobiliary Manifestations of Inflammatory Bowel Disease', *Gastroenteroly Clinics of North America* (1999) 28.491–513

Reeves, Carol, during Robert Winston's programme on Chopin, BBC Radio 4, 27 March 2012

Reichsmann, F.: 'Life Experiences and Creativity of Great Composers: A Psychosomaticist's View', *Psychosomatic Medicine* (1981) 43.291–3

Reisman, T. N., Leverett, L., Hudson, J. R., and Kaiser, M. H.: 'Syphliitic Gastropathy', *Journal of Digestive Diseases* (1975) 20.588–93

Rietschel, E. T., Rietschel, M., and Beutler, B.: 'How the Mighty have Fallen: Fatal Infectious Diseases of Divine Composers', *Infectious Disease Clinics of North America* (2004) 18.311–39

Roberts, W. C, Ko, J. M., Moore T. R., and Jones, W. H.: 'Causes of Pure Aortic Regurgitation in Patients having Isolated Aortic Valve Replacement at a Single US Tertiary Hospital (1993–2005)', *Circulation* (2006) 114–22

Rold, R. L.: 'Schubert and Syphilis', *Journal of Medical Biography* (1995) 3.232–5

Romandi, F.: 'Re-Examining Syphilis: An Update on Epidemiology, Clinical Manifestation and Management', *Annals of Pharmacotherapy* (2008) 42.226–36

Roses, D. F.: 'Brahms and Billroth', *Surgery, Gynaecology and Obstetrics* (1986) 163.385–98

Rossini, G.: 'I puritani', *La revue et gazette musicale*, 19 April 1835

Rothenberg, R., Becker, G., and Wiet, R.: 'Syphilitic Hearing Loss', *Southern Medical Journal* (1979) 72.118–20

Rothschild, B. M.: 'History of Syphilis', *Clinical Infectious Diseases* (2005) 40.1454–63

Sacks, O.: 'Tourette's Syndrome and Creativity: Exploiting the Ticcy Witticisms and Witty Ticcicisms', *British Medical Journal* (1992) 305.1515–16

Sakula, A.: 'Was Mozart Poisoned?', *History of Medicine* (January–February 1980) 6–9

Sams, E.: 'Schumann's Hand Injury', *Musical Times* (1971) 112.1156–9

Sams, E.: 'Schumann's Hand Injury: Some Further Evidence', *Musical Times* (1972) 113.456

Sams, E.: 'Schubert's Illness Re-Examined', *Musical Times* (1980) 121.15–22

Schievink, W. J.: 'Genetics of Intracranial Aneurysms', *Neurosurgery* (1997) 40.651–63

Schumann, R.: 'Neue Bahnen', *Neue Zeitschrift für Musik* (1853) 39.185–6

Schwartz, D. W.: 'A Psychoanalytical Approach to the Great Renunciation', *Journal of the American Psychoanalytic Association* (1965) 13.551

Schwarz, A.: 'Beethoven's Renal Disease, Based on his Autopsy: A Case of Papillary Necrosis', *American Journal of Kidney Diseases* (1993) 21.643–52

Seeley, W. W., Matthews, B. R., Crawford, R. K., et al.: 'Unravelling *Bolero*, Progressive Aphasia, Transmodal Creativity and Right Posterior NeoCortex, *Brain* (2008) 131.39–49

Sewell, Brian: 'Why I will Never Love my Father', *Daily Mail*, 14 November 2011

Shafar, J.: 'The Brahms-Billroth Friendship', *British Medical Journal* (1981) 282.1775

Shaffer, Peter: 'Paying Homage to Mozart', *New York Times*, 2 September 1984

Sharma, O. P.: 'Beethoven's Illness: Whipple's Disease rather than Sarcoidosis', *Journal of the Royal Society of Medicine* (1994) 87.283–5

Shaw, George Bernard: 'Rossini Centenary', *Illustrated London News*, 5 March 1892

Shearer, P.: 'The Deafness of Beethoven: An Audiologic and Medical Overview', *American Journal of Otolaryngology* (1990) 11.370–4

Silverstein, A.: 'The Brain Tumour of George Gershwin and the Legs of Cole Porter', *Seminars in Neurology* (1999) 19 (Suppl. 1).3–9

Simkin, B.: 'Mozart's Scatological Disorder', *British Medical Journal* (1992) 305.1563–7

Slater, E., and Meyer, A.: 'Contributions to a Pathography of the Musicians: 1. Robert Schumann', *Confinia Psychiatrica* (1959) 2.65–94

Slater, E., and Meyer, A.: 'Contributions to a Pathography of the Musicians: 2. Organic and Psychotic Disorders', *Confinia Psychiatrica* (1960) 3.129–145

Smith, R.: *Alkan: The Enigma*, Kahn & Averill, London, 1977

Solomon, M.: 'Franz Schubert and the Peacocks of Benvenuto Cellini', *19th Century Music* (1989) 12.193–206

Sorsby, M.: 'Beethoven's Deafness', *Journal of Laryngology & Otology* (1930) 45.529–44

Šostar, Z., Vodanović, M., Breitenfeld, D,. et al.: 'Composers – Substance Abusers', *Alcoholism* (2009) 45.127–42

Sparrow, N. L., and Duval, A. J.: 'Hearing Loss and Paget's Disease', *Journal of Laryngology and Otology* (1967) 81.601–11

Squires, P. C.: 'The Problem of Beethoven's Deafness', *Journal of Abnormal and Social Psychology* (1937) 32.11–62

Stanley, J. K.: 'Radial Tunnel Syndrome', *Journal of Hand Therapy* (2006) 19.180–4

Steblin, R.: 'The Peacock's Tale: Schubert's Sexuality Reconsidered', *19th Century Music* (1993) 17.15–33

Steptoe, A., Reivich, K., and Seligman, M. E. P.: 'Composing Mozart's Personality', *The Psychologist* (February 1993) 69–71

Sterndale-Bennett, R.: 'The Death of Mendelssohn', *Music & Letters* (1955) 36.37–46

Stevens, K. M., and Hemenway, W. G.: 'Beethoven's Deafness', *Journal of the American Medical Association* (1970) 210.434–7

Stone, J.: 'Death of Mozart', *Journal of the Royal Society of Medicine*(1991) 84.179

Strohl, E. L.: 'The Unique Friendship of Theodor Billroth and Johannes Brahms', *Surgery, Gynaecology and Obstetrics* (1970) 147.757–61

Stuttaford, Thomas: 'How Did the Great Composer Die?', *The Times*, 4 November1993

Swafford, J.: 'Did the Young Brahms Play Piano in Waterfront Bars?', *19th Century Music* (2001) 24.268–75

Sweeting, Adam: 'How Did Tchaikovsky Die?', *Daily Telegraph*, 15 January 2007

Swerdlow, N. R.: 'Current Controversies and the Battlefield Landscape', *Current Neurology and Neuroscience Reports* (2005) 5.329–31

Talwalkar, J. A., and Lindor, K. D.: 'Primary Sclerosing Cholangitis', *Inflammatory Bowel Diseases* (2005) 11.62–72

Tondreau, R.: 'Egas Moriz (1874–1955)', *Radiographics* (1985) 5.996–7

Tramont, E. C.: Syphilis: 'From Beethoven to HIV', *Mount Sinai Journal of. Medicine* (1990) 57.192–6

Travers, R.-C.: 'Une mise au point sur la maladie de Vivaldi', *Informazioni e studi Vivaldiani* (1982) 3.52–60

Treves, R.: 'Mozart's Death', *Annals of the Rheumatic Diseases*(1991) 50.963–4

Turner, M. R., Parton, M. J., Shaw, C. E., et al.: 'Prolonged Survival in Motor Neurone Disease: A Descriptive Study of the King's Database, 1990–2002', *Journal of Neurology, Neurosurgery, and Psychiatry* (2003) 74.995–7

Vincent, R. W., Ryan, R. F., and Longenecker, C. G.: 'Malformation of Ear Associated with Urogenital Abnormalities', *Plastic and Reconstructive Surgery* (1961) 28.214–20

Waddell, C.: 'Creativity and Mental Illness – is There a Link?', *Canadian Journal of Psychiatry* (1998) 43.166–72

Wainapel, S. F.: 'Frederick Delius: Medical Assessment', *New York State Journal of Medicine.* (1980) 80.1886–7

Waivers, L. E.: 'Did Columbus Discover More than America?', *North Carolina Medical Journal* (1989) 50.687–90

Walker, F.: 'Schubert's Last Illness', *Monthly Musical Record* (1947) 27.232

Walkup, J. T., Mink, J. W., and Hollenbeck, P. J. (eds.): 'Tourette Syndrome', *Advances in Neurology* (2006*)* 99.1–16

Warren, J. D., and Rohrer, J. D.: 'Ravel's Last Illness: A Unifying Hypothesis', *Brain* (2008) 132.114

Wassermann, A. von, Neisser, A., and Bruch, C.: 'Eine serodiagnostische Reaktion bei Syphilis', *Deutsche Medizinische Wochenschrift* (1906) 32.745–6

Westerhagen, C. von: 'Wagner's Last Day', *Musical Times* (1979) 120.395–7

Wheater, M.: 'Mozart's Last Illness –a Medical Diagnosis', *Journal of the Royal Society of Medicine*(1990) 83.586–9

White, Michael: 'One Ring to Rule Them All', *Daily Telegraph*, 19 July 2013

Wilks, S.: 'Morbid Appearances in the Intestines of Miss Banks', *Medical Times Gazette* (1859) 2.264–5

Winternitz, E.: Gnagflow Trazom: 'An Essay on Mozart's Script, Pastimes and Nonsense Letters', Journal *of the American Musicological Society* (1958) 11.200–16

Woodside, M.: 'Comment and Chronicle', *19th Century Music* (1990) 13.273–4

Young, D. A. B.: 'Rachmaninov and Marfan's Syndrome', *British Medical Journal* (1986) 23.1625–6

Yu, A. S. L., and Brenner, B. M.: 'Diagnosing Mozart's Mortal Illness: An Exercise in Cranio-Nephrology', *Journal of the American. Society of Nephrology* (1992) 2.1666–70

Zajaczkowski, H.: 'The Quest for the Inner Man' (book review), *Musical Times* (1992) 133.574

Zegers, R. H. C., Weighl, A., Steptoe, A.: 'The Death of W. A. Mozart: An Epidemiological Perspective', *Annals of Internal Medicine* (2009) 151.274–8

Index

Health issues listed here are not necessarily those from which the composer suffered, but include alleged illnesses.